GENES AND AUTOIMMUNITY - INTRACELLULAR SIGNALING AND MICROBIOME CONTRIBUTION

Edited by **Spaska Angelova Stanilova**

Genes and Autoimmunity - Intracellular Signaling and Microbiome Contribution
http://dx.doi.org/10.5772/45733
Edited by Spaska Angelova Stanilovau

Contributors

Hiroshi Tanaka, Ekua Weba Brenu, Lotti Tajouri, Kevin Ashton, Don Staines, Sonya Marshall-Gradisnik, Ramona Tallone, Giuseppe D'Annunzio, Andrea Accogli, Sara Bolloli, Renata Lorini, Natalie Cherepahina, Zaur Shogenov, Jamiliya Tabaksoeva, Murat Agirov, Sergey Suchkov, Mariya Bocharova, Mikhail Paltsev, Yuji Hiromatsu, Sergey Krynskiy, Artem Kostyakov, Dmitry Sergeevich Kostyushev, Dmitrii Gnatenko, Seunghee Cha, Adrienne Gauna, Iwona Ben-Skowronek, Irena Manolova, Spaska Stanilova, Stephen Pennington, Stella Ademowo, Oliver FitzGerald, Lisa Staunton

Published by InTech
Janeza Trdine 9, 51000 Rijeka, Croatia

Publishing Process Manager Dejan Grgur
Technical Editor InTech DTP team
Cover InTech Design team

Additional hard copies can be obtained from orders@intechopen.com

Genes and Autoimmunity - Intracellular Signaling and Microbiome Contribution, Edited by Spaska Angelova Stanilova
p. cm.
ISBN 978-953-51-1028-6

For EU product safety concerns:
IN TECH d.o.o., Prolaz Marije Krucifikse Kozulić 3, 51000 Rijeka, Croatia,
info@intechopen.com or visit our website at intechopen.com.

Meet the editor

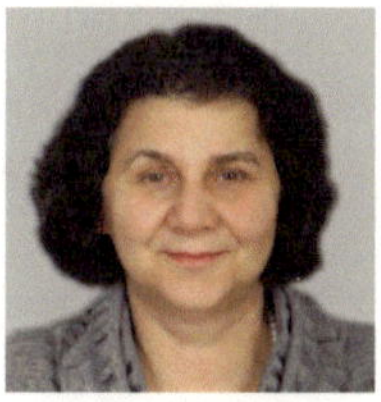

Dr Spaska Angelova Stanilova started her career in Medical Biology and received her PhD in Immunology at Higher Medical Institute in 1991. She is currently a full professor of Molecular Biology and Dcs in Immunology, and Head of Department of Molecular Biology, Immunology and Medical Genetics at the Faculty of Medicine, Trakia University. At the department, she leads the Molecular Immunology research unit at the crossroad of genetics and immune regulation. Their main research goals are to gain an insight into the molecular mechanisms of gene expression with an emphasis on implication of cytokine gene polymorphisms and intracellular signaling in immune mediated and cancer diseases. Dr Stanilova is a member of the European Federation of Immunological Society and has reviewed for several scientific journals.

Contents

Preface

Recently, it has been a great challenge to acquire an in-depth knowledge in regards to the inner workings and interactions between the immune system and environmental factors along with their impact on human health.

Environmental factors like growing pollution, changes in lifestyle habits, dietary components, as well as various microorganisms are interfering with components of our immune system driving a normal immune response to hyper- or hypo-reactivity.

When the immune system becomes hyper-reactive it targets one's own healthy cells leading to the destruction of tissues in the body, a process which is known as the onset of autoimmune disease. The common target organs include the thyroid, adrenal, stomach, liver, pancreas, kidneys, skin, joints, muscles and the nervous system. The organ specific autoantibodies often occur together with non-organ specific antibodies such as anti-DNA and anti-nucleoproteins in Systemic Lupus Erythematosus (SLE).

Autoimmune disorders are known to affect a substantial number of people worldwide, demonstrating a gender bias and it is the second largest cause of chronic illness. They represent the fifth leading cause of death among women in age groups up to 60.

The main feature of the human immune system is the fine discrimination between self components from foreign antigens. Immunological tolerance is a state of unresponsiveness induced by prior exposure to a particular antigen, mostly self antigens. Thus, the body must establish self-tolerance mechanisms in order to avoid reactivity towards self components.

One theory explains that breaking of self-tolerance is when some microorganisms (such as bacteria or viruses) or xenobiotics trigger the changes in immune regulation which results in autoimmune disorders. Recognition of the molecular pattern of a pathogen, which is distinguishable from the host molecules is important for protective immune response and when mistaken, could often lead to autoimmunity. This process strongly depends on the individual genetics background in a person. Certain individuals are genetically susceptible to developing autoimmune diseases. There are a number of genes that may plausibly be involved in the development of autoimmunity. It is known that genetics predisposition is associated with three main sets of genes, including immunoglobulins, T-cell receptors and major histocompatibility complex (MHC), but are not restricted to them. The development of autoimmunity is also strongly influenced by inherited disease-associated single nucleotide polymorphisms rather than deletion or rearrangements. Cytokine, cytokine receptors and TLR-associated genes have recently attracted great interest as candidate genes for autoimmune diseases. Over the past decade there has been great interest in testing candidate gene polymorphisms for evidence of their association with various autoimmune diseases. The genetic hallmarks of autoimmunity are undoubted, however particular genes and triggering intracellular signaling pathway remains elusive. Genes of cytokine and immune cell receptors regulating function of immune system are expressed under control of intracellular signaling pathway such as TLR signaling pathway, Fc receptors, receptors and ligands of immunological synapses, vitamin D receptors and other immune related genes.

Two opposite hypothesis are currently under investigation. One of them (hygiene hypothesis) discusses whether the reduced exposure to certain infections, as a result of improved hygiene and living conditions, may be responsible for the increased incidence in autoimmune conditions. The other hypothesis is that autoimmune diseases might be a consequence of post-infections conditions. Despite this contradiction, infection agents and their antigens obviously play a pivotal role in the development of autoimmunity through interaction with the immune system. Arguments that support the role of infection in specific autoimmune diseases come from clinical, epidemiological and laboratory studies. New data demonstrates that the gut flora compositions can also influence the development of autoimmune diseases. For example, the use of probiotics containing lactobacilli decreases the incidence of diabetes in NOD mice. At the same time, a range of differing factors such as dietary supplements, hormones, alcohol consumption, vitamins and drugs, cigarette smoking, etc. implicated in autoimmune disease onset. Dietary antigens also stimulate antigen receptors and aberrant immune response can progress to autoimmunity.

According to the afore discussed, it seems obvious that neither genetic predisposition nor environmental factors alone are sufficient to cause the disease. The triggering factors and intracellular signaling pathway crosstalk are currently under extensive investigation with high hopes for revealing the autoimmunity clue.

In conclusion, autoimmune diseases develop in genetically predisposed organisms as a result of a specific triggering agent (infectious or noninfectious), causing dysfunction in the immune system activity with subsequently developed abnormal autoimmune mechanism affecting its own cells and tissues of the organism.

This book attempts to seize the new opportunities for moving research forward, leading to a new approach for the prevention and treatment of autoimmune diseases. The first section of this book is focused on genes, gene expression and signaling pathways involved in autoimmune pathogenesis. The second one attempts to present current data for interaction of microbiota with human immune system, which are implicated in the development of autoimmune disease.

We hope the book will be useful for anyone wanting to expand their knowledge of the occurrence and mechanisms of autoimmunity.

Dr Spaska Angelova Stanilova, PhD, Dsc
Professor of Molecular Biology and Immunology
Head of Department of Molecular Biology, Immunology and Medical Genetics
Faculty of Medicine, Trakia University
Bulgaria

Section 1

Genes and Intracellular Signaling

Chapter 1

Genetic Susceptibility to Graves' Ophthalmopathy

Junichi Tani and Yuji Hiromatsu

Additional information is available at the end of the chapter

http://dx.doi.org/10.5772/53441

1. Introduction

Graves' disease (GD) is an autoimmune thyroid disorder (AITD) with aberrant antibody production resulting in hyperthyroidism [1]. It is characterized by T cell and B cell reactivity to the thyrotropin (thyroid stimulating hormone; TSH) receptor (TSHR) located on the endothelial surface of thyroid follicular cells, and the presence of abundant serum antibodies against TSHR (TRAb) is used as a specific marker of GD. Follicular hyperplasia, intracellular colloid droplets, cell thinning and patchy T cell-predominant lymphocytic infiltrations can be observed in thyroid gland histology of GD patients. GD is considered primarily a T helper-2 (Th2) autoimmune disease, as TRAb stimulates TSHR as an agonist, resulting in the excessive production of thyroid hormones. The pathogenesis of GD has been studied for decades and several risk factors have been identified. Similar to other autoimmune diseases, GD is believed to develop because of a combination of genetic susceptibility and environmental triggers. Often there is a familial history of disease and it is prevalent in women [2]. These facts support a role for genetic susceptibility in the pathogenesis of GD. Environmental factors are also considered important for the susceptibility and onset of disease. Infections have been predicted to have a pivotal role in triggering autoimmune reactions and the breakdown of tolerance leading to GD, although evidence is scarce. Often, patients with GD frequently have a history of some type of psychological and/or physiological stress [3]. Recently, epigenetic factors have also been demonstrated to be involved in autoimmune pathogenesis [4]. Classical GD was described as a syndrome consisting of tachycardia, goiter and orbitopathy, called "Merseburg triad". Most GD patients develop tachycardia and goiter; however, GD patients with orbitopathy, named Graves' ophthalmopathy (GO), occur in up to 60% of all GD patients [5]. In particular, GO worsens the patients quality of life because of its intractable symptoms, including diplopia, proptosis, chemosis and retro-orbital pain. With severe GO patients may risk visual loss. Moreover, GO is also experienced in patients with Hashimoto's thyroiditis (HT) across ethnic backgrounds [6, 7]. HT is another common AITD, which is thought to develop from a combination of genetic susceptibility and environmental factors. Many studies have investigated the genetic predisposition of HT, and suggest that GO patients may have partially different genetic backgrounds from GD patients and HT patients without GO.

In this review, we describe the pathogenesis and genetic predisposition of GD and HT first, followed by illustrating those of GO. Finally, we discuss the upcoming problems in future research.

2. The pathogenesis of Graves' disease

As described above, GD is considered a Th2 autoimmune disease. Generating TRAb is the essential for development of the disease, as TRAb signals through TSHR as an agonist, resulting in the overproduction of T4 that induces symptoms such as tachycardia, sweating and body weight loss (thyrotoxicosis) [8]. However, how TRAb is induced remains unknown.

GD is thought to have genetic predisposition. In 1967, Hall et al. published on the frequent familial occurrence of AITD, illustrating that a third of siblings of GD patients developed AITD and over half of asymptomatic children had thyroid antibodies in their blood [9]. Similar observations have been made for decades. Twin studies on GD have also provided persuasive evidence for a role of genetic susceptibility. Monozygotic (MZ) twins with completely identical genes would be expected to have full concordance in a monogenic disease. For diseases with more complex inheritance patterns, the concordance rate in MZ twins would be reduced, although still higher than for dizygotic (DZ) twins. Brix et al. conducted a twin cohort study and determined that the probandwise concordance rates of MZ pairs were much higher than for DZ pairs [10] and estimated that 79% of predisposition to the development of GD arose from genetic factors [11]. These results of family and twin studies demonstrated that GD had genetic predisposition(s) that were not due to a single gene, but rather to multiple interactions among genes [12]. Such genetic factors increase the susceptibility to GD and the development of GD may be triggered by individual environmental factors such as infection, iodine intake, psychological and/or physiological stress, smoking or pollution [13]. Iodine can induce thyroid autoimmunity by increasing the immunogenicity of thyroglobulin and/or releasing free oxygen radicals, resulting in immune attack against thyroid tissue [14]. Establishment of autoimmunity against the thyroid gland is mediated by dendritic cells (DCs), macrophages and/or B lymphocytes that present the antigen(s) to T lymphocytes through an immunological synapse. Furthermore, thyroid follicular cells can also present antigen by expressing major histocompatibility complex (MHC) class I and II molecules. Thus, autoimmune reactions against TSHR are established under such circumstances with the appropriate cytokine conditions. Once the stimulating anti-TSHR antibodies are produced, they continue to provide impetus to the thyroid follicular cells via TSHR to produce thyroid hormone uncontrollably. As will be discussed, many studies have been conducted in the development of GD over the last few decades, identifying numerous genes, of which some have proven to be significant genetic factors in GD pathogenesis. In the next section, we describe these susceptibility loci.

3. Genetic susceptibility to Graves' disease

The establishment and development of immunological reactions specific to TSHR are hallmarks of GD. Therefore, GD susceptibility genes are likely to be involved in immune reactions, immunological regulation and thyroid specific proteins. The main methodological approaches for identification of susceptibility loci are based on linkage or association analysis, detecting single-nucleotide polymorphisms (SNPs). The majority of loci involved in the development of GD that have been identified confer only a low risk for disease, except one or two loci (odds ratio: ~1.2–1.5), suggesting gene-gene interactions among genes involved in GD and/or subset effects of GD should be further investigated. Recently, because of advances in high throughput genotyping technologies, it has become possible to conduct genome wide association studies (GWAS). However, only a few GWAS for GD have been conducted to date and published new findings from these are scarce. Currently, several groups are conducting GWAS studies for GD from various points of view.

Next, we will discuss the susceptibility loci for GD according to its pathogenesis, such as genes involved in immune reactions, immunological regulation and thyroid specific proteins.

3.1. Immunological synapse genes

The immunological synapse is the interface between T lymphocytes and antigen-presenting cells (APC) that is formed during peripheral T lymphocyte activation. It consists of a peptide antigen bound between human leukocyte antigen (HLA) class II molecules and the T-cell receptor (TCR), costimulatory molecules including cytotoxic T-lymphocyte-associated protein 4 (CTLA-4), B7 (CD80 and CD86), CD40 and other molecules [15]. Variations of molecules in the immunological synapse have been elucidated as genetic risk factors for GD. The MHC region, encoding the HLA glycoproteins, is a highly polymorphic genetic region [2]. HLA molecules play pivotal roles in the function of the immune system, binding fragments of antigens in the form of peptides and presenting them to T lymphocytes. HLA molecules are divided into HLA class I (HLA-A, B, C) and class II (HLA-DR, DQ, DP). HLA class I molecules interact with $CD8^+$ T lymphocytes which have cytotoxic effector functions. As host tissues are surveyed by $CD8^+$ T lymphocytes, HLA class I molecules are widely expressed throughout the body, including the thyroid follicular cells. HLA class II molecules, permanently expressed on the surface of cells involved in antigen presentation, present antigens to $CD4^+$ T lymphocytes, which initiate and regulate specific immune responses. Therefore, binding of an antigen fragment to HLA class II is an integrant of the development of immune responses. Apart from peripheral immunologic reactions, HLA molecules are necessary for ontogenesis of the immune system since they participate in the maturation and selection of lymphocytes in the thymus [15]. HLA genes and molecules display polymorphisms to ensure immunological diverseness. Such polymorphisms are particularly extensive in regions, known as pockets, which directly bind peptide residues and have extremely important functional significance because different HLA variants bind a distinctly different repertoire of peptides.

3.1.1. HLA class I

From the early reports of Farid et al. [16] and Grumet et al. [17], HLA class I antigens are thought to be primarily involved in the pathogenesis of GD. HLA-C*07 in particular was suggested to associate with GD susceptibility [18]. Simmonds et al. tested other loci and concluded that HLA-C and to a lesser extent HLA-B, were primarily associated with GD. However, the observed associations to HLA class I alleles could not be attributed to linkage disequilibrium (LD) within this haplotype. To date, many studies have evaluated other HLA class I alleles [19], and some demonstrated significant association to GD susceptibility. While the association between GD and HLA class I antigens has been evaluated, how they are involved in the pathology of GD is unclear. As cytotoxic pathogenesis is thought to be involved during the early stages of GD, they may alter immunological responses.

3.1.2. HLA class II

HLA-DR3 was the first candidate gene to be associated with AITD in Caucasians [20]. It has been identified as a major susceptibly gene for GD, although this is not the case for all ethnic populations. This association was originally demonstrated in a mixed Brazilian population, but the association was not observed in a Japanese population [19]. HLA-DR3 is also associated with the presence of GO and disease course of GD [2]. In other ethnic groups, different alleles were shown to associate with GD [19]. Recent studies on the variants of HLA class II antigens, especially HLA-DR3, focused on the binding pocket that interacts directly with antigenic peptides. Specifically, these studies concluded that the substitution of the neutral amino acids Ala or Gln for positively charged Arg at position 74 of the DR beta 1 chain (DRb1–Arg74) resulted in a structural change in the HLA-DR peptide binding pocket that conferred an increased risk for the development of GD [21]. Conversely, glutamine at this peptide binding pocket position was proven protective against GD. This change of amino acid at the pocket of the peptide binding cleft alters its three-dimensional structure that likely allows pathogenic peptides to bind to the HLA molecule so that subsequently auto-reactive T cells recognize the antigenic peptide and induce an autoimmune response.

3.1.3. CTLA-4

CTLA-4 is a major negative regulator of T cell activation [22]. While APCs activate T cells by interactions between HLA antigen and the TCR, CTLA-4 acts as an accessory molecule to the TCR and suppresses T cell activation to control normal T cell responses. Therefore, it is postulated that CTLA-4 polymorphisms reduce their own expression and/or function, resulting in increased predisposition to autoimmunity. Indeed, CTLA-4 polymorphisms have been identified in various autoimmune conditions [23] including both GD [24] and HT [19], across ethnic and geographic groups. CTLA-4 loci are shown to regulate T cell activation in a complicated manner. Vieland et al. recently showed CTLA-4 played a role in the susceptibility to high levels of thyroid specific antibodies (TAb), and clinical AITD when interacting with other loci [25]. They also demonstrated that both the G allele and the A allele of the A/G49 SNP of CTLA-4 might predispose to AITD when interacting with different loci. At present, three main variants of CTLA-4 have been evaluated: an AT-repeat microsatellite at the 3'UTR of the

CTLA-4 gene; an A/G SNP at position 49 in the signal peptide resulting in an alanine/threonine substitution (A/G49); and an A/G SNP located downstream and outside of the 30UTR of the CTLA-4 gene (designated CT60) [19]. To identify which is the causative variant for AITD including GD, many functional studies are currently being conducted.

3.1.4. CD40

CD40 expressed primarily on B cells and other APCs, plays a crucial role in B cell activation and antibody secretion as a co-stimulatory molecule [26]. It is associated with GD as a positional candidate on the basis of a genome-wide linkage study [27, 28]. Further sequencing studies of the CD40 gene have shown a C/T SNP in the CD40 gene, likely to be the causative variant in Caucasian, Korean and Japanese populations [19]. The CC genotype of this SNP was demonstrated to associate with development of GD in many ethnic populations [29]. The CC genotype, located in the Kozak sequence of CD40, can alter CD40 translation and expression [28]. The C-allele of the SNP was shown to increase the translation of CD40 mRNA transcripts by 20–30% compared to the T-allele [28, 30]. CD40 is expressed on B cells [26] and on thyroid follicular cells [31], and so the C-allele-induced increase in CD40 expression on B cells and/or thyrocytes may predispose to the disease. Increased expression of CD40 on B cells may result in the enhanced production of anti-TSHR-stimulating antibodies, whereas increased expression of CD40 on thyrocytes can trigger an autoimmune response to the thyroid.

3.1.5. The protein tyrosine phosphatase-22 (PTPN-22) gene

Lymphoid tyrosine phosphatase, encoded by the protein tyrosine phosphatase-22 (PTPN22) gene, is shown to be a negative regulator of T cell activation [32]. The PTPN22 gene is associated with AITD, including both GD and HT. Differences in the ethnic contribution of the PTPN22 SNP have also been identified [19, 33]. PTPN22 is involved in limiting the adaptive immune response to antigen by dephosphorylating and inactivating TCR-associated kinases and their substrates. The best documented association of PTPN22 variants to autoimmune disorders including GD is rs2476601 (C1858T). This C1858T SNP, encoding an Arg to Trp substitution at residue 620 (R620W), is located in the P1 proline-rich motif of PTPN22, which binds with high affinity to the Src homology 3 (SH3) domain of Csk [34]. This disease-associated variant is a gain-of-function variant, resulting in suppression of TCR signaling more efficiently than wild type protein. *In vitro* experiments have shown hyper-responsiveness of T cells expressing the W620 allele, indicating that carriers of this allele may be prone to autoimmunity [35]. While many experiments have been conducted to evaluate the immunological pathway of PTPN-22 polymorphisms, they are still controversial. Many complicated immunological pathways concerning T cell activation are expected to be involved. Further studies are required to elucidate the role of PTPN-22 polymorphisms in susceptibility to disease.

3.2. T cell regulation

Natural regulatory T (Treg) cells are an important subset of T cells that regulate T cell activation [36]. They play a pivotal role in peripheral tolerance to self-antigens. In murine studies, up-regulation of Treg cells suppressed experimental autoimmune thyroiditis [37], while depletion of Tregs increased their susceptibility to experimental GD [38]. Treg cells are characterized by constitutively expressing CD25, CTLA-4, and glucocorticoid-induced tumor necrosis factor receptor. Their development is regulated by a master gene, FOXP3 [36]. Interestingly, both FOXP3 and CD25 are associated with AITD [19, 39].

3.2.1. FOXP3

Ban Y. et al. tested the FOXP3 gene in two cohorts of AITD patients, including U.S. Caucasians and Japanese. They demonstrated an association of a microsatellite in the FOXP3 gene with AITD in Caucasians but not in the Japanese, suggesting ethnic differences in disease susceptibility [39]. The estimated pathogenesis of the FOXP3 variant is thought to mediate pathogenesis by weakening suppression of autoimmune effector T cell activity.

3.2.2. CD25

Treg cells are characterized by the constitutive expression of high levels of CD25, the alpha chain of the IL-2 receptor [36]. Similar to FOXP3, recent studies have found an association between the CD25 gene and GD [19]. While the variant of CD25 is thought to alter the suppressive effects on self-reactive T cells, the detailed mechanisms are still unclear.

3.3. Thyroid specific genes

As GD is a thyroid specific autoimmune disease, it is highly likely that polymorphisms of genes coding for thyroid-specific proteins affect the susceptibility to GD, similar to other AITD such as HT.

3.3.1. Thyroglobulin

Thyroglobulin (Tg) is a main target of the immune response in AITD [40]. A whole-genome linkage study identified the Tg gene as a major AITD susceptibility gene [41]. Moreover, several groups also have reported similar findings for Tg gene predisposition to AITD in Caucasian, Japanese and Taiwanese populations [19]. Tg variants may predispose to GD by altering Tg degeneration in endosomes with slight changes in amino-acid sequences. This may result in the production of a pathogenic Tg peptide repertoire that interacts with HLA-DRb-Arg74 and leads to a high prevalence of GD [42]. Recently, a newly identified TG promoter SNP (-1623A/G) was found to associate with AITD in another pathway [43]. The disease-associated G allele in -1623A/G SNP confers increased promoter activity through the binding of the interferon regulatory factor-1 (IRF-1), a major interferon-induced transcription factor. Murine studies indicated that IRF-1 was associated with AITD [44]. These results suggest that variants of Tg itself possibly alter the reactivity of cytokines through IRF-1.

3.3.2. TSH receptor

Regarding the pathology of GD, it is not surprising that TSHR gene variants predispose to GD. Indeed, TSHR was the first gene after HLA to be tested for association with GD. Early studies tested three non-synonymous SNPs in the TSHR gene for association with GD, D36H and P52T that are located in the extracellular domain and D727E which in present in the intracellular domain [19]. However, conflicting results on the association of SNPs in the TSHR gene to GD were reported. This encouraged increasing research for susceptibility loci to non-coding sequences within the TSHR gene. Japanese large scale analyses of SNPs showed evidence for three haplotypes within TSHR intron 7 that were strongly associated with GD. In contrast, a Caucasian study showed evidence for a SNP (rs2268458) located in intron 1 associated with GD. Moreover, Brand et al. investigated a combined panel of 98 SNPs in intron 1 of TSHR [45], showing 2 SNPs associated with GD. Functional analyses suggested that SNPs in the intron region could be associated with reduced expression of full length TSHR mRNA and in turn lead to increased shedding of the A-subunit of the TSHR receptor, which is an important molecule for the induction of autoantibodies against TSHR [46]. Recently, a non-synonymous SNP in the distal part of the gene, rs3783941, was indicated to be associated with GD in a large GWAS study of non-synonymous variants among 4500 subjects [47]. However, this might represent a false positive because this association was not replicated. However, there remains the possibility that the lack of replication was due to insufficient power.

3.4. Other genes

Many other genes, apart from the three categories described above, have been associated with the development of GD. Fc receptor-like 3 (FCRL3) is a receptor of unknown function with structural homology to immunoglobulin constant chains (Fc receptors). Allele C of rs7528684 located at position –169 in the promoter region was demonstrated to associate with GD in the Japanese [48] and UK population [47]. In contrast, a negative association between GD and FCRL3 was also reported [49]. FCRL3 is expressed in lymphoid tissues especially on the surface of B cells and a subset of Treg cells [50]. This suggested a function of FCRL3 in the regulation of autoimmunity, although its functions remain unknown. Variants of the promoter of the Secretoglobin 3A2 (SCGB3A2) gene encoding secretory Uteroglobin-Related Protein 1 (UGRP1) have been reported to associate with GD in an extensive study of 2500 patients and controls from the Chinese population [51]. This finding was confirmed in a UK population and Russian population study [19]. UGRP1 is a ligand for macrophage scavenger receptor with collagenous structure, which is predominantly expressed in the lung, although low-level expression is also present in the thyroid [52]. While SNPs in SCGB3A2 were found to reduce promoter activity by 24% [53], their function in the pathogenesis of GD is unclear. The variant rs1990760 present as A946T in the interferon-induced helicase C domain 1 (IFIH1) C domain was demonstrated to associate with GD in a UK population [54]. However, no statistically significant association was found in subsequent German [55], Chinese [56] and Japanese studies [57]. IFIH1 is part of a family of intracellular proteins involved in innate immunity through recognition of viral RNA [58], although it is unknown how polymorphisms in IFIH1 affect the pathogenesis of GD. The variant rs763361, which is a non-synonymous SNP in the intracellular tail of the CD226 molecule, was also reported to be associated with GD [54]. This variant possibly alters splicing of the CD226 transcript, suggesting an association with GD. There are also a number of other genes reported to be associated with GD, such as vitamin D receptor (VDR), type II iodothyronine deiodinase, IL23 receptor (IL23R), estrogen receptor beta (ESR2) and a promoter variant of a gene encoding nuclear factor-kappaB (NF-κB) [19, 59]. To examine the significance of these polymorphisms on the predisposition of GD, further studies with significant power and a variety of ethnic groups are required.

4. Genetic susceptibility to Hashimoto's thyroiditis (HT)

Although HT is less commonly involved in GO patients, it is the most prevalent autoimmune thyroid disorder. Lymphocytic infiltration within the thyroid gland is often followed by a gradual destruction and fibrous replacement of the thyroid parenchymal tissue. The principal biochemical characteristic of the disease is the presence in the patients' sera of autoantibodies against two major thyroid antigens (TAbs), thyroid peroxidase (TPO) and Tg. Antibodies against TPO (TPOAbs) and Tg (TgAbs) cause damage to thyroid cells because of antibody dependent cell cytotoxicity [60]. TPOAbs are prevalent in nearly all patients and TgAbs are present in approximately 80% of HT patients. TSHR antibodies are the principal biochemical characteristics of GD, and generally do not exist among HT patients. While TSHR antibodies are of primary importance in developing GO, it is unclear how GO develops in certain HT patients who do not have TSHR antibodies. With increasing knowledge of the etiology and pathology of AITD, including HT and GD, HT has been shown to develop in genetically susceptible individuals triggered by environmental cues similar to patients with GD [61]. In the following section, we shall discuss the genetic predisposition of HT. The genetic susceptibility of HT is similar to that of GD described above. Despite the disease outcomes being opposite, hypothyroidism and hyperthyroidism, respectively, the immunopathology and genetic predisposition are shown to be common. Indeed, a report describes monozygotic twins where one developed HT and the other GD, indicating commonality between the genetic factors of HT and GD [62]. On the basis of familial and twin studies, a strong genetic predisposition to AITD has been identified. Familial clustering of AITD including HT and GD has been confirmed [61]. The sibling risk ratio for AITD was calculated as 28, which indicated the highly significant contribution of genetic factors to disease development [63].

4.1. HLA genes

In HT, aberrant expression of HLA class II molecules on thyrocytes has been demonstrated. Presumably, thyrocytes may act as APCs capable of presenting thyroid autoantigens and initiating autoimmune thyroid disease [64]. In Caucasians, associations between HT and various HLA alleles, including DR3, DR5, DQ7, DQB1*03, DQw7 or DRB1*04-DQB1*0301 haplotype were reported. In Japanese, associations with DRB4*0101, HLA-A2 and DRw53 were demonstrated, while in Chinese patients association with DRw9 was observed [61].

4.2. CTLA-4

Several polymorphisms of the CTLA-4 gene in HT patients have been studied. The initially reported (AT)n microsatellite CTLA-4 polymorphism in the 3' untranslated region (UTR) was found to be associated with HT in Caucasian and Japanese patients, but not in an Italian population [61]. The exon 1 located 49A/G SNP results in a threonine to alanine substitution and is associated with HT [65]. The exact mechanism conferring susceptibility to HT has not been elucidated yet and further studies are needed to find out which CTLA-4 polymorphism is causative.

4.3. PTPN22

As is for GD, the C1858T SNP of the PTPN22 gene was also demonstrated to be a risk factor for HT [66]. However, the mechanism is not clear. This observation was not confirmed in German, Tunisian and Japanese population studies [61].

4.4. Vitamin D receptor (VDR) gene

Vitamin D, which acts via VDR, is classically involved in the metabolism of calcium. However, recent studies have revealed it possesses immunomodulatory properties and its deficiency is implicated in the development of autoimmune diseases [67]. Many immune cells, particularly DCs, express VDR, whose stimulation has been shown to enhance tolerogenicity. Tolerogenic DCs promote the development of Treg cells, inducing peripheral tolerance. Therefore, modulation of VDR may affect the ability of DCs to alter the induction ability of Treg cells. To date the association between VDR-FokI SNP in exon 2 and HT has been identified in Japanese and Taiwanese populations [61]. In a Croatian study, the VDR gene 3′ region polymorphisms were related to HT [68], possibly by affecting VDR mRNA expression.

4.5. Thyroglobulin genes

Considering the pathogenesis of HT, it is reasonable that Tg gene polymorphisms genetically predispose individuals to HT. As described in the previous section, there have been reported many genetic regions related to AITD [69]. The association of HT with Tgms2, a microsatellite marker in intron 27 of the Tg gene was confirmed in Japanese and Caucasian populations [61]. However, these observations were not confirmed in a larger data set of UK Caucasian patients or in a Chinese population.

4.6. TPO genes

TPO is also considered an important gene in the pathogenesis of HT, because antibodies against TPO are characteristic of HT. To date, the T1936C, T2229C and A2257C TPO gene polymorphisms have been tested for association with TPOAb levels [61].

4.7. Cytokine genes, immune related genes and others

According to recent advances in the understanding of immune cell subsets and cytokines, several genes encoding different inflammatory cytokines have been studied in HT, and some have shown the ability to influence the severity of disease. As HT is thought to be a cytotoxic T cell-mediated autoimmune disease, cytokines produced by T-helper type 1 (Th1) cells, including interferon (IFN)-γ, have been well studied among HT patients. The T allele of the +874A/T IFN-γ SNP, which causes an increased production of IFN-γ, was reported to be associated with the severity of hypothyroidism in HT patients [70]. However, a higher frequency of severe hypothyroidism was also observed in Japanese patients with a CC genotype of -590C/T interleukin (IL)-4 SNP [71]. IL-4 is a key Th2 cytokine that can suppress cell-mediated autoimmunity, and this polymorphism was thought to lead to reduced IL-4 production. These studies demonstrated the complexity of HT pathogenesis. Gene polymorphisms of transforming growth factor (TGF)-β, an inhibitor of cytokine production, were also associated with HT [72]. The T allele of +369T/C SNP causes reduced secretion of TGF-β, and was more frequent in severe hypothyroidism than in mild hypothyroidism. SNPs of the gene encoding FOXP3, an essential regulatory factor for Treg cell development, was shown to associate with a severe form of HT [61]. The C allele of tumor necrosis factor (TNF)-α, 1031T/C SNP, was shown to associate with the development of HT by an over-production of TNF-α [61].

5. Genetic susceptibility to Graves' ophthalmopathy

In the previous sections we described genetic susceptibility to GD and HT because GO develops in GD and occasionally in HT patients. While GD and HT patients in the previously described studies included those with and without GO, the research described in this section will focus on the genetic factors of GO compared to the possession rate of the polymorphism among normal controls, GD without GO patients and GD with GO patients.

5.1. The pathogenesis of GO

GO is an orbital manifestation of AITDs, mainly GD, and develops in 25-50% of GD patents and up to 5% of HT patients. The pathogenesis of GO has been studied for several decades, but remains controversial. At present, it is presumed to occur through the same underlying immune processes as GD, such as the involvement of TRAbs [73]. TSHR was expressed in the orbit tissues, especially on fibroblasts. When TRAbs interact with TSHR, inflammatory immune cells and cytokines become activated and cause inflammation in the retrobulbar tissues. Inflammation in the muscles that direct eyeball movement upsets the coordination of their movements, resulting in enlargement of the involved muscles and double vision. Inflammation in retro-orbital fat tissue enlarges its volume, leading to protrusion of the eyeball (proptosis). Some patients develop inflammation of the eyelids and/or lachrymal gland. However, such pathways are unable to expound why GO can develop in some HT patients who do not possess TRAbs. Moreover, the level of TSHR expression in the orbital tissue, including fibroblasts and eye muscles, is so low that it is unlikely to induce sufficient inflammation to affect tissues such that they lose function. One hypothesis suggests that the thyroid and orbit tissues share antigens, and that when autoantibodies are induced during autoimmune thyroid disease, concurrent inflammation in the orbit(s) may also occur [74]. Potential shared antigens include Fp, G2S, calsequestrin (CSQ) 1 and 2 and collagen XIII [74]. However these results have not been confirmed. Although it is difficult to regard such antigens as primary antigens for GO because Fp, G2s, and CSQ1 and 2 are proteins located inside the cell, they may emerge as a consequence of destruction of the thyroid gland and/or orbit tissues through autoimmune or other immune reactions. TRAb titers were positively correlated with clinical features of GO, whereas thyroid stimulating immunoglobulin (TSI) and TPO antibody were not [75]. Recently a new TSI testing method showed a significant correlation between TSI and the clinical features of GO [76].

5.2. The genetics of GO

While the pathogenesis of GO is thought to share similar genetic factors with GD and HT, it is unknown what divides GD patients with GO from GD patients without GO. Much research has focused on inflammatory factors because the inflammation present in orbital tissues in GO patients is believed to be disease-specific. In the following section, we provide a detailed review of the immunogenetic associations of GO. A summary of the relevant studies is provided in Table 1.

Categories		GD including GO	GO	HT
Immunological	HLA class I	HLA-C*07		
synapse genes		HLA-B*08		HLA-A2
	HLA class II	HLA-DR3	HLA-DPB 2.1/8	HLA-DR3
			HLA-DR4	HLA-DR5
			HLA-DR7	HLA-DR7
			HLA-DRB1	HLA-DQB1*03
			HLA-DRB3	HLA-DQw7
				HLA-DRB1*04
				HLA-DQB1*0301
				HLA-DRB4*0101
				HLA-DRw53
				HLA-DRw9
		CTLA-4	CTLA-4	CTLA-4
		PTPN22		PTPN22
			PTPN12	
		CD40		
T cell regulation		FOXP3		FOXP3
		CD25		
Thyroid specific genes		Thyroglobulin		Thyroglobulin
		DIO 2		
		TSHR		

Categories	GD including GO	GO	HT
Cytokines or		TNF-α	TNF-α
Cytokine receptors		IL-1α	IL-4
		IL-1β	TGF-β
		IL-1RA	
		IFN-©	IFN-γ
	IL-23R		
Other immunological	NF-κB	NF-κB	
molecules	CD226	ICAM-1	
	FCRL3	TLR-9	
	SCGB3A2	CD86	
	IFIH1	CD103	
Others	VDR	GR	VDR
	ESR2		

Each genetic locus is referenced in the body of the manuscript.

GD: Graves' disease; GO: Graves' ophthalmopathy; HT: Hashimoto's thyroiditis; HLA: Human leukocyte antigen; CTLA: Cytotoxic T-lymphocyte-associated protein; CD: Cluster of Differentiation; PTPN: Protein tyrosine phosphatase; FOXP: forkhead box P; TSHR: Thyroid stimulating hormone receptor; FCRL: Fc receptor-like; SCGB3A2: Secretoglobin 3A2; IFIH1: Interferon-induced helicase C domain 1; VDR: Vitamin D receptor; GR: Glucocorticoid receptor; DIO 2: Type II iodothyronine deiodinase; IL: Interleukin; ESR2: Estrogen receptor beta; NF-κb: Nuclear factor-kappa B; IFN: Interferon; TGF: Transforming growth factor; TPO: Thyroid peroxidase; TNF: Tumor necrosis factor; ICAM: Intercellular Adhesion Molecule; TLR: Toll-like receptor.

Table 1. Genetic predisposition to Graves' disease, Graves' ophthalmopathy and Hashimoto's thyroiditis

5.3. Cytokines

Similar to GD, disease in GO is thought to involve an imbalance between the production of pro- and anti-inflammatory cytokines [77]. Therefore, SNPs in cytokine related genes that participate in the GO pathogenesis could promote or protect from its development. As shown in Table 1, the association between various pro- and anti-inflammatory cytokine gene polymorphisms in GO have been identified. Cytokines released mainly by leukocytes infiltrating into the retro-orbital tissues are likely to play key roles in the cascade of autoimmune reactions in the orbit [78]. Although several significant associations between genetic polymorphisms of cytokine genes and GO have been reported, the immediate consequences of cytokine gene polymorphisms are not well studied. Thus, how polymorphisms of cytokine genes relate to biological changes such as serum and local tissue concentration and functional activity are unknown. Moreover, publication of polymorphisms suggested to have a positive correlation with GO provokes many unpublished and/or published contradictory reports performed by other research groups. This might reflect the presence of different genetic patterns of susceptibility among different ethnic groups, or might be an outcome of the product of chance. Among cytokines studied, the association of genetic susceptibility to GO with cytokine gene polymorphisms from the family of IL-1 and TNF-α-related cytokines seems to be the strongest. Recently a specific TNF-α inhibitor, Infliximab, was demonstrated to be effective for treatment of severe GO [79]. Several groups showed positive associations between the development of GO and TNF-α polymorphisms, including -863C/A region in Japanese and Chinese, -238G/A in Polish and -1031T/C in Japanese populations [80]. As regards the IL-1 superfamily, IL-1α and-β are pro-inflammatory cytokines, and the IL-1receptor antagonist (RA) competes for receptor binding with IL-1α and-β [81]. Retro-orbital fibroblasts derived from GO patients expressed and secreted significantly reduced levels of intracellular and soluble IL-1RA [82]. Thus, an imbalance between IL-1 and IL-1RA may play an important role in the pathogenesis of GO and gene polymorphisms in IL-1α, -1β and/or IL-1RA may have a causal relationship with such an imbalance. IL-1 is a key cytokine in many inflammatory reactions. It stimulates retro-orbital fibroblasts to proliferate, synthesize glycosaminoglycans and express immunomodulatory molecules [83] including adhesion molecules, cytokines, complement regulatory proteins and stress proteins. Reports on polymorphisms of IL-1α and -β genes are conflicting, with some showing positive [84] and negative [85] associations.

IFN-γ is a type II interferon involved in Th1 immune responses and can regulate Th2 immune reactions. We studied IFN-γ gene polymorphisms in Japanese GD patients and 2 out of 8 polymorphisms were associated with GO [86]. An Iranian group also demonstrated a significant association between GO and an IFN-γ polymorphism at UTR 5644A/T [87].

5.4. CTLA-4

As shown in previous sections, CTLA-4 gene polymorphisms, especially the A/G49 SNP of CTLA-4, are strongly associated with GD and HT. A UK study showed the A/G49 SNP of CTLA-4 was associated with an increased risk of GO [88] and was confirmed by an Iranian group [80]. However, the association between the CTLA-4 gene polymorphism and the development of GO is still controversial [89]. First, the same polymorphism was shown to be associated with HT and GD with or without GO. Second, many follow-up studies have been performed, and while some studies confirmed such an association the others did not [80].

5.5. HLA

As GD is believed to be a Th2 related disease, HLA class II is thought to have an association with GD. GO is one of many symptoms of GD, and thus it is justifiable to regard GO as a Th2 related disease. However, this is still controversial because no antibodies have been confirmed to have a causal association with GO except TSHR antibodies. Moreover, not all GD patients develop GO; the prevalence of GO among GD patients is only 25-50%. Thus, there is a limitation in studying autoimmune associations of different HLA alleles because of the strong LD between HLA alleles and alleles of undefined neighboring loci, which may exert primary effects [90]. Therefore, functional studies of the biological effects of different HLA alleles are needed to determine the true effects of these potential genetic associates of GO. Several studies support a role for HLA-DRB1, which has a critical role in antigen presentation, in the development of GO [80]. However, contradictory reports also exist [80, 90]. HLA-DR7 alleles are also reported to have an association with the development of GO [91], and several isolated studies have shown a weak association between HLA-DR4, HLA-DPB 2.1/8 and HLA-DRB3 alleles and GO [80, 92]. However, the opposite outcome has also been shown for HLA-DR3, -DR4 and -DR7 alleles [89]. Several HLA class I and class II lesions were shown to be genetic susceptibility genes for GO [80], although they are still controversial because of a lack of confirmation of the results.

5.6. Other genes

GO has reported to be associated with several genes involved in immunopathogenesis. Polymorphisms in intracellular adhesion molecule (ICAM)-1, which is a pivotal molecule in leukocyte migration and circulation, was recently reported to be a predisposition for GO [93]. Interactions between CD40 and CD40 ligand were demonstrated to induce the expression of ICAM-1 on the surface of retro-orbital fibroblasts [94]. Thus, the polymorphism of ICAM-1 could alter its expression levels resulting in the modification of leukocyte migration to the orbits. Similar to GD and HT, PTPN22 is a candidate genetic factor for GO [95], although the connection between PTPN22 and GO has not been confirmed. However, a polymorphism in PTPN12, an important regulator of T cell receptor signal transduction other than PTPN22, was demonstrated to have an association with the presence of mild to moderate GO in a Caucasian population through interactions with TSHR [80]. NF-κB, toll-like receptor (TLR)-9, glucocorticoid receptor, CD86 and CD103 have also been reported to be associated with the clinical course of GO [59, 80]. While TSHR gene polymorphisms are major genetic factors of GD, they have been demonstrated to play a role in the development of GO among GD patients.

The evaluation of genetic predisposition to GO is complicated. As described above, studies on the association of GO and cytokines or CTLA-4 are still controversial. The polymorphisms of HLA genes have unsolved problems because they tend to be in LD with neighboring genes. Unfortunately, functional analysis of candidate genes is not performed often enough, and so the genetic predisposition to GO is often not validated. Despite many studies, there is often a bias towards certain ethnic groups, whereas for example those containing African populations are scant. The clinical features of GO between ethnic groups can be different. For example, the severity and activity of GO in Asian populations tend to be milder than in Caucasian patients [96]. This suggests that genetic factor(s) are important in the development of GO severity. Moreover, the ratio of females/males with GO is lower than that of GD without GO and HT [1, 97], suggesting that GO is less dependent on the X chromosome. Thus, it is reasonable to regard GO as a disease that has genetic predispositions. On the contrary, Yin et al. recently showed that there was no association between both the development of GO and the severity GO and genetic polymorphisms of HLA-DR3, CTLA-4, TSHR and IL-23R, which are well-established GD susceptibility genes [98]. They also showed that any combination of genetic polymorphisms among these four genes did not contribute to GO, suggesting an absence of distinct genetic predisposition to GO. Indeed, the strongest influencing factor in the development of GO is smoking, which is a typical environmental factor [97]. Does this mean then that the effects of different ethnic backgrounds and sex ratio on the clinical phenotype of GO can be explained by environmental factors only? This is a fundamental issue that should be resolved.

	Class	Grade
0	**N**o physical signs or symptoms	
I	**O**nly signs, no symptoms (lid retraction, lid lag)	Lid retraction **a**:<2mm **b**: 2-5mm **c**: "/>5mm
II	**S**oft tissue involvement (sandy sensation, lacrimation, photophobia, lid fullness, conjunctival injection, chemsis, lid edema)	**0**: Absent **a**: Mild **b**: Moderate **c**: Marked
III	**P**roptosis	**0**: < 17mm **a**: 17 - 18mm **b**: 18 - 21mm **c**: "/>21mm
IV	**E**xtraocular muscle involvement	**0**: Absent **a**: Limitation of motion in extremes of gaze **b**: Evident restriction of motion **c**: Fixation of a globe or globes
V	**C**orneal involvement	**0**: Absent **a**: Stippling of the cornea **b**: Ulceration **c**: Clouding, necrosis, perforation
VI	**S**ight loss (optic nerve involvement)	**0**: Absent **a**: Visual acuity 0.63-0.5 **b**: 0.4-0.1 **c**: <0.1 - no light perception

Table 2. Modified "NOSPECS" classification. Grades a, b and c within class I, class II, class III and class IV are largely undefined. Severity should be scored by skillful experts in GO. The classification score should be expressed as the largest each class and the subclass, e.g. class II_a, III_b, IV_b.

5.7. Subtypes of Graves' ophthalmopathy

The most important issue is the definition of GO. Currently, ophthalmopathy related to AITD is described as GO, although there is no evidence to suggest that GO accompanied by GD and GO with HT are the same disease despite, having almost the same clinical phenotype. Moreover, GO has diverse symptoms and clinical features. For example, some lesions are unilateral, others are bilateral, and some effects are observed in the extra-ocular muscle and others in the retro-orbital fat tissue without any lesions in the extra-ocular muscles. Observations in patients with GO indicate the presence of subtypes, although there have been few descriptions published to date.

For half a century, clinicians have sorted GO patients for treatment by clinical grade. Werner SC has classified GO into 7 classes as shown in Table 2 [99]. This classification is termed "NOSPECS" classification and has been adopted as the "official" classification of the American

Thyroid Association. Clinicians use this as a clinical stratification of GO. Indeed, the prognosis of eye function of the patient tends to worsen in the order of this classification. Intriguingly, there exist many GO patients who develop a certain class of symptoms do not develop symptoms that belong to a lower class. For instance, it is not rare for a patient with GO who has an extra-ocular muscle symptom (class VI) to have no symptoms of proptosis (class III). This suggests that there are several symptoms involved in GO, which could progress independently each other. Although these facts have encouraged researchers to analyze the clinical course and patterns of affected lesions in GO patients, such reports are scarce. El-Kaissi et al. classified the clinical features of GO into three subtypes [100] containing: 1) congestive ophthalmopathy that mainly affects the retro-orbital fat tissue; 2) myopathic ophthalmopathy affecting the extra-ocular muscle(s); and 3) mixed congestive and myopathic ophthalmopathy. From the clinical point of view, this classification is useful because eye muscle involvement is a key factor for the aggressive treatment for GO that consists of intravenous glucocorticoid therapy and/or irradiation of the retro-orbital lesion. Furthermore, there are also other symptoms of GO including inflammation of the lachrymal glands and/or eyelids and eyelid retraction. To identify and diagnose extra-ocular muscle lesions precisely and accurately, magnet resonance imaging (MRI) of the retro-orbital area is an efficient tool for clinicians. It is useful to make detailed graphics to measure the volume of extra-ocular muscles and the grade of proptosis, and to discriminate the affected lesion inside the orbit from normal tissue. MRI can be used to obtain a variety of subtracted images useful for making decisions on the condition of GO [101, 102]. While MRI has several undesirable aspects (i.e. time-consuming, expensive, difficulty in comparison of images taken at different times and/or by different machines), it is still the most useful device for the evaluation of GO. The progress of MRI technology has contributed to the treatment of GO.

Examples of MRI for GO are shown. Figure 1 shows an 83-year-old male affected with GO. MRI imaging indicates the enlargement of all bilateral extra-ocular muscles with compression of the optic nerves. This patient has a rapidly progressing disorder in bilateral visual function. However, he has no proptosis. This case is NOSPECS class I_b, II_a, III_0, IV_b, V_0, VI_b and "myopathic ophthalmopathy" type. With bilateral lower eyelid retraction and mild lid edema, this can be sorted as "mixed ophthalmopathy" type. Figure 2 shows a 42-year-old female with bilateral proptosis. She has right lid retraction in primary gaze (Darylmple's sign) and lid edema. MRI imaging indicates her disease does not affect extra-ocular muscles. This case is NOSPECS class is I_a, II_a, III_b IV_0, V_0, VI_0 and "congestive ophthalmopathy." Figure 3 shows a 51-year-old female with GD. She has bilateral eyelids swelling without proptosis or diplopia. MRI shows the prominent swelling of upper eyelid and slight enlargement of the superior levator muscles. There is no enlargement of the rectus muscles nor retro-orbital fat expansion. This case is classified as NOSPECS class I_0, II_c, III_0 IV_0, V_0, VI_0. With examining without MRI, this case is regarded as "congestive ophthalmopathy." However the findings on MRI images suggest it is "mixed congestive and myopathic ophthalmopathy." Figure 4 shows a 65-year-old male with HT. While he has no TRAb, he has evident proptosis (left side > right side) and deviation of the left eyeball. MRI imaging shows marked enlargement of the inferior and medial rectus muscles of the left eye. The MRI STIR imaging suggests intense inflammation in these muscles. This case is classified as NOSPECS class I_0, II_a, III_a IV_c, V_0, VI_0 and "mixed congestive and myopathic ophthalmopathy."

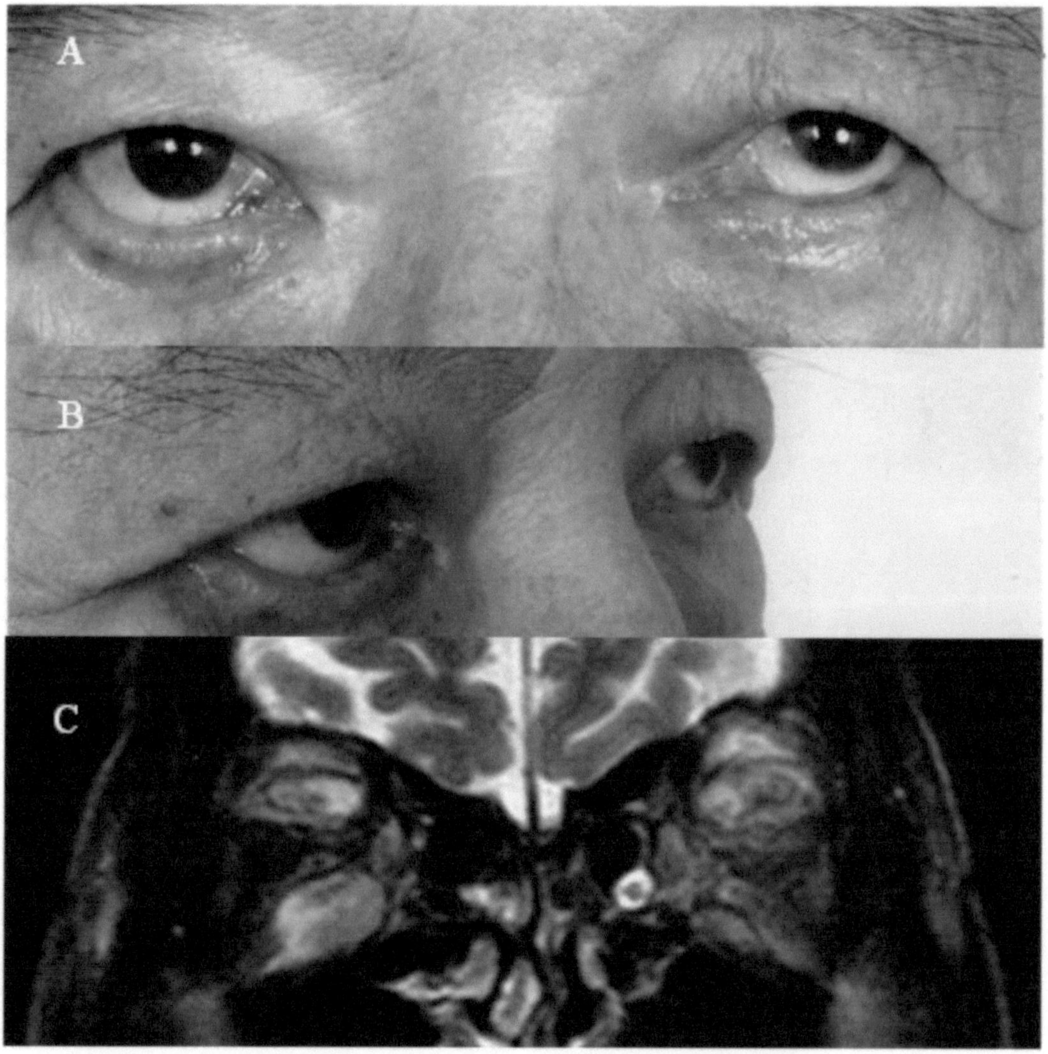

Figure 1. An 83-year-old male with GD. A) He has bilateral lower eyelid retraction and mild lid edema. B) He has no proptosis suggesting NOSPECS class III_0. C) MRI imaging indicates the enlargement of all bilateral extra-ocular muscles with compression of the optic nerves. The STIR (Short TI Inversion Recovery) imaging, which suppresses the signal from fat, shows high intensity inside the bilateral eye muscles indicating the inflammation of eye muscles. This case is NOSPECS class I_b, II_a, III_0, IV_b, V_0, VI_b.

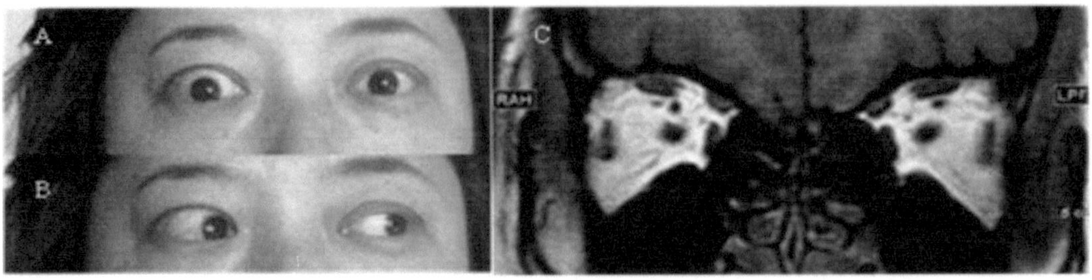

Figure 2. A 42-year-old female with bilateral proptosis. A). She has right lid retraction in primary gaze (Darylmple's sign) and lid edema. B) However her eye movement was normal. C) MRI imaging shows all her extraocular muscles are intact. This case is NOSPECS class is I_a, II_a, III_b IV_0, V_0, VI_0.

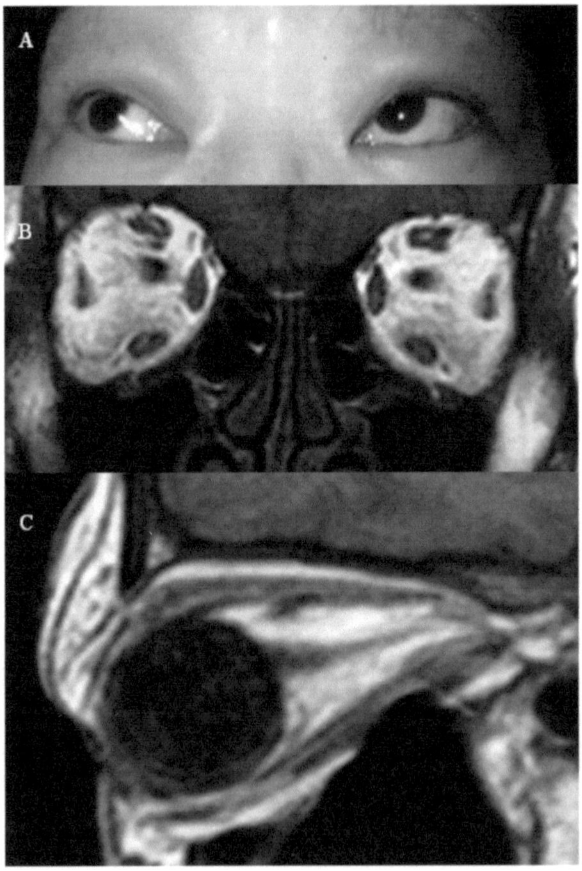

Figure 3. A 51-year-old female with GD. A) She has bilateral eyelids swelling without proptosis or diplopia. B, C) MRI shows the prominent swelling of upper eyelid and the enlargement of the superior levator palpebrae muscle. There is no enlargement of the rectus muscles or retro-orbital fat expansion. This case is classified as NOSPECS class I_0, II_c, III_0 IV_0, V_0, VI_0.

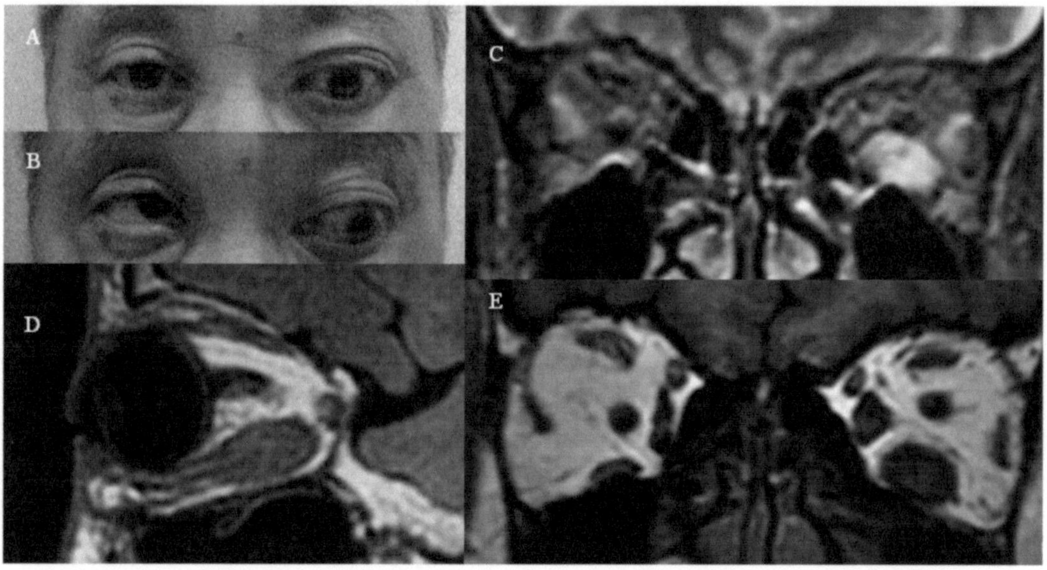

Figure 4. A 65-year-old male with HT. He has hypothyroidism and needs thyroid hormone replacement therapy. His eye symptoms, which are mainly diplopia, commenced when he had a traffic accident. They worsened in a few months and came to see us. A) He has evident proptosis (left side > right side) and deviation of the left eye ball. B) His left eye movement is seriously impaired when gazing in left to upward direction. His left inferior and medial rectus muscles are shown to be enlarged in the MRI imaging (C, D, E). The MRI STIR imaging shows intense inflammation in muscles involved (C). This case is classified as NOSPECS class I_0, II_a, III_a IV_c, V_0, VI_0.

Recent progress in imaging inspection including MRI introduces a new concept of the disease. Volpe et al. demonstrated that 55% of GD patients without clinical evidence of GO were diagnosed with GO by ocular echography [103]. They named this type of GO as "occult thyroid eye disease." If MRI is performed for all GD patients, a large number of patients with "occult thyroid eye disease" would likely be diagnosed. Thus, we have to consider such GO patients for further evaluation of the pathogenesis and immunogenetics of GO. Furthermore, we could sort GO phenotypes in order of timing of development of disease (simultaneous onset with GD, later onset and earlier onset than GD). Thus, further investigation and discussions by experts are needed to establish more accurate definitions of the subtypes of GO.

6. Conclusion

GO is a manifestation related to AITD, although the immunogenetic component of disease susceptibility is still controversial. The strongest factor which affects the presence and/or severity of GO is smoking, a common environmental factor. From these studies and/or experimental data, some researchers have concluded that there is no genetic susceptibility component in GO. In contrast, many studies investigating the effects of ethnic background on the presence and severity of GO and differences in the male/female ratio between GO patients and GD without GO patients suggest the possibility of a genetic predisposition to GO. To solve such discrepancies, there should be an emphasis on reconsideration of the determination of GO. The disease we all recognize as GO might not be a single disease. At present, GO has many manifestations during the course of the disease, including associated diseases (GD, HT and sometimes thyroid cancer), differences in onset timing, MRI findings and location of lesions. Therefore, reclassification of GO into several patterns using MRI will be of great help. Using state-of-the-art imaging equipment and immunological and biological technology, we should classify GO into more ideal and probable subtypes, which might help research focused on the pathogenesis and/or genetics of GO. To date, several studies have tested genetic susceptibility from the view point of NOSPECS severity classification, resulting in a failure to establish evidence for genetic factors of GO. High quality research should be conducted by experts of GO, allowing discussion on the probable and appropriate genetic susceptibility of GO. Moreover, ongoing GWAS studies and genetic mapping of SNPs studies on GD and HT will accumulate evidence and new findings on genetic susceptibility to the diseases, contributing to the establishment of genetic predispositions to GO, which can be appropriately classified into subtypes. Further studies are required for this purpose.

Author details

Junichi Tani and Yuji Hiromatsu

Division of Endocrinology and Metabolism, Department of Medicine, Kurume University School of Medicine, Kurume, Fukuoka, Japan

References

[1] Hasham, A, & Tomer, Y. Genetic and epigenetic mechanisms in thyroid autoimmunity. Immunol Res. (2012). Mar 29 in press.

[2] Jacobson, E. M, Huber, A, & Tomer, Y. The HLA gene complex in thyroid autoimmunity: from epidemiology to etiology. J Autoimmun. (2008). , 30, 58-62.

[3] Mizokami, T. Wu Li A, El-Kaissi S, Wall JR. Stress and thyroid autoimmunity. Thyroid. (2004). , 14(12), 1047-55.

[4] Karouzakis, E, Gay, R. E, Gay, S, & Neidhart, M. Epigenetic control in rheumatoid arthritis synovial fibroblasts. Nat Rev Rheumatol. (2009). , 5(5), 266-72.

[5] Gillespie, E. F, Smith, T. J, & Douglas, R. S. Thyroid eye disease: towards an evidence base for treatment in the 21st century. Curr Neurol Neurosci Rep. (2012). , 12(3), 318-24.

[6] Tomer, Y. Unilateral ophthalmopathy in a patient with Hashimoto's thyroiditis. Thyroid (2000). , 10, 99-100.

[7] Yoshihara, A. Yoshimura Noh J, Nakachi A, Ohye H, Sato S, Sekiya K, Kosuga Y, Suzuki M, Matsumoto M, Kunii Y, Watanabe N, Mukasa K, Inoue Y, Ito K, Ito K. Severe thyroid-associated orbitopathy in Hashimoto's thyroiditis. Report of 2 cases. Endocr J. (2011). , 58(5), 343-8.

[8] Prabhakar, B. S, Bhn, R. S, & Smith, T. J. Current perspective on the pathogenesis of Graves' disease and ophthalmopathy. Endocr. Rev. (2003). , 24, 802-835.

[9] Hall, R, & Stanbury, J. B. Familial studies of autoimmune thyroiditis.Clin. Exp. Immunol. (1967). Suppl-25.

[10] Brix, T. H, Christensen, K, Holm, N. V, Harvald, B, & Hegedus, L. A population-based study of Graves' disease in Danish twins. Clin. Endocrinol. (Oxf), (1998). , 48, 397-400.

[11] Brix, T. H, Kyvik, K. O, Christensen, K, & Hegedus, L. Evidence for a major role of heredity in Graves' disease: a population-based study of two Danish twin cohorts. J. Clin. Endocrinol. Metab. (2001). , 86, 930-934.

[12] Stenszky, V, Kozma, L, Balazs, C, Rochlitz, S, Bear, J. C, & Farid, N. R. The genetics of Graves' disease: HLA and disease susceptibility. J. Clin. Endocrinol. Metab. (1985). , 61, 735-740.

[13] Brent, G. A. Environmental exposures and autoimmune thyroid disease. Thyroid. (2010). , 20, 755-761.

[14] Papanastasiou, L, Vatalas, I. A, Koutras, D. A, & Mastorakos, G. Thyroid autoimmunity in the current iodine environment. Thyroid. (2007). , 17, 729-739.

[15] DustinML T-cell activation through immunological synapses and kinapsesImmunol Rev. (2008). , 221, 77-89.

[16] Farid, N. R, Barnard, J. M, & Marshall, W. H. The association of HLA with autoimmune thyroid disease in Newfoundland. The influence of HLA homozygosity in Graves' disease. Tissue Antigens. (1976). , 8, 181-189.

[17] Grumet, F. C, Payne, R. O, Konishi, J, & Kriss, J. P. HL-A antigens as markers for disease susceptibility and autoimmunity in Graves' disease. J. Clin. Endocrinol. Metab. (1974). , 39, 1115-1119.

[18] Simmonds, M. J, Howson, J. M. M, Heward, J. M, Carr-smith, J, Franklyn, J. A, Todd, J. A, & Gough, S. C. L. A novel and major association of HLA-C in Graves' disease that eclipses the classical HLA-DRB1 effect. Hum. Mol. Genet. (2007). , 16, 2149-2153.

[19] Ploski, R, Szymanski, K, & Bednarczuk, T. The Genetic Basis of Graves' Disease. Curr Genom. (2011). , 12, 542-563.

[20] Tomer, Y. Genetic susceptibility to autoimmune thyroid disease: past, present, and future. Thyroid. (2010). , 20, 715-725.

[21] Ban, Y, Davies, T. F, Greenberg, D. A, Concepcion, E. S, Osman, R, Oashi, T, & Tomer, Y. Arginine at position 74 of the HLA-DR beta1 chain is associated with Graves' disease. Genes Immun. (2004). , 5, 203-208.

[22] Teft, W. A, Kirchhof, M. G, & Madrenas, J. A molecular perspective of CTLA-4 function. Annu Rev Immunol. (2006). , 24, 65-97.

[23] Ueda, H, Howson, J. M, Esposito, L, Heward, J, Snook, H, Chamberlain, G, Rainbow, D. B, Hunter, K. M, & Smith, A. N. Di Genova G, Herr MH, Dahlman I, Payne F, Smyth D, Lowe C, Twells RC, Howlett S, Healy B, Nutland S, Rance HE, Everett V, Smink LJ, Lam AC, Cordell HJ, Walker NM, Bordin C, Hulme J, Motzo C, Cucca F, Hess JF, Metzker ML, Rogers J, Gregory S, Allahabadia A, Nithiyananthan R, Tuomilehto-Wolf E, Tuomilehto J, Bingley P, Gillespie KM, Undlien DE, Ronningen KS, Guja C, Ionescu-Tirgoviste C, Savage DA, Maxwell AP, Carson DJ, Patterson CC, Franklyn JA, Clayton DG, Peterson LB, Wicker LS, Todd JA, Gough SC. Association of the T-cell regulatory gene CTLA4 with susceptibility to autoimmune disease. Nature. (2003). , 423, 506-511.

[24] Bednarczuk, T, Hiromatsu, Y, Fukutani, T, Jazdzewski, K, Miskiewicz, P, Osikowska, M, & Nauman, J. Association of cytotoxic T-lymphocyte-associated antigen-4 (CTLA-4) gene polymorphism and non-genetic factors with Graves' ophthalmopathy in European and Japanese populations. Eur J Endocrinol. (2003). , 148, 13-8.

[25] Vieland, V. J, Huang, Y, Bartlett, C, Davies, T. F, & Tomer, Y. A multilocus model of the genetic architecture of autoimmune thyroid disorder, with clinical implications. Am J Hum Genet. (2008). , 82, 1349-1356.

[26] Banchereau, J, Bazan, F, Blanchard, D, Briere, F, Galizzi, J. P, Van Kooten, C, Liu, Y. J, Rousset, F, Saeland, S, & The, C. D. antigen and its ligand. Annu Rev Immunol. (1994). , 12, 881-922.

[27] Tomer, Y, Concepcion, E, & Greenberg, D. A. A C/T Single-nucleotide polymorphism in the region of the CD40 gene is associated with Graves' Disease. Thyroid. (2002). , 12, 1129-1135.

[28] Jacobson, E. M, Concepcion, E, Oashi, T, & Tomer, Y. A Graves' disease-associated kozak sequence single-nucleotide polymorphism enhances the efficiency of CD40 gene translation: A case for translational pathophysiology. Endocrinology. (2005). , 146, 2684-2691.

[29] Kurylowicz, A, Kula, D, Ploski, R, Skorka, A, Jurecka- Lubieniecka, B, Zebracka, J, Steinhof-radwanska, K, Hasse- Lazar, K, Hiromatsu, Y, Jarzab, B, & Bednarczuk, T. Association of CD40 gene polymorphism (C-1T) with susceptibility and phenotype of Graves' disease. Thyroid. (2005). , 15, 1119-1124.

[30] Park, J. H, Chang, H. S, Park, C. S, Jang, A. S, Park, B. L, Rhim, T. Y, Uh, S. T, Kim, Y. H, Chung, I. Y, & Shin, H. D. Association analysis of CD40 polymorphisms with

asthma and the level of serum total IgE. Am J Respir Crit Care Med. 20076; , 175, 775-782.

[31] Jacobson, E. M, Huber, A. K, Akeno, N, Sivak, M, Li, C. W, Concepcion, E, Ho, K, & Tomer, Y. A CD40 Kozak sequence polymorphism and susceptibility to antibodymediated autoimmune conditions: the role of CD40 tissuespecific expression. Genes Immun. (2007). , 8, 205-214.

[32] Cloutier, J. F, & Veillette, A. Cooperative inhibition of T-cell antigen receptor signaling by a complex between a kinase and a phosphatase. J Exp Med. (1999). , 189, 111-121.

[33] Ichimura, M, Kaku, H, Fukutani, T, Koga, H, Mukai, T, Miyake, I, Yamada, K, Koda, Y, & Hiromatsu, Y. Associations of protein tyrosine phosphatase nonreceptor 22 (PTPN22) gene polymorphisms with susceptibility to Graves' disease in a Japanese population. Thyroid. (2008). , 18, 625-30.

[34] Vang, T, Congia, M, Macis, M. D, Musumeci, L, Orru, V, Zavattari, P, Nika, K, Tautz, L, Tasken, K, Cucca, F, Mustelin, T, & Bottini, N. Autoimmune-associated lymphoid tyrosine phosphatase is a gain-of-function variant. Nat Genet. (2005). , 37, 1317-1319.

[35] Bottini, N, Musumeci, L, Alonso, A, Rahmouni, S, Nika, K, & Rostamkhani, M. MacMurray J, Meloni GF, Lucarelli P, Pellecchia M, Eisenbarth GS, Comings D, Mustelin T. A functional variant of lymphoid tyrosine phosphatase is associated with type I diabetes. Nat Genet. (2004). , 36, 337-338.

[36] Josefowicz, S. Z, Lu, L. F, & Rudensky, A. Y. Regulatory T cells: mechanisms of differentiation and function. Annu Rev Immunol. (2012). , 30, 531-64.

[37] Gangi, E, Vasu, C, Cheatem, D, & Prabhakar, B. S. I. L-10-p. r. o. d. u. c. i. n. g C. D4+C. D Regulatory T cells play a critical role in granulocyte-macrophage colony-stimulating factor induced suppression of experimental autoimmune thyroiditis. J Immunol. (2005). , 174, 7006-7013.

[38] Saitoh, O, & Nagayama, Y. Regulation of Graves' hyperthyroidism with naturally occurring CD4+CD25+ regulatory T cells in a mouse model. Endocrinology. (2006). , 147, 2417-2422.

[39] Ban, Y, Tozaki, T, Tobe, T, Ban, Y, Jacobson, E. M, Concepcion, E. S, & Tomer, Y. The regulatory T cell gene FOXP3 and genetic susceptibility to thyroid autoimmunity: an association analysis in Caucasian and Japanese cohorts. J Autoimmun. (2007). , 28, 201-207.

[40] Czarnocka, B. Thyroperoxidase, thyroglobulin, Na(+)/I(-) symporter, pendrin in thyroid autoimmunity. Front Biosci. (2011). , 16, 783-802.

[41] Tomer, Y, Ban, Y, Concepcion, E, Barbesino, G, Villanueva, R, Greenberg, D. A, & Davies, T. F. Common and unique susceptibility loci in Graves and Hashimoto dis-

eases: results of whole-genome screening in a data set of 102 multiplex families. Am J Hum Genet. (2003). , 73, 736-747.

[42] Hodge, S. E, Ban, Y, Strug, L. J, Greenberg, D. A, Davies, T. F, Concepcion, E. S, Villanueva, R, & Tomer, Y. Possible interaction between HLA-DRbeta1 and thyroglobulin variants in Graves' disease. Thyroid. (2006). , 16, 351-355.

[43] Stefan, M, Jacobson, E. M, Huber, A. K, Greenberg, D. A, Li, C. W, Skrabanek, L, Conception, E, Fadlalla, M, Ho, K, & Tomer, Y. A novel variant of the thyroglobulin promoter triggers thyroid autoimmunity through an epigenetic interferon alpha-modulated mechanism. J. Biol. Chem. (2011). , 286, 31168-79.

[44] Tani, J, Mori, K, Hoshikawa, S, Nakazawa, T, Satoh, J, Nakagawa, Y, Ito, S, & Yoshida, K. Prevention of lymphocytic thyroiditis in iodide-treated non-obese diabetic mice lacking interferon regulatory factor-1. Eur J Endocrinol. (2002). , 147, 809-14.

[45] Brand, O. J, Barrett, J. C, Simmonds, M. J, Newby, P. R, Mccabe, C. J, Bruce, C. K, Kysela, B, Carr-smith, J. D, Brix, T, Hunt, P. J, Wiersinga, W. M, Hegedus, L, & Connell, J. Wass JAH, Franklyn JA, Weetman AP, Heward JM, Gough SCL. Association of the thyroid stimulating hormone receptor gene (TSHR) with Graves' disease. Hum. Mol. Genet. (2009). , 18, 1704-1713.

[46] Chen, C. R, Pichurin, P, Nagayama, Y, Latrofa, F, Rapoport, B, & Mclachlan, S. M. The thyrotropin receptor autoantigen in Graves disease is the culprit as well as the victim. J. Clin. Invest. (2003). , 111, 1897-1904.

[47] Wellcome Trust Case Control ConsortiumAustralo-Anglo- American Spondylitis Consortium (TASC). Association scan of 14,500 nonsynonymous SNPs in four diseases identifies autoimmunity variants. Nat. Genet. (2007). , 39, 1329-1337.

[48] Kochi, Y, Yamada, R, Suzuki, A, Harley, J. B, Shirasawa, S, Sawada, T, Bae, S. C, Tokuhiro, S, Chang, X, Sekine, A, Takahashi, A, Tsunoda, T, Ohnishi, Y, Kaufman, K. M, Kang, C. P, Kang, C, Otsubo, S, Yumura, W, Mimori, A, Koike, T, Nakamura, Y, Sasazuki, T, & Yamamoto, K. A functional variant in FCRL3, encoding Fc receptor-like 3, is associated with rheumatoid arthritis and several autoimmunities. Nat. Genet. (2005). , 37, 478-485.

[49] Gu, L. Q, Zhu, W, Zhao, S. X, Zhao, L, Zhang, M. J, Cui, B, Song, H. D, Ning, G, & Zhao, Y. J. Clinical associations of the genetic variants of CTLA-4, Tg, TSHR, PTPN22, PTPN12 and FCRL3 in patients with Graves' disease. Clin. Endocrinol. (Oxf). (2010). , 72, 248-55.

[50] Swainson, L. A, Mold, J. E, Bajpai, U. D, & Mccune, J. M. Expression of the autoimmune susceptibility gene FcRL3 on human regulatory t cells is associated with dysfunction and high levels of programmed cell death-1. J. Immunol. (2010). , 184, 3639-3647.

[51] Song, H. D, Liang, J, Shi, J. Y, Zhao, S. X, Liu, Z, Zhao, J. J, Peng, Y. D, Gao, G. Q, Tao, J, Pan, C. M, Shao, L, Cheng, F, Wang, Y, Yuan, G. Y, Xu, C, Han, B, Huang, W, Chu,

X, Chen, Y, Sheng, Y, Li, R. Y, Su, Q, Gao, L, Jia, W. P, Jin, L, Chen, M. D, Chen, S. J, Chen, Z, & Chen, J. L. Functional SNPs in the SCGB3A2 promoter are associated with susceptibility to Graves' disease. Hum. Mol. Genet. (2009). , 18, 1156-1170.

[52] Areschoug, T, & Gordon, S. Scavenger receptors: role in innate immunity and microbial pathogenesis. Cell Microbiol. (2009). , 11, 1160-1169.

[53] Niimi, T, Munakata, M, Keck-waggoner, C. L, Popescu, N. C, Levitt, R. C, Hisada, M, & Kimura, S. A polymorphism in the human UGRP1 gene promoter that regulates transcription is associated with an increased risk of asthma. Am. J. Hum. Genet. (2002). , 70, 718-725.

[54] Todd, J. A, Walker, N. M, Cooper, J. D, Smyth, D. J, Downes, K, Plagnol, V, Bailey, R, Nejentsev, S, Field, S. F, Payne, F, Lowe, C. E, Szeszko, J. S, Hafler, J. P, & Zeitels, L. Yang JHM, Vella A, Nutland S, Stevens HE, Schuilenburg H, Coleman G, Maisuria M, Meadows W, Smink LJ, Healy B, Burren OS, Lam AAC, Ovington NR, Allen J, Adlem E, Leung HT, Wallace C, Howso, JMM, Guja C, Ionescu-Tirgoviste C, Simmonds MJ, Heward JM, Gough SCL, Dunger DB, Wicker LS, Clayton DG. Robust associations of four new chromosome regions from genome-wide analyses of type 1 diabetes. Nat. Genet. (2007). , 39, 857-864.

[55] Penna-martinez, M, Ramos-lopez, E, Robbers, I, Kahles, H, Hahner, S, Willenberg, H, Reisch, N, Seidl, C, Segni, M, & Badenhoop, K. The rs1990760 polymorphism within the IFIH1 locus is not associated with Graves' disease, Hashimoto's thyroiditis and Addison's disease. BMC Med. Genet. (2009).

[56] Zhao, Z. F, Cui, B, Chen, H. Y, Wang, S, Li, I, Gu, X. J, Qi, L, Li, X. Y, Ning, G, Zhao, Y. J, & The, A. T polymorphism in the interferon induced helicase gene does not confer susceptibility to Graves' disease in Chinese population. Endocrine. (2007). , 32, 143-147.

[57] Ban, Y, Tozaki, T, Taniyama, M, Nakano, Y, Ban, Y, & Hirano, T. Genomic polymorphism in the interferon-induced helicase (IFIH1) gene does not confer susceptibility to autoimmune thyroid disease in the Japanese population. Horm. Metab. Res. (2010). , 42, 70-72.

[58] Chistiakov, D. A. Interferon Induced with Helicase C Domain 1 (IFIH1) and Virus-Induced Autoimmunity: A Review. Viral Immunol. (2010). , 23, 3-15.

[59] Kurylowicz, A, Hiromatsu, Y, Jurecka-lubieniecka, B, Kula, D, Kowalska, M, Ichimura, M, Koga, H, Kaku, H, Bar-andziak, E, Nauman, J, Jarzab, B, Ploski, R, & Bednarczuk, T. Association of NFKB1-94ins/del ATTG promoter polymorphism with susceptibility to and phenotype of Graves' disease. Genes Immun. (2007). , 8, 532-8.

[60] Mclachlan, S. M, & Rapoport, B. Why measure thyroglobulin autoantibodies rather than thyroid peroxidase autoantibodies? Thyroid. (2004). , 14, 510-520.

[61] Zaletel, K, & Gaberscek, S. Hashimoto's Thyroiditis: From Genes to the Disease. Curr Genom. (2011). , 12, 576-588.

[62] Tani, J, Yoshida, K, Fukazawa, H, Kiso, Y, Sayama, N, Mori, K, Aizawa, Y, Hori, H, Nakasato, N, & Abe, K. Hyperthyroid Graves' disease and primary hypothyroidism caused by TSH receptor antibodies in monozygotic twins: case reports. Endocri J. (1998). , 45, 117-121.

[63] Villanueva, R, Greenberg, D. A, Davies, T. F, & Tomer, Y. Sibling recurrence risk in autoimmune thyroid disease. Thyroid. (2003). , 13, 761-764.

[64] Tandon, N, Zhang, L, & Weetman, A. P. HLA associations with Hashimoto's thyroiditis. Clin. Endocrinol. (Oxf). (1991). , 34, 383-386.

[65] Kavvoura, F. K, Akamizu, T, Awata, T, Ban, Y, Chistiakov, D. A, Frydecka, I, Ghaderi, A, Gough, S. C, Hiromatsu, Y, Ploski, R, Wang, P. W, Ban, Y, Bednarczuk, T, Chistiakova, E. I, Chojm, M, Heward, J. M, Hiratani, H, Juo, S. H, Karabon, L, Katayama, S, Kurihara, S, Liu, R. T, Miyake, I, Omrani, G. H, Pawlak, E, Taniyama, M, Tozaki, T, & Ioannidis, J. P. Cytotoxic T lymphocyte associated antigen 4 gene polymorphisms and autoimmune thyroid disease: a meta-analysis. J. Clin. Endocrinol. Metab. (2007). , 92, 3162-3170.

[66] Criswell, L. A, Pfeiffer, K. A, Lum, R. F, Gonzales, B, Novitzke, J, Kern, M, Moser, K. L, Begovich, A. B, Carlton, V. E, Li, W, Lee, A. T, Ortmann, W, Behrens, T. W, & Gregersen, P. K. Analysis of families in the multiple autoimmune disease genetics consortium (MADGC) collection: the PTPN22 620W allele associates with multiple autoimmune phenotypes. Am J Hum Genet. (2005). , 76, 561-571.

[67] Toubi, E, & Shoenfeld, Y. The role of vitamin D in regulating immune responses. Isr. Med. Assoc. J. (2010). , 12, 174-175.

[68] Stefani, M, Papi, S, Suver, M, Glavas-obrovac, L, & Karner, I. Association of vitamin D receptor gene 3'-variants with Hashimoto's thyroiditis in the Croatian population. Int. J. Immunogenet. (2008). , 35, 125-131.

[69] Ban, Y, Greenberg, D. A, Concepcion, E, Skrabanek, L, Villanueva, R, & Tomer, Y. Amino acid substitutions in the thyroglobulin gene are associated with susceptibility to human and murine autoimmune thyroid disease. Proc Natl Acad Sci USA. (2003). , 100, 15119-15124.

[70] Ito, C, Watanabe, M, Okuda, N, Watanabe, C, & Iwatani, Y. Association between the severity of Hashimoto's disease and the functional +874A/T polymorphism in the interferon-gamma gene. Endocr. J. (2006). , 53, 473-478.

[71] Nanba, T, Watanabe, M, Akamizu, T, & Iwatani, Y. The-590CC genotype in the IL4 gene as a strong predictive factor for the development of hypothyroidism in Hashimoto disease. Clin. Chem. (2008). , 54, 621-623.

[72] Yamada, H, Watanabe, M, Nanba, T, Akamizu, T, Iwatani, Y, & The, T. C polymorphism in the transforming growth factor- beta1 gene is associated with the severity

and intractability of autoimmune thyroid disease. Clin. Exp. Immunol. (2008)., 151, 379-382.

[73] Bahn, R. S. Graves' ophthalmopathy. N. Engl. J. Med. (2010)., 362, 726-738.

[74] Tani, J, Gopinath, B, Nguyen, B, & Wall, J. R. Extraocular muscle autoimmunity and orbital fat inflammation in thyroid-associated ophthalmopathy. Expert Rev Clin Immunol. (2007)., 3, 299-311.

[75] Gerding, M N, Van Der Meer, J W, Broenink, M, Bakker, O, Wiersinga, W. M, & Prummel, M. F. Association of thyrotrophin receptor antibodies with the clinical features of Graves' ophthalmopathy. Clin. Endocrinol. (Oxf). (2000)., 52, 267-271.

[76] Ponto, K. A, Kanitz, M, Olivo, P. D, Pitz, S, Pfeiffer, N, & Kahaly, G. J. Clinical relevance of thyroid-stimulating immunoglobulins in Graves' ophthalmopathy.Ophthalmology. (2011)., 118, 2279-85.

[77] Hunt, P. J, Marshall, S. E, Weetman, A. P, Bell, J. I, Wass, J. A, & Welsh, K. I. Cytokine gene polymorphisms in autoimmune thyroid disease. J. Clin. Endocrinol. Metab. (2000)., 85, 1984-1988.

[78] Kumar, S, & Bahn, R. S. Relative overexpression of macrophage derived cytokines in orbital adipose tissue from patients with Graves' ophthalmopathy. J. Clin. Endocrinol. Metab. (2003)., 88, 4246-4250.

[79] Durrani, O. M, Reuser, T. Q, & Murray, P. I. Infliximab: a novel treatment for sight-threatening thyroid associated ophthalmopathy. Orbit. (2005)., 24, 117-119.

[80] Khalilzadeh, O, Noshad, S, Rashidi, A, & Amirzargar, A. Graves' Ophthalmopathy: A Review of Immunogenetics. Curr Genom. (2011)., 12, 564-575.

[81] Sims, J. E, Smith, D. E, & The, I. L. family: regulators of immunity. Nat. Rev. Immunol. (2010)., 10, 89-102.

[82] Muhlberg, T, Joba, W, Spitzweg, C, Schworm, H. D, Heberling, H. J, & Heufelder, A. E. Interleukin-1 receptor antagonist ribonucleic acid and protein expression by cultured Graves' and normal orbital fibroblasts is differentially modulated by dexamethasone and irradiation. J. Clin. Endocrinol. Metab. (2000)., 85, 734-742.

[83] Tan, G. H, Dutton, C. M, Bahn, R. S, & Interleukin-1, I. L. receptor antagonist and soluble IL-1 receptor inhibit IL-1-induced glycosaminoglycan production in cultured human orbital fibroblasts from patients with Graves' ophthalmopathy. J. Clin. Endocrinol. Metab. (1996)., 81, 449-452.

[84] Cuddihy, R. M, & Bahn, R. S. Lack of an association between alleles of interleukin-1 alpha and interleukin-1 receptor antagonist genes and Graves' disease in a North American Caucasian population. J.Clin. Endocrinol. Metab. (1996)., 81, 4476-4478.

[85] Liu, N, Li, X, Liu, C, Zhao, Y, Cui, B, & Ning, G. The association of interleukin-1alpha and interleukin-1beta polymorphisms with the risk of Graves' disease in a case-control study and meta-analysis. Hum. Immunol. (2010). , 71, 397-401.

[86] Fukutani, T, Hiromatsu, Y, Kaku, H, Miyake, I, Mukai, T, Imamura, Y, Kohno, S, Takane, N, Shoji, S, Otabe, S, & Yamada, K. A polymorphism of interferon-gamma gene associated with changes of anti-thyrotropin receptor antibodies induced by antithyroid drug treatment for Graves' disease in Japanese patients. Thyroid. (2004). , 14-93.

[87] Anvari, M, Khalilzadeh, O, Esteghamati, A, Esfahani, S. A, Rashidi, A, Etemadi, A, Mahmoudi, M, & Amirzargar, A. A. Genetic susceptibility to Graves' ophthalmopathy: the role of polymorphisms in proinflammatory cytokine genes. Eye (Lond). (2010). , 24, 1058-1063.

[88] Vaidya, B, Imrie, H, Perros, P, Dickinson, J, Mccarthy, M. I, Kendall-taylor, P, & Pearce, S. H. Cytotoxic T lymphocyte antigen-4 (CTLA-4) gene polymorphism confers susceptibility to thyroid associated orbitopathy. Lancet. (1999). , 354, 743-744.

[89] Bednarczuk, T, Gopinath, B, Ploski, R, & Wall, J. R. Susceptibility genes in Graves' ophthalmopathy: searching for a needle in a haystack? Clin. Endocrinol. (Oxf). (2007). , 67, 3-19.

[90] Bednarczuk, T, Hiromatsu, Y, Seki, N, Ploski, R, Fukutani, T, Kurylowicz, A, Jazdzewski, K, Chojnowski, K, Itoh, K, & Nauman, J. Association of tumor necrosis factor and human leukocyte antigen DRB1 alleles with Graves' ophthalmopathy. Hum. Immunol. (2004). , 65, 632-639.

[91] Lavard, L, Madsen, H. O, Perrild, H, Jacobsen, B. B, & Svejgaard, A. HLA class II associations in juvenile Graves' disease: indication of a strong protective role of the DRB1*0701,DQA1*0201 haplotype. Tissue Antigens. (1997). , 50, 639-641.

[92] Weetman, A. P, Zhang, L, Webb, S, & Shine, B. Analysis of HLADQB and HLA-DPB alleles in Graves' disease by oligonucleotide probing of enzymatically amplified DNA. Clin. Endocrinol. (Oxf). (1990). , 33, 65-71.

[93] Kretowski, A, Wawrusiewicz, N, Mironczuk, K, Mysliwiec, J, Kretowska, M, & Kinalska, I. Intercellular adhesion molecule 1 gene polymorphisms in Graves' disease. J. Clin. Endocrinol. Metab. (2003). , 88, 4945-4949.

[94] Zhao, L. Q, Wei, R. L, Cheng, J. W, Cai, J. P, & Li, Y. The expression of intercellular adhesion molecule-1 induced by CD40-CD40L ligand signaling in orbital fibroblasts in patients with Graves' ophthalmopathy. Invest Ophthalmol Vis Sci. (2010). , 51, 4652-60.

[95] Skórka, A, Bednarczuk, T, Bar-andziak, E, Nauman, J, & Ploski, R. Lymphoid tyrosine phosphatase (PTPN22/LYP) variant and Graves' disease in a Polish population: association and gene dose-dependent correlation with age of onset. Clin Endocrinol (Oxf). (2005). , 62, 679-82.

[96] Chng, C. L, Seah, L. L, & Khoo, D. H. Ethnic differences in the clinical presentation of Graves' ophthalmopathy. Best Pract Res Clin Endocrinol Metab. (2012). , 26, 249-58.

[97] Stan, M. N, & Bahn, R. S. Risk factors for development or deterioration of Graves' ophthalmopathy. Thyroid. (2010). , 20, 777-83.

[98] Yin, X, Latif, R, Bahn, R, & Davies, T. F. Genetic Profiling in Graves' Disease: Further Evidence for Lack of a Distinct Genetic Contribution to Graves' Ophthalmopathy. Thyroid. (2012). , 7, 730-736.

[99] Werner, S. C. Classification of the eye changes of Graves' disease. American Journal of Ophthalmology. (1969). , 68, 646-648.

[100] El-Kaissi, S, Frauman, A. G, & Wall, J. R. Thyroid-associated ophthalmopathy: a practical guide to classification, natural history and management. Intern Med J. (2004). , 34, 482-91.

[101] El-Kaissi, S, & Wall, J. R. Determinants of extraocular muscle volume in patients with Graves' disease. J Thyroid Res. (2012).

[102] Hiromatsu, Y, Kojima, K, Ishisaka, N, Tanaka, K, Sato, M, Nonaka, K, Nishimura, H, & Nishida, H. Role of magnetic resonance imaging in thyroid-associated ophthalmopathy: its predictive value for therapeutic outcome of immunosuppressive therapy. Thyroid. (1992). , 2, 299-305.

[103] Volpe, N. J, & Sbarbaro, J. A. Gendron Livingston K, Galetta SL, Liu GT, Balcer LJ. Occult thyroid eye disease in patients with unexplained ocular misalignment identified by standardized orbital echography. Am J Ophthalmol. (2006). , 142, 75-81.

Chapter 2

Gene Polymorphisms of Immunoregulatory Cytokines IL-10 and TGF-β1 in Systemic Lupus Erythematosus

Irena Manolova, Mariana Ivanova and Spaska Stanilova

Additional information is available at the end of the chapter

http://dx.doi.org/10.5772/53799

1. Introduction

Systemic lupus erythematosus (SLE) is a complex multifactorial autoimmune disease characterized by loss of immune tolerance and defective immune regulatory mechanisms that leads to B cell hyperactivity and the production of pathogenic autoantibodies directed against a wide range of autoantigens, and particularly nuclear antigens [Liossis et al., 1996; Yurasov et al., 2006; Mandik-Nayak et al., 2008]. In common, the complex interaction of genetic, environmental, as well as immunological factors causes the breaking of self-tolerance of the immune system and leads to development of autoimmunity. The immune system has various mechanisms at the cellular and molecular level that negatively regulate immune responses and counteract establishment of chronic and destructive immunity [Nakken et al., 2012]. A number of circulating cytokine abnormalities have been reported in SLE and recent advances have revealed new insights in cytokine regulation of autoimmune inflammatory responses [Diveu et al., 2008]. In particular, the production of Interleukin-10 (IL-10) and transforming growth factor-β1 (*TGF*-β1), the two main Treg cytokines that suppress the inflammatory response, has been found to be deeply deregulated in SLE patients, so they have been considered essential elements in the etiopathology of the disease.

Given the importance of cytokines in immune system regulation, these molecules are of high interest not only in the "effector phase" of autoimmune disease in which self-tolerance has already been broken, but also in the "initiation phase" of autoimmunity, in which a lasting immune response against self antigens is first generated. Recently, it has been suggested that initial susceptibility to autoimmune disease lies at least partly in the genetics of cytokine regulation, and that many genetic polymorphisms affecting cytokine patterns could alter thresholds for immune responses, resulting in pro-inflammatory presentation of self antigens and the subsequent misdirection of adaptive immunity against self which is observed in autoimmune disease [Kariuki et al., 2010]

Genetic polymorphisms have emerged in recent years as important determinants of disease susceptibility and severity. Polymorphisms are naturally occurring DNA sequence variations, which differ from gene mutations in that they occur in the normal healthy population and have a frequency of at least 1%. Approximately 90% of DNA polymorphisms are single nucleotide polymorphisms (SNPs) due to single base substitutions. Others include insertion/deletion polymorphisms, minisatellite and microsatellite polymorphisms. Although most polymorphisms are functionally neutral, some have effects on regulation of gene expression or on the function of the coded protein. These functional polymorphisms, despite being of low penetrance, could contribute to the differences between individuals in susceptibility to and severity of disease. Many studies have examined the relationship between certain cytokine gene polymorphism, cytokine gene expression in vitro, and the susceptibility to and clinical severity of diseases [Bidwell et al., 1999; Hollegaard and Bidwell, 2006]. Some genetic polymorphisms at the promoter regions of IL-10 and TGF-β1 genes have been associated with cytokine production. Given that the production of these molecules is controlled at genetic level, functional polymorphisms in their promoters could influence the development and severity of the disease. In the present review, we summarize the information about involvement of IL-10 and TGF-β1 genetic variants on SLE appearance and clinical presentation.

2. Role of IL-10 and *TGF*-β1 in immune regulation and autoimmunity

2.1. IL-10

IL-10 is a pleiotropic cytokine with important immunoregulatory functions, which can be produced by both leukocytes and structural cells within tissues, being produced in particular by Tregs *in vivo* [Wakkach et al., 2008]. It is pivotal in inhibiting inflammation and suppresses Th1-mediated immune response through down regulation of proinflmamatory cytokine secretion from both Th1 and activated macrophages (De Waal Malefyt et al., 1993; Fiorentino et al., 1998]. It also inhibits antigen presenting cells by downregulating major histocompatibility complex class II (MHC-II) and B7 expression [Ding et al., 1993]. In addition to these inhibitory actions, IL-10 promotes B-cell-mediated functions, enhancing survival, proliferation, differentiation, and antibody production [Rousset et al., 1992]. Hence, increased production of IL-10 could thus explain B cell hyperactivity and autoantibody production, two main features of the immune dysregulation in SLE. In fact, high serum levels of IL-10 have been reported in patients with SLE and they correlated positively with the disease activity [Park et al., 1998].

The role of IL-10 in the pathogenesis of lupus remains controversial. The abnormally elevated amounts of IL-10 detected in serum of patients with SLE [Houssiau et al.,1995] and the observation that anti-IL-10 therapy can down-modulate disease in such patients [Llorente and Riehaud-Patin, 2003] suggest that this cytokine may promote disease. In contrast, mouse models have suggested a preventive role for IL-10 in the pathogenesis of lupus [Yin et al.,

2002]. In particular, IL-10 knockout mice were demonstrated to develop severe lupus, with earlier appearance of skin lesions, increased lymphadenopathy, more severe glomerulonephritis, and higher mortality than their IL-10-intact littermate controls [Yin et al., 2002]. Interestingly, the injection of IL-10 could prevent the occurrence of the disease in such models [Yin et al., 2002]. The authors of the study suggested that the contradictory role of IL-10 in lupus could be explained taking into account the phase of the disease. IL-10 deficiency enhanced IFN-γ production in the CD4 and CD8 lineages, and that, in turn, was associated with increased production of IgG2a anti-dsDNA antibodies, especially at the early stages of disease development. In contrast, at later phases of disease, excessive amounts of IL-10 production led to enhanced autoantibody production and subsequent formation of pathogenic autoantibody–antigen complexes [Yin et al., 2002]. However, Llorente and colleagues demonstrated that constitutive IL-10 production by monocytes and B cells in healthy members of multicase families with SLE was significantly higher than that of healthy unrelated controls, but was similar to that of SLE patients, thus suggesting that a genetically controlled high innate IL-10 production may predispose to SLE development. [Llorente et al.,1997]

2.2. *TGF-β1*

Recently, experimental studies have demonstrated an association between *TGF*-β1 and the development of autoimmunity [Aoki et al., 2005]. TGF-β1 belongs to a large family of multifunctional proteins, secreted by a variety of cell types that act as signal molecules in controlling a great number of biological processes. Like IL-10, it is a highly pleiotropic cytokine with an important role in maintaining immune homeostasis [Li et al., 2006]. There are three TGF-β isoforms in mammalian cells, TGF-β1, 2 and 3, which use similar signaling pathways and exert overlapping, albeit not identical biological functions. TGF-β1 is involved in many critical cellular processes, including cell growth, extracellular matrix formation, cell motility, hematopoiesis, apoptosis and immune function (Moustakas et al., 2002; Schuster & Krieglstein, 2002). The cells of immune system, including B, T and dendritic cells as well as macrophages, mostly produce TGF-β1, an isoform that is also found in large amounts in the plasma [Flanders and Roberts, 2001]. TGF-β1 has pronounced anti-inflammatory and immunosuppressive functions, the latter being realized by controlling the activation, proliferation, differentiation and survival of all effector immune cells [Rubtsov et al., 2007; Wahl, 1992]. Importantly, TGF-β1 inhibits maturation of dendritic cells and modulates the functions of antigen-presenting cells, reducing the macrophage production of IL-1, IL-6, and TNF-α [Fainaru et al., 2007]. However, immunosuppressive effect of TGF-β1 was most pronounced for T cells [Rubtsov et al., 2007; Li et al., 2006]. It inhibits T cell proliferation and production of IL-2, differentiation of Th1, Th2, and cytotoxic T lymphocytes (CTL). TGF-β1 suppresses IFN-γ production from Th1, NK cells and CTL, as well as their cytotoxic activity. TGF-β1 plays an essential role in the functioning and survival of regulatory T cells (Treg), and *de novo* generation of Foxp3$^+$ Treg from naive CD4$^+$ CD25$^-$ T lymphocytes in the periphery [Pyzik et al., 2007; Selvaraj et al., 2007; Zheng et al., 2007]. Furthermore, recent study reveals a role for TGF-β1 as effector molecule of Foxp3$^+$ Treg cells [Li et al., 2007]. In contrast to IL-10, TGF-β1 is also an important negative regulator of B cell differentiation and proliferation, inhibiting the production of most immunoglobulin isotypes except IgA [Lebman and Edmiston, 1999].

There are strong evidences to suggest the great importance of this cytokine in the control of autoimmunity [Aoki et al., 2005]. An association between *TGF-β1* and the development of autoimmunity is clearly demonstrated in studies with complete knockout of *TGF-β1* in mice or genetic manipulation of its receptors in T cells. TGF-β1 knockout mice and those with impaired TGF-β1 signaling in T cells develop an autoimmune syndrome with multiple organ involvement and death [Shull et al., 1992; Dang et al., 1995; Gorelik et al., 2000; Marie et al., 2006;]. This syndrome resembles SLE and Sjogren's syndrome in humans [Dang et al., 1995] and is characterized by multifocal inflammatory process affecting the heart, brain, lungs, skeletal muscle, liver, stomach, pancreas, salivary glands and other organs, lymfoproliferation, spontaneous activation of autoreactive T lymphocytes and production of autoantibodies [Dang et al., 1995; Shull et al., 1992].

3. Functional IL-10 and TGF-β1 genetic polymorphisms

3.1. IL-10 genetic polymorphisms and IL-10 production

Human IL-10 is secreted mostly by antigen-presenting cells and Treg lymphocytes subset in response to several activation stimuli. This cytokine could be also constitutively produced at low levels by immune cells, mainly monocytes, macrophages and dendritic cells. IL-10 is a non-covalent homodimer of 36 kDa with two polypeptide chains and its gene, with GeneBank accession number: X78437, is located on chromosome 1 at 1q31- q32 and a number of polymorphisms in the promoter region have been characterized. In contrast to many other cytokines, the synthesis of IL-10 is regulated by the transcription factors Sp1 and Sp3, which are constitutively expressed by different cell types [Moore et al. 2001]. It has been recently shown that c-Jun binds to a highly conserved noncoding sequences (CNS-3) in the IL10 locus, enhancing the expression of IL-10, and AP-1 signaling pathway particularly through c-jun transcription and activity strongly affects IL-10 expression in the Th2 cells and monocytes [Wang Z et al., 2005; Dobreva et al., 2009]. Large interindividual differences in the IL-10 inducibility have been observed, which has shown to have a genetic component of over 70%. The IL-10 gene comprises 5 exons, and to date, at least 49 IL10–associated polymorphisms have been reported, and an even larger number of polymorphisms are recorded in SNP databases (Ensembl Genome Browser, 2006). Promoter polymorphisms have been subject to the most studies, particularly with regard to possible influences on gene transcription and protein production. Three SNPs at -1082(A/G), -819(C/T), -592(C/A) upstream from the transcription start site [D'Alfonso et al., 1995; Turner et al., 1997] have been described as well as additional two microsatellite (CA)n repeats, termed IL10.G (-1.1Kb) and IL10.R (-4Kb) and located at -1151 and -3978 respectively (Eskdale and Galager, 1995; Eskdale et al., 1997).

A complete linkage disequilibrium exists between the alleles present at positions -1082, -819 and -592; so these polymorphisms occurred in tandem These SNPs have been associated with variability in IL-10 production [Eskdale et al., 1998; Turner et al., 1998]. In particular, SNP at position -1082A/G of IL-10 gene has been associated with IL-10 production alone or in haplotypes with other distal SNPs. Turner et al.,1997 have shown that

http://dx.doi.org/10.5772/53799

-1082A allele is associated with lower in vitro IL-10 production by Con A-stimulated PBMC from normal subjects. In our studies, the functional effect of -1082 A/G polymorphism was demonstrated among the Bulgarian population in both healthy volunteers and in patients with sepsis (Stanilova et al., 2006). In Caucasian populations, only three haplotypes have been found (GCC, ACC and ATA), the individuals GCC/GCC being considered as genetically high IL-10 producers [Suarez et al., 2005; Suarez et al., 2003; Turner et al., 1997]. Although the functional effects of polymorphisms in IL-10 have not yet been fully elucidated, obviously that they may play a significant role in modulating susceptibility, development and clinical fetures of autoimmune disease and particularly SLE. The observation of increased circulating levels of IL-10 in active SLE patients which revealed positive correlation with SLEDAI and anti-double-stranded DNA (dsDNA) titer has been reported (Park et al., 1998; Hye-Young et al., 2007). Moreover, a trend toward SLE patients having hypomethylated IL-10 promoter region accompanied by greater disease activity of SLE was recently observed (Lin et al., 2012).

3.2. TGF-β1 genetic polymorphisms and plasma concentrations of TGF-β1

The TGF-β1 gene is located on chromosome 19 (q13.1-13.3) and several SNPs were described so far in promoter region, in the non-translated region (introns), in the coding region (exons), and in the 3'-UTR region of the gene. They include three polymorphisms in the promoter region (-988C/A, -800G/A, and -509C/T), two polymorphisms located in exon 1 +869T/C (codon 10) and +915G/C (codon 25), one on exon 5 +11929C/T (codon 263), and one in 3'-UTR region of the gene at position +72 [Cambien et al., 1996]. Certain inherited variants in the promoter region of the TGF-β gene (-800G/A and -509C/T) have been associated with higher cytokine circulating concentrations. The -800G/A SNP is located in a consensus cyclic AMP response element binding protein (CREB) half site and may cause reduced affinity for CREB transcription factors whose binding is important for transcription control [Grainger at al. 1999]. The -509C/T is located within a YY1 consensus binding site and -509T allele has been associated with increased TGF-β1 plasma level [Grainger at al. 1999] and reduced T-cell proliferation [Meng et al., 2005] and a study of twins estimated that the -509C/T polymorphism explained approximately 8% of the genetic variation in TGF-β1 plasma levels (Grainger at al.,1999). Two SNPs, the +868T/C SNP, and the +915G/C SNP, give rise to amino acid substitutions at positions 10 (Leu10Pro) and 25 (Arg25Pro) in the signal peptide of TGF-β1, respectively (Cambien et al.,1996; Awad et al. 1998). The +868T/C SNP was reported to influence steady-state concentrations of *TGFB1* mRNA in peripheral blood mononuclear cells and serum levels of TGF-β1, and the +915G/C SNP was found to be related to TGF-β1 production in peripheral blood leukocytes (Awad et al., 1998). Another nonsynonymous SNP of *TGFB1*, the +11929C/T SNP ($Thr^{263}Ile$) is located in exon 5 (Cambien et al.,1996; Awad et al.1998). The 11929C/T SNP is located closely to the site where the latency-associated peptide is cleaved from the active part of the protein (Dubois et al., 1995) and therefore, this SNP may be related to the activation process of TGF-β1, as suggested previously (Cambien et al. 1996). A high degree of linkage disequilibrium was observed between pairs of the −509C/T, 868T/C, 913G/C, and 11929C/T SNPs in white populations (Cambien et al.,1996; Grainger at al. 1999).

Although immunosuppressive effects of TGF-β1 have been well established, few studies have investigated serum TGF-β1 levels in autoimmune disorders. In fact, patient with SLE have reduced TGF-β1 production by their peripheral blood lymphocytes (Oshtuka et al., 1998). Hence, reduced TGF-β1 production by immune cells might contribute to the characteristic T cell disregulation, aberrant stimulation of autoreactive B cell, and autoantibody production in SLE patients. Also, it has been reported that decreased serum levels of TGF-β1 in patients with systemic lupus are the most pronounced and constant abnormality in the cytokine levels in these patients [Becker-Merok et al., 2010]. In attempt to elucidate the importance of TGF-β1 for the development of SLE we measured serum levels of TGF-β1 in 53 patients with SLE recruited from 'St Ivan Rilski' University Hospital, Sofia and in 66 healthy controls [unpublished data]. Serum samples were routinely collected and stored frozen at -20 C until assayed. At the time of sampling, neither of the patients and control subjects had clinical signs or symptoms of intercurrent illness. The concentrations of activated TGF-β1 protein in the serum samples of patients and controls were measured by quantitative sandwich ELISA technique, using commercially available kits (Qantakine®, R&D systems, Abingdon, UK). Before assay, the latent TGF-β1 contained in sera was activated to the immunoreactive form using acid activation and neutralization. The results were calculated by reference to the standard curve and expressed as ng/ml. Table 1 presents the serum concentrations of TGF-β1 in patients and healthy controls.

	TGF-β1 concentrations (mean±SD)	**Significance**
SLE		
total (n=53)	8.88 ± 3.79	
male (n=7)	8.57 ± 2.72	
female (n=46)	8.93 ± 3.95	male *vs* female p = 0.82
Healthy controls		
total (n=66)	32.99 ± 24.84	
male (n=13)	60.98 ± 31.32	
female (n=53)	26.12 ± 17.34	male *vs* female p <0.001
Significance	SLE *vs* HC p<0.001	

Table 1. *TGF*-β1 concentrations (ng/ml 9) in SLE patients and healthy controls.

Our results showed significantly lower levels of active TGF-β1 in lupus patients compared with healthy individuals (p<0.001). These data are in principal agreement with other studies [Jin et al., 2011; Lu et al., 2004]. In addition to the decreased TGF-β1 serum concentrations in SLE patients, the authors of these studies also reported an association between lower TGF-β1 and disease activity, as well as the development of organ damage [Jin et al., 2011; Lu et al., 2004]. Taken together, these observations support the role of TGF-β1 in SLE pathogenesis and modulation of disease expression. In our study, we also observed a large interindividual variation in serum TGF-β1 levels among healthy subjects. This variation might be partly due to the possible influence of some endogenous factors, such as *gender* and age on the production of *TGF*-β1. Given this supposition, we examined *TGF*-β1 levels in the context of age and gender in both healthy and affected individuals. The highest levels of *TGF*-β1 were found in men among the healthy subjects. In SLE patients such a correlation between serum levels of *TGF*-β1 and gender was not observed (Table 1), which could be explained with fact, that only men individuals with genetic predisposition to lower *TGF*-β1 production developed SLE or down regulation of *TGF*-β1 by disease progress. Additionally, age was positively correlated with serum *TGF*-β1 in healthy controls. *TGF*-β1 serum levels were lower in individuals under 45 years and higher in those aged over 45 years (P<0.001) among healthy controls as shown in Figure 1. In SLE patients, there was not a relationship between age and serum *TGF*-β1 levels. Thus, healthy individuals showed a pattern in which serum *TGF*-β1 was higher in men and elder people. It seems likely that age- or gender-specific cytokine differences could play a role in the observed age- and gender-related incidence patterns observed in SLE [Petri M, 2002].These data allow us to hypothesis that high levels of serum TGF-β1 may protect against autoimmunity in men as well as low levels of serum TGF-β1 may predispose to the onset of autoimmunity in younger individuals.

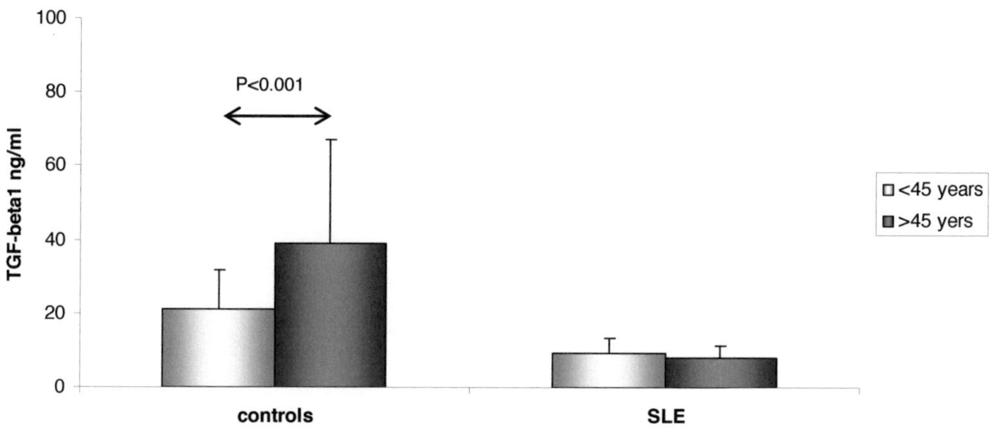

Figure 1. Mean (±SD) serum *TGF*-β1 concentrations (pg/ml) in SLE patients and healthy controls according to the age of individuals.

Nowadays, it is considered that the control of TGF-β1 production is complex, but it has been estimated that 54% of its production is under genetic control [Grainger et al., 1999]. In this regard, we analyzed the serum levels of TGF-β1 in relation to various genotypes of -509C/T polymorphism of TGFB1 in 52 healthy controls (n = 21 for CC, 15 for CT, and16 for TT) and in 48 SLE patients (n = 17 for CC, 24 for CT, and 7 for TT). As the mean TGF-β1 levels varied significantly by case-control status (P < 0.001), patients and controls were proceeded separetly for the genotype-serum levels analysis. The results are presented on Figure 2. Among healthy individuals the highest TGF-β1 concentration was detected in individuals with TT genotype (mean ± SD, 56.9 ± 28.6 ng/ml) compared to those with CC genotype (mean ± SD, 29.5 ± 21.1

ng/ml; p = 0.001) and those with CT genotype (mean ± SD, 25.7 ± 18.8; p = 0.002). Besides the level of serum TGF-β1 in patients was found to be lower than in control subjects (Figure 1), significantly higher TGF-β1 levels were observed in SLE patients having the TT genotype (mean ± SD, 9.8 ± 2.6 ng/ml) compared to patients with CC genotype (mean ± SD, 6.7 ± 2.6 ng/ml; p=0.023). Overall, individuals with TT homozygous genotype had higher serum TGF-β1 concentration in comparison to those with either CC homozygous genotype or CT heterozygous genotype.

The study of Awad and colleagues related the carriage of GG homozygous genotype in position +915 of TGFB1 to significantly higher TGF-β1 production in peripheral blood leukocytes [Awad et al., 1998]. However, Lu et al., 2004 also, analyzing the serum levels of TGF-β1 as well as the TGF-β1 production of unstimulated and stimulated peripheral blood mononuclear cells, did not observe functional correlations with TGF-β1 production and -509 and codon10 alleles. The authors raise the question whether the lower serum TGF-β1 level that cause defective immune regulation in SLE is primarily under genetic control or secondary to the influence of ongoing cellular interactions in the cytokine context. The data from our preliminary study shown that a number of factors such as age, sex, presence of disease, and allele variants of -509 C/T SNP in the gene for TGF-β1 influence the level of this cytokine in the serum. Thus, a genetically controlled low production of TGF-β1 is a predisposing factor for the loss of negative regulation found in SLE and may constitute an important component of the genetically determined susceptibility to this disease and the autoimmune events responsible for its pathogenesis, developed under appropriate environmental stimuli.

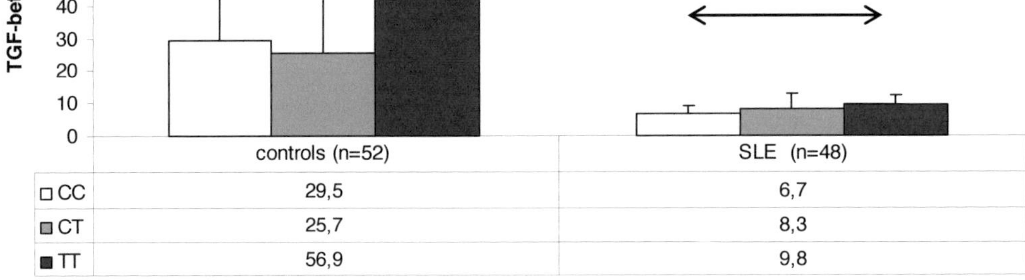

Figure 2. Mean (± SD) serum *TGF*-β1 concentrations (ng/ml) in SLE patients and healthy controls according to the genotypes of -509 C/T polymorphism of *TGFB1*. * p < 0.05, ** p <.01

4. Role of IL-10 and TGF-β1 genotypes as risk factor for appearance of SLE

4.1. Role of IL-10 promoter polymorphism in susceptibility and clinical manifestation of SLE

Several evidences suggest that IL-10 could be a strong candidate gene influencing SLE susceptibility. IL-10 gene has been mapped to chromosome 1q31-32, which is a susceptibility region for SLE (LOD=3.79) [Johanneson et al., 2002]. It is also homologous to a murine SLE susceptibility region [Tsao et al., 1997]. More recently, Gateva et al., 2010 performed a large-scale replication study involving 1,310 cases and 7,859 controls, and identified 21 additional candidate susceptibility loci for SLE. Among the newly identified SLE loci is IL-10.

However, in spite of the considerable number of genetic studies performed, no definitive result about its involvement in SLE susceptibility was achieved. Some works showed significant associations between IL-10 microsatellites or SNPs with SLE susceptibility or with the development of certain clinical or immunological features [Rood et al., 1999; D'Alfonso et al., 2002; Schotte et al., 2004; Chen et al., 2006; Sung et al., 2006; Chong et al., 2006; Rosado et al., 2008] while other studies indicated that these polymorphisms did not appear to have any relevance in the disease [Alarcón-Riquelme et al., 1999; Van der Linden et al., 2000; Dijstelbloem et al., 2002; Guarnizo-Zuccardi et al., 2007]. The role of IL-10 genotypes has been recently reviewed by Lopez et al., 2010. The more recent association studies dealing IL-10 promoter polymorphisms for SLE susceptibility are summarized on Table 2.

With respect to microsatellite variants, different alleles of IL10.G have been reported to be associated with SLE incidence in various populations. Thus, frequency of IL10.G9 allele (21 CA repeats) was significantly decreased in European [D'Alfonso et al., 2000, D'Alfonso et al., 2002, Eskdale et al., 1997] and Mexican-American [Mehrian et al., 1998] SLE patients, whereas the long alleles IL10.G10, G11 and G13 (with a CA repeat number greater than 21) were significantly increased in Mexican-American [Mehrian et al., 1998], Italian [D'Alfonso et al., 2000, D'Alfonso et al., 2002] and British [Eskdale et al., 1997] patients respectively. On the contrary, an increase in IL10.G4 (short allele) was reported in Chinese patients [Chong et al., 2004] whereas no significant differences in IL10.G alleles were detected in other cohorts [Schotte et al., 2004, Alarcon-Riquelme et al., 1999; Johansson et al., 2002]. Recently, a large meta-analysis summarized the results focused on the role of IL-10 promoter polymorphisms for SLE susceptibility from 16 published case-control studies involving a total of 2391 SLE patients and 3483 controls (Nath et al., 2005). The results of the meta-analysis performed by Nath et al., 2005 showed a significant association between SLE and the G11 allele of IL10.G (OR=1.279, 95% CI; 1.027±1.593, P=0.028) in whole populations, and IL-10 promoter -1082G allele was associated with SLE in Asians (OR=1.358, 95% CI; 1.015±1.816, P=0.039). It has been reported that LPS-stimulated cells from individuals carriers of the IL10.G allele with 26 CA repeats presented higher IL-10 production than those from carriers of short alleles [Eskdale et al., 1998], suggesting that long alleles might be responsible for a high IL-10 production. Thus, accordingly to these data, high IL-10 producer genotypes (with more than 21 CA repeats) could be associated with SLE susceptibility, while presence of short alleles could confer a protective effect [Chen et al., 2006; D'Alfonso et al., 2002].

Polymoprhisms	Association	SLE/contr.	Population	References
IL10G, IL10R -1082; -819; -592	Association of IL10.G11 allele in whole populations; Association of -1082G allele with SLE in Asians	2391/3483	Meta-analysis	Nath et al., 2005
-592 A/C	No association with susceptibility Association of -592C with SLE activity	350/330	Korean	Sung et al., 2005
IL10G	Increased G9 and decreased G8 in SLE Association of G13 with ACLA-IgM Association of G8 with CNS lupus	237/304	Taiwanese	Chen et al., 2006
-1082, -819, -592	Association of ACC/ACC with susceptibility to SLE	195/159	Thai	Hirankarn et al., 2006
-1082; -819; -592	No association	120/102	Colombian	Guarnizo-Zuccardi et al., 2007
IL10G, IL10R -1082; -819; -592	No association of microsatellites Increased GCC in SLE	116/51	Spanish	Rosado et al., 2008
-1082; -819; -592	Increased GCC in SLE	103/300	Polish	Sobkowiak et al., 2009
-1082; -819; -592 -592 A/C	No association	110/138	Chinese	Yu et al., 2010
-1082; -819; -592	Increased ATA haplotype in sLE	172/215	Taiwanese	Lin et al., 2010
-1082	No association	157/126	Bulgarian	Miteva et al., 2010

Table 2. Association of IL-10 promotor polymorphisms - IL10G, IL10R, -1082G/A (rs1800896), -819C/T (rs1800871), -592A/C (rs1800872), with SLE. Association studies published after 2005 years are given only.

Conflicting results were also obtained after examining the possible association between SLE susceptibility and SNPs at -1082, -819, and -592 positions of IL-10 gene in the different populations in which they were investigated. The frequency of high IL-10 producers (carriers of -1082G allele or GCC haplotype) has been found to be increased in several works with Asian [Nath et al., 2005; Hirankarn et al., 2006] or European [Rosado o et al., 2008; Sobkowiak et al., 2009] patients, although most of the studies performed in Caucasian populations did not show significant associations [Lazarus et al. 1997, Guarnizo-Zuccardi et al, 2007;, Koss et al., 2000; Suárez et al., 2005; Dijstelbloem et al., 2002; Van der Linden et al., 2000; Crawley et al., 1999].

Rosado et al., 2008 found that the GCC haplotype frequency was significantly higher in Spanish patients with SLE. To assess the functional role of genotypes, they also quantified serum IL-10 levels from patients and controls and found higher serum IL-10 levels in patients. On the basis of these data, they suggest that the IL-10 promoter haplotype that produces higher levels of cytokine is associated with SLE in Spanish population. Similar are the results and final conclusion of the study performed by Sobkowiak et al., 2009; despite the higher prevalence of the GCC/GCC, GCC/ATA and ATA/ATA genotypes in SLE patients than in controls, they observed that only GCC/GCC genotype was significant more frequent in SLE. Hence, the conclusion suggests the GCC/GCC promoter genotype may contribute to SLE incidence in Polish patients. A very recent study investigated the association between of IL-10 promoter polymorphisms (-1082, -819 and -592) with SLE in a total of 172 Taiwanese patients and 215 controls reported an association of IL-10 ATA haplotype with SLE in Taiwanese population [Lin et al., 2010]. In another Asian population, an association of ACC/ACC haplotype of IL-10 in susceptibility to SLE has been observed by Hirankarn et al., 2006.

In this regard, we investigated the role of -1082A/G promoter polymorphism of IL-10 gene as risk factor for development and clinical manifestations of SLE in Bulgarian population. Our preliminary results did not reveal a significant association of -1082 SNP in IL-10 with SLE [Miteva et al., 2010]. New data for the distribution and the frequencies of the -1082A/G alleles and genotypes among the SLE patients and healthy controls are presented on Table 3. The results of our case-control study based on 157 patients with SLE and 166 unaffected control individuals showed that the genotype distribution is consistent with those published for other Caucasian type control cohorts [Lopez et al., 2010). We also found the prevalence of homozygous GG genotype in SLE cases (27%) compared to the controls (13%) with OR = 1.185 (95% CI = 0.58÷2.45), although the difference did not reach statistical significance (p=0.548). In addition, we observed an increased frequency of GG genotype compared to the reference AA genotype in patients with antiphospholipid synrom (APS) (27%) compared with patients without APS (14%) with OR = 2.750, 95% CI = 0.910 ÷ 8.347, p = 0.074). This suggests that carriage of a higher IL-10 producing genotype is a risk factor for antiphospholipid autoantibody production and APS appearance, thus having a modifying effect on the clinical presentation of the disease.

rs1800896-10		**Genotype**						**Allele**	
82 A/G		**AA**	**AG**	**AG+AA**	**AG+GG**	**GG**		**A**	**G**
IL10		**n (%)**	**n (%)**	**n (%)**	**n (%)**	**n (%)**		**n (%)**	**n (%)**
SLE (n=157)		56	74	130	101	27		186	128
		(36%)	(47%)	(73%)	(74%)	(27%)		(59%)	(41%)
							χ^2=0.203		
HC (n=166)		59	83	142	107	24	p=0.934	201	131
		(36%)	(50%)	(86%)	(64%)	(14%)		(61%)	(39%)
OR (95% CI)		0.844	0.793	0.814		1		0.947	1
		(0.41±1.72)	(0.40±1.56)	(0.43±1.54)	-	*ref.*		(0.68±1.31)	*ref.*
	p		*0.614*	*0.471*	*0.5*	-			*0.735*
OR		1.	0.939	-	0.994	1.185		1	1.056
(95% CI)		*ref*	(0.56±1.57)		(0.61±1.61)	(0.58±2.42)		*ref.*	(0.76±1.47)
p			*0.799*	-	*0.981*	*0.614*			*0.735*

Table 3. Genotypic and allelic frequency of gene polymorphism at position -1082 A/G in IL-10 gene in SLE patients and controls

The presence of autoantibodies, mainly directed against nuclear antigens (ANAs), is one of the most characteristic features of SLE. The effect of IL-10 genotypes did not seem to be especially relevant, although it has been reported an increased prevalence of antibodies against several extractable nuclear antigens (anti-ENA) in patients with the allele IL-10.G9 [Eskdale, et al., 1997], and the presence of anti-Sm antibodies was found significantly overrepresented among patient carriers of G14 and G15 alleles and R2-G15 and R2-G14 haplotypes [Schotte et al., 2004]. An association of the carriage of low IL-10 producer alleles such as IL10.G13 allele with the presence of anticardiolipin IgM antibodies and IL10.G8 allele with neurological affectation has been reported in Taiwanese patients with SLE [Chen et al., 2006], results very similar to the data from our study.

Considering increased circulating levels of IL-10 have been consistently reported in the sera of patients with SLE, it is possible that different cytokine production may not only influence the autoantibody production, but also the clinical presentation of the disease. However, there were no definitive data on the association of IL-10 polymorphisms and specific clinical manifestations, probably due to the heterogeneity of the disease. For instance, renal involvement has been associated with both high (GCC) [Lazarus et al., 1997, Zhu et al., 2005] and low (ATA) [Mok et al., 1999] IL-10 producer genotypes. High prevalence of neuropsychiatric [Rood et al., 1999; Chen et al. 2006] and cardiovascular disorders [Fei et al., 2004] has been reported in patients with low genetic production whereas high IL-10 production has been linked to an increased incidence of serositis, hematological disorder [Chong et al.], SLICC/ACR Damage Index [Sung et al., 2006] and presence of discoid or mucocutaneous lesions [Suárez et al., 2005; Alarcón-Riquelme et al.,1999]. This last association was supported by the increased frequency of the high producer -1082G allele observed in patients with discoid lupus erythematosus [Suárez et al., 2005; Van der Linden et al., 2000] and by the fact that cutaneous manifestations improved in SLE patients under anti IL-10 monoclonal antibody treatment [Llorente et al., 2000]. In conclusion IL-10 promoter SNPs alone have not exhibits strong association with SLE susceptibility, but their role cant' be excluded. Each polymorphism in regulatory regions of gene, may either directly influence gene expression or indirectly via tight linkage with other polymorphisms occurring elsewhere in the same or in other cytokine gene. A particular combination of SNPs on cytokine genes in individual genotype has different impacts on induced cytokine production. Miteva and Stanilova investigate the combined effect of -1082A*G in IL10 and +16974A*C in IL12B SNPs on induced cytokine production by stimulated peripheral blood mononuclear cells isolated from healthy donors (Miteva, Stanilova, 2008). Results demonstrated that the production of IL-10 from PBMC depended on both, -1082A*G in IL10 and +16974A*C in IL12B polymorphisms and the presence of high producer IL-12p40 genotype led to diminished production of IL-10 determined by -1082*G-allele of SNP in IL10. In the same vein, we suppose that individuals with genotype which combine SNPs responsible for higher production of IL-10 simultaneously with lower production of TGF-β1 should be more susceptible to SLE.

http://dx.doi.org/10.5772/53799

4.2. Role of TGB-β1 genetic polymorphisms in susceptibility and clinical manifestation of SLE

Regarding the association between decreased *TGF*-β1 serum levels and the development of autoimmunity, the mechanisms which control the concentration of *TGF*-β1 in plasma are under extensive investigations. The concentration of both latent complex and active *TGF*-β1 in plasma has been shown to be predominantly under genetic control [Grainger et al., 1999]. In light of these findings TGF-β1 gene is a functional candidate gene for genetic predisposition in systemic lupus erythematosus.

The presence of polymorphisms in the *TGFB1* locus may indicate predisposition to diseases, such as systemic lupus erythematosus that have been linked here and elsewhere [Caserta et al., 2004; Lu et al., 2004] to the circulating levels of TGF-β1. To test this hypothesis, we performed a population based case-control study to investigate the association of -509C/T polymorphism of the *TGFB1* gene with susceptibility to SLE [Manolova et al., 2012]. In this investigation, the change at position -509C/T in the *TGFB1* gene (rs1800469) was studied using RFLP-PCR among 147 cases with SLE and 134 normal Bulgarian subjects. The genotype distribution and allele frequencies of -509C/T SNP in gene promoter of *TGFB1* among SLE patients and healthy donors are presented in Table 4.

rs1800469 -509C/T TGFB1	**Genotype**						**Allele**	
	CC n (%)	**CT n (%)**	**CT+CC n (%)**	**CT+TT n (%)**	**TT n (%)**		**C n (%)**	**T n (%)**
SLE (n=149)	48	79	127	101	22		175	123
	(32.2%)	(53%)	(85.2%)	(67.8%)	(14.8%))		(58.7%)	(41.3%)
HC (n=134)	48	57	105	86	29	χ^2=3.735 p=0.155	153	115
	(35.8%)	(42.5%)	(78.3%)	(64.1%)	(21.6%)		(57.1%)	(42.9%)
OR (95% CI)	*1.318*	1.827	1.59	-	1		1.069	1
	(0.63-2.77)	(0.91±3.69)	(0.83±3.07)		*ref.*		(0.76±1.5)	*ref.*
p	*0.428*	*0.068*	*0.133*	-			*0.694*	
OR (95% CI)	1	1.386	-	1.17	0.759		1	0.935
	ref.	(0.79±2.43)		(0.7±1.98)	(0.36±1.59)		*ref.*	(0.66±1.33)
p		*0.223*	-	*0.522*	*0.428*			*0.694*

Table 4. Genotypic and allelic frequency of gene polymorphism at position -509 in *TGFB1* gene in SLE patients and controls

The genotype distribution for TGFB1 -509C/T polymorphism was in agreement with Hardy-Weinberg equilibrium among cases ($\chi 2$=2.00; p=0.367) and controls ($\chi 2$=2.237; p=0.326). Homozygous CC genotype was found in 32.2% of patients and 36.8% of control subjects, heterozygous CT genotype was observed in 53% of SLE patients and 42.5% of controls, homozygous TT genotype was detected in 14.8% of cases and 21.6% of controls. There were no significant differences in the genotype (p=0.155) and allele (p=0.694) frequencies of -509C/T polymorphism of the TGFB1 gene between SLE patients and controls. However, we observed a higher frequency of heterozygous CT genotype (OR = 1.827; 95% CI 0.91±3.69; p = 0.068) and lower frequency of TT genotype (OR = 0,759; 95% CI: 0.36±1.59; p=0.428) in SLE patients compared to healthy controls. In logistic regression analysis the presence of allele C in the genotype (CT + CC versus TT) was associated with a 1.6 times higher risk of developing systemic lupus erythematosus.

Genotype and allele frequencies of -509C/T polymorphism in *TGFB1* which we established in Bulgarian population were comparable to those found in other populations. However, the available data in the literature reveal the existence of ethnic differences in frequencies of the allele variants of this polymorphic marker (Table 5). C allele had the higher representation among Europeans in French [Cambien et al., 1996], German [Wu et al., 2008] and British [Awad et al., 1998] studies with a frequency of 65 to 76 percent, while among healthy individuals from different Asian ethnicities T allele occurs more frequently or almost equally with the C allele [Amirghofran Z, 2009; Zhang et al., 2009; Chung et al.,, 2007]. In Bulgarian population allele C is slightly more common and was found in 57% of healthy subjects and in 59% of cases with SLE.

Locus	Allele	Frequency (%) among healthy controls				
		Bulgarian study Data from this study	French study Cambien et al., 1996	British study Awad et al., 1998	German study Wu et al., 2009	Asian study Lu et al., 2004
-509	C	57	66	76	70	48
	T	43	34	24	30	52

Table 5. Interethnic differences in allele frequencies of -509C/T SNP in *TGFB1* in healthy controls.

According to our knowledge there are only a limited number of studies aiming to evaluate the possible role of polymorphisms in the TGF-β1 gene as predisposing factors for SLE, but the results of these studies are contradictory. The polymorphisms in of -509C/T SNP in TGF-β1 have been explored in SLE only by three research teams [Lu et al., 2004; Caserta et al., 2004; Vuong et al., 2010]. In overall, the contradictory results in the literature could be explained by the genetic heterogeneity of SLE in different populations and possible sample stratification. Table 6 summarizes the association studies dealing TGF-β1 gene polymorphisms for SLE susceptibility.

Polymoprhisms	Association	SLE/contr.	Population	References
+915G/C (rs1800471)	No association	203/158	German	Schotte et al., 2003
-988C/A (rs2241712), -800G/A (rs1982072), -509C/T (rs1800469), +869T/C (rs1982073), +915G/C (rs1800471)	No association	138/182	Taiwanese	Lu et al., 2004
-509C/T (rs1800469)	No association	23/32	North America	Caserta et al., 2004
+869T/C (rs1982073), +915G/C (rs1800471)	Association of +869C allele with SLE; decreased high TGF-β1 producers haplotypes in SLE (codon10 T allele/25 G allele) No association with clinical manifestations	120/102	Colombian	Guarnizo-Zuccardi et al., 2007
+869T/C (rs1982073)	No association with susceptibility +869TT associated with aseptic necrosis and anti-Ro antibodies	196/102	Japan	Wang et al., 2007
-509C/T (rs1800469) +869T/C (rs1982073) intron G/T (rs2241715) 3'-UTR A/G (rs6957)	No association	272/307	Sweden	Vuong et al., 2010
-509C/T (rs1800469)	Decreased frequency of TT (OR = 0,759; 95% CI: 0.36±1.59) allele C (CT+CC vs TT) risk factor for SLE (OR=1.59; 95% CI: 0.83±3.07)	149/134	Bulgarian	Manolova et al. 2012

Table 6. Association of TGF-β1 gene polymorphisms with SLE.

Lu et al. conducted a case-control study involving 134 patients and 182 healthy individuals of Taiwanese origin to evaluate the association of -509C/T SNP in *TGFB1* with susceptibility to systemic lupus erythematosus [Lu et al., 2004]. In the same study, authors investigated also association of some others TGFβ1 single nucleotide polymorphisms, including -988C/A, -800G/A, +869T/C (Leu10Pro), and +915 G/C (Arg25Pro) with susceptibility to SLE and shown that none of the TGFβ1 SNPs was strongly associated with SLE in Taiwanese patients. They conclude that these polymorphisms do not represent a genetic predisposition to SLE. In another study, Schotte and colleagues investigated the +915G/C polymorphism at codon25 and did not found any association between this polymorphism and SLE in German population [Schotte et al., 2003]. In addition, authors found no association of major disease manifestations or specific autoantibodies with TGFB1 genotypes or alleles. The authors conclude that +915G/C polymorphism in TGFB1 neither significantly contributes to the disease susceptibility, nor predisposes to clinical and immunological manifestations typical of SLE. Also, there were no significant associations between several SNPs from the TGFβ1 including -509C/T, +869T/C, intronic G/T (rs2241715), and3'-UTR A/G(rs6957) with SLE or with lupus nephritis in Sweden population [Vuong et al., 2010].

In contrast to these data are the results obtained by Guarnizo-Zuccardi et al., 2007 for several cytokine gene polymorphisms in Colombian patients with SLE. They analyze the relation between the +868T/C and the +915G/C SNP in *TGFB1* with the development and clinical manifestations of SLE. The authors found a strong association of SLE with the TGF-β1 codon25 C allele, associated with decreased TGF-β1 production and found lower rates of higher-producing GG genotype and a higher frequency of heterozygous genotypes in this polymorphic marker in patients with SLE. As for the +868T/C polymorphism at codon10, Guarnizo-Zuccardi et al., 2007 did not observe association between SLE and codon10 when analyzing independently, but they found a significant association when the haplotypes codon10/20 were evaluated, which could be because of the linkage disequilibrium between the two SNPs. This extended genotypic analysis revealed a lower frequency of high TGF-β1 producers – haplotype 10/25 T/T-G/G in Colombian patients with SLE. Unlike the relationship of +868T/C and +915G/C SNPs of the *TGFB1* gene to disease susceptibility, they found no association between clinical features of the disease and the polymorphisms studied. As opposed to this report, Wang et al., 2007 did not find an impact of +869T/C polymorphism in TGF-β1 gene on disease susceptibility in population-based case-control study involving 196 patients with SLE and 106 healthy controls in Japan. However, they found an association between +869T/C *TGFB1* polymorphism and several clinical features of SLE. The carriage of TT genotype of +869T/C polymorphism which is associated with a lower serum TGF-β1 level was related to the occurrence of aseptic necrosis and higher incidence of anti-SSA/Ro antibodies in SLE patients. Consistent with the last finding, the children with the TT +869T/C genotype of *TGFB1* gene have been reported to be more susceptible to anti-SSA/Ro antibody-associated congenital hear block [Clancy et al., 2003].

Systemic lupus erythematosus is a heterogeneous disease with diverse clinical manifestations that range could be due to genetic factors. In this regard, we also analyzed the effect of the -509C/T polymorphism in TGFB1 the clinical manifestations evolved in the course of the disease [Manolova et al., 2012]. The results of our study demonstrated a weak association of -509C/T polymorphism of TGFB1 with clinical manifestations of SLE. The carriage of the heterozygous genotype was associated with about 2-fold higher risk for the occurrence of hematological manifestations (OR=2.41; 95%CI: 1.10±5.32; p=0.016) and antibodies against dsDNA (OR = 2.0; 95% CI: 0.96±4.2, p = 0.045) in lupus patients, while the CC genotype is a protective factor for these events. Based on our and others data, we could assume the TGFβ1 gene polymorphisms as one of the genetic factors that explain the heterogeneity seen in SLE.

5. Conclusions

In recent years, efforts have been made to identify genes involved in the genetic predisposition and severity of SLE. During the last two decades, many of the 'candidate' cytokine genes implicated in SLE development have been identified and was summarized in this review. SLE is clinically heterogeneous and genetically complex, and we expect that individual genes and cytokine patterns will be more or less important to different disease manifestations and subgroups of patients. Defining these genotype-cytokine-phenotype relationships will increase our understanding of both initial and progression disease pathogenesis.

In ours and others studies have been analyzed the association of IL-10 and TGF-β1genetic variants with susceptibility to and outcome of SLE, showing variable results in most cases. However, it is known that the actions of cytokines may be profoundly conditioned by the presence of other cytokines, this being particularly true in the case of IL-10 and TGF-β1. New studies of particular combinations of SNPs on these cytokine genes in individual genotype and their impacts on the induced cytokine production could reveal the relation with susceptibility and clinical presentation of autoimmunity diseases.

Author details

Irena Manolova[1], Mariana Ivanova[2] and Spaska Stanilova[3]

1 Department of Health Care, Medical Faculty, Trakia University, Stara Zagora, Bulgaria

2 Clinic of Rheumatology, University Hospital, Medical University, Sofia, Bulgaria

3 Department of Molecular Biology, Immunology and Medical Genetics, Medical Faculty, Trakia University, Stara Zagora, Bulgaria

References

[1] Alarcón-Riquelme ME, Lindqvist AK, Jonasson I, Johanneson B, Sandino S, Alcocer-Varela J, Granados J, Kristjánsdóttir H, Gröndal G, Svenungsson E, Lundberg I, Steinsson K, Klareskog L, Sturfelt G, Truedsson L, Alarcón-Segovia D, Gyllensten UB. Genetic analysis of the contribution of IL10 to systemic lupus erythematosus. J Rheumatol 1999;26(10):2148-52.

[2] Amirghofran, Z, Jalali, S. A, Ghaderi, A, & Hosseini, S. V. Genetic polymorphism in the transforming growth factor beta1 gene (-509 C/T and-800 G/A) and colorectal cancer. Cancer Genet Cytogenet (2009). , 190(1), 21-5.

[3] Aoki, C. A, Borchers, A. T, Li, M, Flavell, R. A, Bowlus, C. L, Ansari, A. A, & Gershwin, M. E. Transforming growth factor beta (TGF-beta) and autoimmunity. Autoimmun Rev (2005). , 4(7), 450-9.

[4] Awad, M. R, Gamel, A, Hasleton, P, Turner, D. M, Sinnott, P. J, & Hutchinson, I. V. Genotypic variation in the transforming growth factor-beta1 gene: association with

transforming growth factor-beta1 production, fibrotic lung disease, and graft fibrosis after lung transplantation. Transplantation (1998). , 66(8), 1014-20.

[5] Becker-merok, A, Eilertsen, G. Ø, & Nossent, J. C. Levels of transforming growth factor-beta are low in systemic lupus erythematosus patients with active disease. J Rheumatol (2010). , 37(10), 2039-2045.

[6] Bidwell, J, Keen, L, Gallagher, G, Kimberly, R, Huizinga, T, Mcdermott, M. F, Oksenberg, J, Mcnicholl, J, & Pociot, F. Hardt C & D'Alfonso S. Cytokine gene polymorphism in human disease: on-line databases. Genes and immunity (1999). , 1, 3-19.

[7] Cambien, F, et al. Polymorphisms of the transforming growth factor-beta 1 gene in relation to myocardial infarction and blood pressure. The Etude Cas-Témoin de l'Infarctus du Myocarde (ECTIM) Study. Hypertension (1996). , 28(5), 881-7.

[8] Caserta, T. M, Knisley, A. A, Tan, F. K, Arnett, F. C, & Brown, T. L. Genotypic analysis of the TGF beta-509 allele in patients with systemic lupus erythematosus and Sjogren's syndrome. Ann Genet (2004). , 47(4), 359-63.

[9] Chen, J. Y, Wang, C. M, Lu, S. C, Chou, Y. H, & Luo, S. F. Association of apoptosis-related microsatellite polymorphisms on chromosome 1q in Taiwanese systemic lupus erythematosus patients. Clin Exp Immunol (2006). , 143(2), 281-7.

[10] Chong, W. P, Ip, W. K, Wong, W. H, Lau, C. S, Chan, T. M, & Lau, Y. L. Association of interleukin-10 promoter polymorphisms with systemic lupus erythematosus. Genes Immun (2004). , 5(6), 484-92.

[11] Chung, S. J, Kim, J. S, Jung, H. C, & Song, I. S. Transforming growth factor-[beta]1-509T reduces risk of colorectal cancer, but not adenoma in Koreans. Cancer Sci (2007). , 98(3), 401-4.

[12] Clancy, R. M, Backer, C. B, Yin, X, Kapur, R. P, Molad, Y, & Buyon, J. P. Cytokine polymorphisms and histologic expression in autopsy studies: contribution of TNF-alpha and TGF-beta 1 to the pathogenesis of autoimmune-associated congenital heart block.J Immunol. (2003). Sep 15;, 171(6), 3253-61.

[13] Crawley, E, Woo, P, & Isenberg, D. A. Single nucleotide polymorphic haplotypes of the interleukin-10 5' flanking region are not associated with renal disease or serology in Caucasian patients with systemic lupus erythematosus. Arthritis and Rheumatism (1999). , 42(9), 2017-2018.

[14] Alfonso, D, Giordano, S, Mellai, M, Lanceni, M, Barizzone, M, Marchini, N, Scorza, M, Danieli, R, Cappelli, M. G, Rovere, M, Sabbadini, P, & Momigliano-richiardi, M. G. P. Association tests with systemic lupus erythematosus (SLE) of IL10 markers indicate a direct involvement of a CA repeat in the 5' regulatory region. Genes Immun (2002). , 3(8), 454-63.

[15] Alfonso, D, Rampi, S, Bocchio, M, Colombo, D, Scorza-smeraldi, G, & Momigliano-richardi, R. P. Systemic lupus erythematosus candidate genes in the Italian popula-

tion: evidence for a significant association with interleukin-10. Arthritis Rheum (2000). , 43(1), 120-8.

[16] Alfonso, D, Rampi, S, Rolando, M, Giordano, V, & Momigliano-richiardi, M. New polymorphisms in the IL-10 promoter region. Genes Immun 2000;1:231-233., 2000.

[17] Dang, H, Geiser, A. G, Letterio, J. J, Nakabayashi, T, Kong, L, Fernandes, G, & Talal, N. SLE-like autoantibodies and Sjögren's syndrome-like lymphoproliferation in TGF-beta knockout mice. J. Immunol (1995).

[18] De Waal Malefyt RDYssel H, de Vries JE. Direct effects of IL-10 on subsets of human CD4+ T cell clones and resting T cells. Specific inhibition of IL-2 production and proliferation. J. Immunol (1993). , 150(11), 4754-65.

[19] Dijstelbloem, H. M, Hepkema, B. G, et al. The R-H polymorphism of Fcγ receptor IIa as a risk factor for systemic lupus erythematosus is independent of single-nucleotide polymorphisms in the interleukin-10 gene promoter. Arthritis and Rheumatism (2002). , 46(4), 1125-1126.

[20] Ding, L, Linsley, P. S, Huang, L-Y, Germain, R. N, & Shevach, E. M. IL-10 inhibits macrophage costimulatory activity by selectively inhibiting the up-regulation of B7 expression. Journal of Immunology (1993). , 151(3), 1224-1234.

[21] Diveu, C, Mcgeachy, M. J, & Cua, D. J. Cytokines that regulate autoimmunity. Curr Opin Immunol (2008). , 20(6), 663-8.

[22] Dobreva, Z. G, Miteva, L. D, & Stanilova, S. A. The inhibition of JNK and MAPKs downregulates IL-10 and differentially affects c-Jun gene expression in human monocytes. Immunopharmacol Immunotoxicol (2009). , 38.

[23] Dubois, C. M, Laprise, M-H, Blanchette, F, Gentry, L. E, & Leduc, R. Processing of transforming growth factor β1 precursor by human furin convertase. J Biol Chem (1995). , 270, 0618-10624.

[24] Eskdale J & Galager GA polymorphic dinucleotide repeat in the human IL- 10 promoter region. Immunogenetics (1995). , 42, 444-445.

[25] Eskdale, J, Gallagher, G, Verweij, C. L, & Keijsers, V. Westendorp RGJ, and. Huizinga TWJ. Interleukin 10 secretion in relation to human IL-10 locus haplotypes. Proc Natl Acad Sci U S A (1998). , 95(16), 9465-70.

[26] Eskdale, J, Kube, D, Tesch, H, & Gallagher, G. Mapping of the human IL10 gene and further characterization of the 5′ flanking sequence. Immunogenetics (1997). , 46, 120-128.

[27] Eskdale, J, Wordsworth, P, Bowman, S, Field, M, & Gallagher, G. Associations between polymorphism at the human IL-10 locus and systemic lupus erythematosus. Tissue Antigens (1997). , 49, 635-9.

[28] European Bioinformatics InstituteSanger Institute. SNP database: Ensembl Genome Browser. (2006). Available at: http://www.ensembl.org/index.html.

[29] Fainaru, O, Shay, T, Hantisteanu, S, Goldenberg, D, Domany, E, & Groner, Y. TGFbeta-dependent gene expression profile during maturation of dendritic cells. Genes Immun (2007). , 8(3), 239-244.

[30] Fei, G-Z, Svenungsson, E, Frostegård, J, Padyukov, L, & The, A. IL-10 allele is associated with cardiovascular disease in SLE. Atherosclerosis (2004). , 177(2), 409-414.

[31] Fiorentino, D. F, Bond, M. W, & Mosmann, T. R. Two types of mouse T helper cell. IV. Th2 clones secrete a factor that inhibits cytokine production by Th1 clones. Journal of Experimental Medicine (1993). , 170(6), 2081-95.

[32] Flanders, K. C, & Roberts, A. B. TGF-β. In:Ippenheim JJ, Feldmann M (eds). Cytokine Reference, Academic Press: San Diego, CA, (2001). , 1

[33] Gateva et alA large-scale replication study identifies TNIP1, PRDM1, JAZF1, UHRF1BP1 and IL10 as risk loci for systemic lupus erythematosus. Nat Genet (2009). , 41(11), 1228-33.

[34] Gorelik L Flavell RAAbrogation of TGFbeta signalling in T cells leads to spontaneous T cell differentiation and autoimmune disease. Immunity (2000). , 12(2), 171-181.

[35] Grainger, D. J, Heathcote, K, Chiano, M, Snieder, H, Kemp, P. R, Metcalfe, J. C, Carter, N. D, & Spector, T. D. Genetic control of the circulating concentration of transforming growth factor type β1. Hum Mol Genet (1999). , 8(1), 93-7.

[36] Guarnizo-zuccardi, P, Lopez, Y, Giraldo, M, Garcia, N, Rodriguez, L, Ramirez, L, Uribe, O, Garcia, L, & Vasquez, G. Cytokine gene polymorphisms in Colombian patients with systemic lupus erythematosus. Tissue Antigens (2007). , 70(5), 376-82.

[37] Hirankarn, N, Wongpiyabovorn, J, Hanvivatvong, O, Netsawang, J, Akkasilpa, S, Wongchinsri, J, Hanvivadhanakul, P, Korkit, W, & Avihingsanon, Y. The synergistic effect of FC gamma receptor IIa and interleukin-10 genes on the risk to develop systemic lupus erythematosus in Thai population.Tissue Antigens (2006). , 68(5), 399-406.

[38] Hollegaard MV & Bidwell JL(2006). Cytokine gene polymorphism in human disease: on-line databases, Supplement 3. Genes Immun 2006;, 7, 269-76.

[39] Houssiau, F. A, Lefebvre, C, Vanden, B. M, Lambert, M, Devogelaer, J-P, & Renauld, J-C. Serum interleukin 10 titers in systemic lupus erythematosus reflect disease activity. Lupus (1995). , 4(5), 393-395.

[40] Hye-young, C, Jae-wook, C, Hyoun-ah, K, Jeong-moon, Y, Ja-young, J, Young-min, Y, Seung-hyun, K, Hae-sim, P, Chang-hee, S, & Cytokine, I. L. and IL-10 as Biomarkers in Systemic Lupus Erythematosus. Journal of clinical immunology (2007). , 27, 461-466.

[41] Jin, T, Almehed, K, & Carlsten, H. Forsblad-d'Elia H. Decreased Serum Levels of TGF-β1 are associated with Renal Damages in Female Patients with Systemic Lupus Erythematosus. Lupus (2011). , 21(3), 310-8.

[42] Johanneson, B, Lima, G, Von Salomé, J, & Alarcón-segovia, D. Alarcón-Riquelme ME; Collaborative Group on the Genetics of SLE, The BIOMED II Collaboration on the Genetics of SLE and Sjögrens syndrome. A major susceptibility locus for systemic lupus erythemathosus maps to chromosome1q31. Am J Hum Genet (2002). , 71(5), 1060-71.

[43] Kariuki, S. N, & Niewold, T. B. Genetic regulation of serum cytokines in systemic lupus erythematosus. Transl Res (2010). , 155(3), 109-17.

[44] Koss, K, Fanning, G. C, Welsh, K. I, & Jewell, D. P. Interleukin-10 gene promoter polymorphism in English and Polish healthy controls. Polymerase chain reaction haplotyping using 3' mismatches in forward and reverse primers. Genes and Immunity (2000). , 1(5), 321-324.

[45] Lazarus, M, Hajeer, A. H, Turner, D, Sinnott, P, & Worthington, J. Ollier WER, and Hutchinson IV, Genetic variation in the interleukin 10 gene promoter and systemic lupus erythematosus. Journal of Rheumatology (1997). , 24(12), 2314-2317.

[46] Lebman, D. A, & Edmiston, J. S. The role of TGF-beta in growth, differentiation, and maturation of B lymphocytes. Microbes Infect (1999). , 1(15), 1297-1304.

[47] Li MoWan YY, Flavell RA. T cell-produced transforming growth factor-beta1 controls T cell tolerance and regulates Th1- and Th17-cell differentiation. Immunity (2007). May;, 26(5), 579-91.

[48] Li, M. O, Wan, Y. Y, Sanjabi, S, Robertson, A. K, & Flavell, R. A. Transforming growth factor-beta regulation of immune responses. Annu Rev Immunol (2006). , 24, 99-146.

[49] Lin, Y. J, Wan, L, Huang, C. M, Sheu, J. J, Chen, S. Y, Lin, T. H, Chen, D. Y, Hsueh, K. C, Lai, C. C, Tsai, F. J, & Tnf-alpha, I. L. promoter polymorphisms in susceptibility to systemic lupus erythematosus in Taiwan. Clin Exp Rheumatol (2010). , 28(3), 318-24.

[50] LinS-Y et al., A whole genome methylation analysis of systemic lupus erythematosus: hypomethylation of the IL10 and IL1R2 promoters is associated with disease activity. Genes and Immunity (2012). , 13, 214-220.

[51] Liossis, S. N, Kovacs, B, Dennis, G, Kammer, G. M, & Tsokos, G. C. B cells from patients with systemic lupus erythematosus display abnormal antigen receptor-mediated early signal transduction events. J Clin Invest (1996). , 98(11), 2549-57.

[52] Llorente, L, Richaud-patin, Y, & Richaud-patin, Y. Dysregulation of interleukin-10 production in relatives of patients with systemic lupus erythematosus. Arthritis and Rheumatism (1997). , 40(8), 1429-1435.

[53] Llorente, L, Richaud-patin, Y, Garcia-padilla, C, Claret, E, Jakez-ocampo, J, & Cardiel, M. H. Clinical and biologic effects of anti-interleukin-10 monoclonal antibody administration in systemic lupus erythematosus. Arthritis and Rheumatism (2000). , 43, 1790-1800.

[54] Llorente, L, & Richaud-patin, Y. The role of interleukin-10 in systemic lupus erythematosus. J Autoimmun (2003). , 20(4), 287-9.

[55] López, P, Gutiérrez, C, & Suárez, A. IL-10 and TNFalpha genotypes in SLE. J Biomed Biotechnol (2010).

[56] Lu, L. Y, Cheng, H. H, Sung, P. K, Yeh, J. J, Shiue, Y. L, & Chen, A. Single-nucleotide polymorphisms of transforming growth factor-β1 gene in Taiwanese patients with systemic lupus erythematosus. J Microbiol Immunol Infect (2004).

[57] Mandik-nayak, L, Ridge, N, Fields, M, Park, A. Y, & Erikson, J. Role of B cells in systemic lupus erythematosus and rheumatoid arthritis. Curr Opin Immunol (2008). , 20(6), 639-45.

[58] Manolova, I, Ivanova, M, Aleksandrova, E, Miteva, L, Stoilov, R, Rashkov, R, & Stanilova, S. Association of transforming growth factor promoter polymorphism with systemic lupus erythematosus. Revmatologia (Sofia) (2012).

[59] Marie JC Liggitt DRudensky AY. Cellular mechanisms of fatal early-onset autoimmunity in mice with the T cell-specific targeting of transforming growth factor-beta receptor. Immunity (2006). , 25(3), 441-454.

[60] Mehrian, R, & Quismorio, F. P. Jr, Sstrassmann G, et al. Synergistic effect between IL-10 and bcl-2 genotypes in determining susceptibility to systemic lupus erythematosus. Arthritis Rheum (1998). , 41, 596-602.

[61] Meng, J, Thongngarm, T, Nakajima, M, Yamashita, N, Ohta, K, Bates, C. A, Grunwald, G. K, & Rosenwasser, L. J. Association of transforming growth factor-beta1 single nucleotide polymorphism C-509T with allergy and immunological activities. Int Arch Allergy Immunol (2005). , 138(2), 151-60.

[62] Miteva, L, & Stanilova, S. The combined effect of IL-10 and IL-12 polymorphisms on induced cytokine production. Human Immunology (2008). , 69, 562-566.

[63] Miteva, L, Manolova, I, Ivanova, M, Stoilov, R, Rashkov, R, & Stanilova, S. Lack of association between promoter polymorphism-1082A/G in Interleukin-10 gene and genetic predisposition to systemic lupus erythematosus. Revmatologia (Sofia) (2010). , 18(3), 33-38.

[64] Mok, C. C, Lanchbury, J. S, Chan, D. W, & Lau, C. S. Interleukin-10 promoter polymorphism in southern Chinese patients with systemic lupus erythematosus. Arthritis Rheum (1998). , 41, 1090-5.

[65] Moore, K. W. de Waal Malefyt R, Coffman RL, O'Garra A. Interleukin-10 and the interleukin-10 receptor. Annu Rev Immunol. (2001). , 19, 683-765.

[66] Moustakas, A, Pardali, K, Gaal, A, & Heldin, C. H. Mechanisms of TGF-β signaling in regulation of cell growth and differentiation. Immunol Lett (2002).

[67] Nakken, B, Alex, P, Munthe, L, Szekanecz, Z, & Szodoray, P. Immune-regulatory mechanisms in systemic autoimmune and rheumatic diseases. Clin Dev Immunol (2012).

[68] Nath, S. K, Harley, J. B, & Lee, Y. H. Polymorphisms of complement receptor 1 and interleukin-10 genes and systemic lupus erythematosus: a meta-analysis. Hum Genet (2005). , 118(2), 225-34.

[69] Ohtsuka, K, Gray, J. D, Stimmler, M. M, Toro, B, & Horwitz, D. A. Decreased production of TGF-b by lymphocytes from patients with systemic lupuis erythematosus. The Journal of Immunology (1998). , 160, 2539-2545.

[70] Park, Y. B, Lee, S. K, Kim, D. S, Lee, J, Lee, C. H, & Song, C. H. Elevated interleukin-10 levels correlated with disease activity in systemic lupus erythematosus. Clinical and Experimental Rheumatology (1998). , 16(3), 283-288.

[71] Petri, M. Epidemiology of systemic lupus erythematosus. Best Pract Res Clin Rheumatol (2002). , 16(5), 847-58.

[72] Pyzik M Piccirillo CATGF-beta1 modulates Foxp3 expression and regulatory activity in distinct CD4+ T cell subsets. J Leukoc Biol (2007). , 82(2), 335-346.

[73] Rood, M. J, Keijsers, V, & Keijsers, V. Neuropsychiatric systemic lupus erythematosus is associated with imbalance in interleukin 10 promoter haplotypes of the. Annals Rheumatic Diseases (1999). , 58(2), 85-89.

[74] Rosado, S, Rua-figueroa, I, Vargas, J. A, Garcia-laorden, M. I, Losada-fernandez, I, Martin-donaire, T, Perez-chacon, G, Rodriguez-gallego, C, Naranjo-hernandez, A, Ojeda-bruno, S, Citores, M. J, & Perez-aciego, P. Interleukin-10 promoter polymorphisms in patients with systemic lupus erythematosus from the Canary Islands. Int J Immunogenet (2008). , 35(3), 235-42.

[75] Rousset, F, Garcia, E, & Garcia, E. Interleukin 10 is a potent growth and differentiation factor for activated human B lymphocytes. Proceedings of the National Academy of Sciences of the United States of America (1992). , 89(5), 1890-1893.

[76] Rubtsov, Y. P, & Rudensky, A. Y. TGFbeta signalling in control of T-cell-mediated self-reactivity. Nat Rev Immunol (2007). , 7, 443-453.

[77] Schotte, H, Gaubitz, M, Willeke, P, Tidow, N, Assmann, G, Domschke, W, & Schlüter, B. Interleukin-10 promoter microsatellite polymorphisms in systemic lupus erythematosus: association with the anti-Sm immune response. Rheumatology (Oxford) (2004). , 43(11), 1357-63.

[78] Schotte, H, Willeke, P, Rust, S, Assmann, G, Domschke, W, Gaubitz, M, & Schlüter, B. The transforming growth factor-beta1 gene polymorphism (G915C) is not associated with systemic lupus erythematosus.Lupus. (2003)., 12(2), 86-92.

[79] Schuster, N, & Krieglstein, K. Mechanisms of TGF-hmediated apoptosis. CellTissue Res (2002)., 307(1), 1-14.

[80] Selvaraj, R. K, & Geiger, T. L. A kinetic and dynamic analysis of Foxp3 induced in T cells by TGF-beta. J Immunol (2007)., 179(2), 7667-7677.

[81] Shull, M. M, et al. Targeted disruption of the mouse transforming growth factor-beta 1 gene results in multifocal inflammatory disease. Nature (1992)., 359(6397), 693-699.

[82] Sobkowiak, A, Lianeri, M, Wudarski, M, Lacki, J. K, & Jagodzinski, P. P. Genetic variation in the interleukin-10 gene promoter in Polish patients with systemic lupus erythematosus. Rheumatol Int (2009)., 29(8), 921-5.

[83] Stanilova, S. A, Miteva, L. D, Karakolev, Z. T, & Stefanov, C. S. Interleukin-10-1082 promoter polymorphism in association with cytokine production and sepsis susceptibility. Intensive Care Med (2006)., 32(2), 260-6.

[84] Suarez, A, Castro, P, Alonso, R, Mozo, L, & Gutierrez, C. Interindividual variations in constitutive interleukin-10 messenger RNA and protein levels and their association with genetic polymorphisms. Transplantation (2003). doi:TP. 0000055216.19866.9A., 75, 711-717.

[85] Suarez, A, Lopez, P, Mozo, L, & Gutierrez, C. Differential effect of IL10 and TNF{alpha} genotypes on determining susceptibility to discoid and systemic lupus erythematosus. Ann Rheum Dis (2005). doi:ard.2004.035048., 64, 1605-1610.

[86] Sung, Y. K, Park, B. L, Shin, H. D, Kim, L. H, Kim, S. Y, & Bae, S. C. Interleukin-10 gene polymorphisms are associated with the SLICC/ACR Damage Index in systemic lupus erythematosus.Rheumatology (Oxford). (2006)., 45(4), 400-4.

[87] Tsao, B. P, et al. Evidence for linkage of a candidate chromosome 1 region to human systemic lupus erythematosus. J Clin Invest (1997)., 99(4), 725-31.

[88] Turner, D. M, Williams, D. M, Sankaran, D, Lazarus, M, Sinnott, P. J, & Hutchinson, I. V. An investigation of polymorphism in the interleukin-10 gene promoter. European Journal of Immunogenetics (1997)., 24(1), 1-8.

[89] Van Der Linden, M. Westendorp RGJ, Sturk A, Bergman W, and Huizinga TWJ. High interleukin-10 production in first-degree relatives of patients with generalized but not cutaneous lupus erythematosus. Journal of Investigative Medicine (2000)., 48(5), 327-334.

[90] Vuong, M. T, Gunnarsson, I, Lundberg, S, Svenungsson, E, Wramner, L, Fernström, A, Syvänen, A. C, Do, L. T, Jacobson, S. H, & Padyukov, L. Genetic risk factors in lu-

pus nephritis and IgA nephropathy--no support of an overlap.PLoS One. (2010). e10559

[91] Wahl, S. M. Transforming growth factor-beta (TGF-bet) in inflammation: a cause and a cure. J Clin Immunol 12, (1992).

[92] Wakkach, A, Augier, S, Breittmayer, J. P, Blin-wakkach, C, & Carle, G. F. Characterization of IL-10-secreting T cells derived from regulatory CD4+CD25+ cells by the TIRC7 surface marker. Journal of Immunology (2008). , 180(9), 6054-6063.

[93] Wang, B, Morinobu, A, Kanagawa, S, Nakamura, T, Kawano, S, Koshiba, M, Hashimoto, H, & Kumagai, S. Transforming growth factor beta 1 gene polymorphism in Japanese patients with systemic lupus erythematosus. Kobe J Med Sci (2007).

[94] Wang, Y. Q, Ugai, S, Shimozato, O, Yu, L, Kawamura, K, Yamamoto, H, Yamaguchi, T, Saisho, H, & Tagawa, M. nduction of systemic immunity by expression of interleukin-23 in murine colon carcinoma cells. Int J Cancer (2003). , 105(6), 820-4.

[95] Wu, G. Y, Hasenberg, T, Magdeburg, R, Bönninghoff, R, Sturm, J. W, & Keese, M. Association between EGF, TGF-beta1, VEGF gene polymorphism and colorectal cancer. World J Surg (2009). , 33(1), 124-9.

[96] Yin, Z, Bahtiyar, G, Zhang, N, Liu, L, Zhu, P, Robert, M. E, Mcniff, J, Madaio, M. P, & Craft, J. IL-10 regulates murine lupus. J Immunol (2002). , 169(4), 2148-55.

[97] Yurasov, S, Tiller, T, Tsuiji, M, Velinzon, K, Pascual, V, Wardemann, H, & Nussenzweig, M. C. Persistent expression of autoantibodies in SLE patients in remission. J Exp Med (2006). , 203(10), 2255-61.

[98] Zhang, Y, Liu, B, Jin, M, Ni, Q, Liang, X, Ma, X, Yao, K, Li, Q, & Chen, K. Genetic polymorphisms of transforming growth factor-beta1 and its receptors and colorectal cancer susceptibility: a population-based case-control study in China. Cancer Lett (2009). , 275(1), 102-8.

[99] Zheng, S. G, et al. IL-2 is essential for TGF-beta to convert naive CD4+CD25- cells to CD25+Foxp3+ regulatory T cells and for expansion of these cells. J Immunol (2007). , 178(4), 2018-2027.

[100] Zhu, L-J, Liu, Z-H, Zeng, C-H, Chen, Z-H, Yu, C, & Li, L-S. Association of interleukin-10 gene-592 A/C polymorphism with the clinical and pathological diversity of lupus nephritis. Clinical and Experimental Rheumatology (2005). , 23(6), 854-860.

Chapter 3

Toll-Like Receptor 3 and Retinoic Acid-Inducible Gene-I Implicated to the Pathogenesis of Autoimmune Renal Diseases

Hiroshi Tanaka and Tadaatsu Imaizumi

Additional information is available at the end of the chapter

http://dx.doi.org/10.5772/53026

1. Introduction

The innate and adaptive immune systems have been reported to play an important role in the pathogenesis of glomerular diseases. Since viral infection may sometimes trigger the development of inflammatory renal disease or the worsening of pre-existing renal disease, recent studies have focused on the involvement of toll-like receptors (TLRs) and their signaling pathways in the inflammatory processes of glomerular cells [1]. Recognition of the molecular pattern of a pathogen, which is distinguishable from host molecules, is important in innate immunity, and TLRs are specialized in the pattern recognition of pathogen molecules. The activation of TLRs and their downstream immune responses can be induced not only by infectious pathogens, but also by non-infectious stimulation, such as endogenous ligands, and this mechanism may be involved in the pathogenesis of autoimmune renal diseases [1-3]. Viral double-stranded RNA (dsRNA) can activate not only TLR3 located in intracellular endosomes, but also retinoic acid-inducible gene-I (RIG-I)-like helicases receptors located in the cytosol [4]. RIG-I and melanoma differentiation-associated gene-5 (MDA5) are members of RNA helicase family in the cytosol, and both act as pathogen recognition receptors [5]. Therefore, RIG-I and MDA5 may also involved in the pathogenesis of autoimmune renal diseases [6-8].

Recent studies revealed the expressions of TLRs in resident renal cells, suggesting the involvement of the TLR signaling pathway in the pathogenesis of glomerular diseases [1-3]. Once presumptive antigenic ligands bind to TLRs, the activation of transcriptional factors, such as interferon regulatory factors (IRF) and nuclear factor kappa B (NF-κB) is induced through intracellular signaling cascade activation. The activation results in the release of adhesion molecules, cytokines and chemokines, which play a pivotal role in the innate and adaptive immune responses [1-3]. For example, the activation of mesangial TLR 3 during hepatitis C virus (HCV) infection contributed to chemokine/cytokine release and caused proliferation and apoptosis in the pathogenesis of HCV glomerulonephritis [9]. This is direct evidence of the involvement of TLRs in the inflammatory processes of viral-induced glomerulonephritis. It has been reported that glomerular mesangial cells (MCs) produce a wide variety of pro-inflammatory molecules that play an important role in immune and inflammatory reactions in the kidney [10]. In an experimental setting, the activation of mesangial TLR3 induced by polyinosinic-polycytidylic acid (poly IC), an authentic dsRNA, upregulated the expression of matrix metalloproteinase 9 (MMP9), plasminogen activator inhibitor type 1, and tissue plasminogen activator in human MCs. These findings suggest that viral RNA can influence the generation and degradation of the extracelluar matrix in the mesangium in ways other than through direct viral stimulation, and, subsequently, the possible development of glomerulosclerosis might occur [11, 12]. Furthermore, in another set of experimental studies using poly IC-stimulation, MCs have been reported to express functional molecules such as interleukin (IL)-6 [6], CC chemokine ligand (CCL) 2 (or monocyte-chemoattractant protein-1, MCP-1) [13], and CCL5 (or regulated on activation, normal T-cell expression and secretion, RANTES) [9].

Like TLR3, RIG-I and MDA5 may detect viral RNAs and mediate immune reactions against RNA viruses [4, 14]. It has been reported that RIG-I, and not TLR3, mediated the secretion of type I interferon (IFN) in poly IC/cationic lipid complex-treated glomerular endothelial cells [15]. In contrast, other investigators have reported that, in MCs, RIG-I was not involved in the poly IC-induced expression of IL-6 [13] or MMP9 [11], while TLR3 was involved in that system. In an interesting experiment using TLR3 signaling-deficient mice, it has been reported that MDA5, but not RIG-I, was required for signaling induced by poly IC/cationic lipid complex in murine MCs [6]. The cells transfected with poly IC/cationic lipid complex is thought to be a model of entry of RNA virus into the cytoplasm. However, the precise role of RIG-I in mesangial inflammation remains to be elucidated. Since there are few data on the role of RIG-I, and the interaction between TLR3, MDA5 and RIG-I in human glomerular diseases, we performed several experiments using cultured normal human MCs. We found that the involvement of novel RIG-I-mediated signaling pathways in mesangial inflammation in human MCs [8, 15-17]. These signaling pathways may be involved in the pathogenesis of human glomerular diseases.

2. RIG-I and lupus nephritis

We previously found significant expression of RIG-I in the glomeruli of biopsy specimens from patients with lupus nephritis, and the level of expression correlated with the severity of the acute inflammatory lesions (Figure 1.) [18].

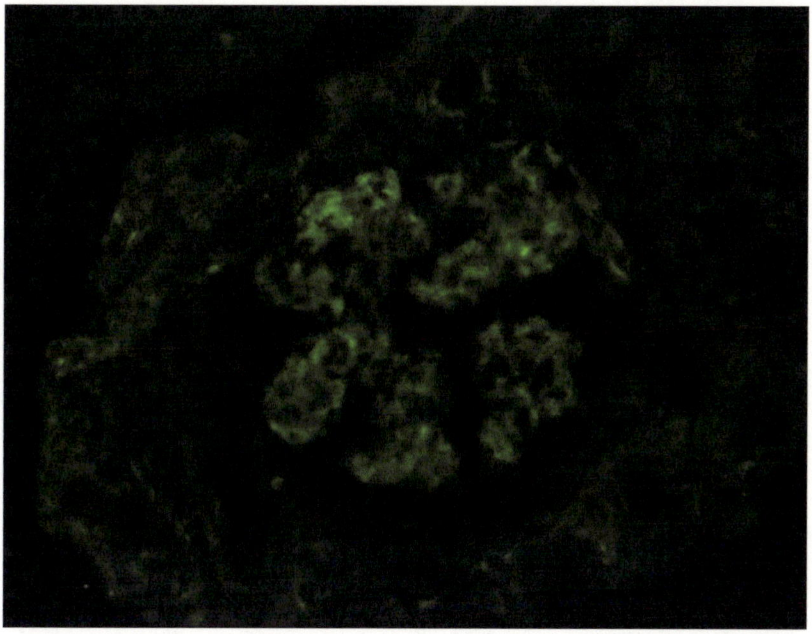

Figure 1. Glomerular immunoreactivity for RIG-I was detectable in cases of diffuse proliferative lupus nephritis, and an intense granular pattern of immunofluorescence was observed in a mesangial area and capillary loop distribution (Suzuki et al. NDT 2007).

In addition, we found that the levels of RIG-I mRNA in the urinary sediment of patients with lupus nephritis were higher than those in patients with IgA nephropathy and controls [19]. Interestingly, repeated measurements of the mRNA expression of RIG-I in the urinary sediment of lupus patients revealed a reduction in the expression following immunosuppressive treatment [19].These findings suggest that RIG-I may be involved in the acute inflammatory process in human lupus nephritis. These clinical observations led us to conduct the following experimental studies.

In order to examine the involvement of RIG-I in lupus nephritis, we conducted experimental studies using human MCs in culture. Because Th1-derived cytokines are known to be key mediators in the progression of lupus-associated renal injury, and IFN-γ is one of the major Th1 type cytokines with potent proinflammatory effects through the upregulation of IFN-inducible genes [3], the effects of IFN-γ on the expression of RIG-I in human MCs in culture were examined. As a result, IFN-γ treatment resulted in a concentration-dependent upregulation of the expression of RIG-I mRNA and protein in human MCs. The treatment of cells with IFN-γ also induced the expression of mRNA for both IRF1 and IRF7, which are important IFN-inducible transcriptional factors [15]. Furthermore, knockdown of RIG-I expression by small interfering RNA (siRNA) inhibited the IFN-γ-induced expression of IRF7, but not that of IRF1. In contrast, IFN-γ did not induce the expression of IFN-β, which is known to be a target gene of IRF-7, in MCs (Figure 2.) [15].

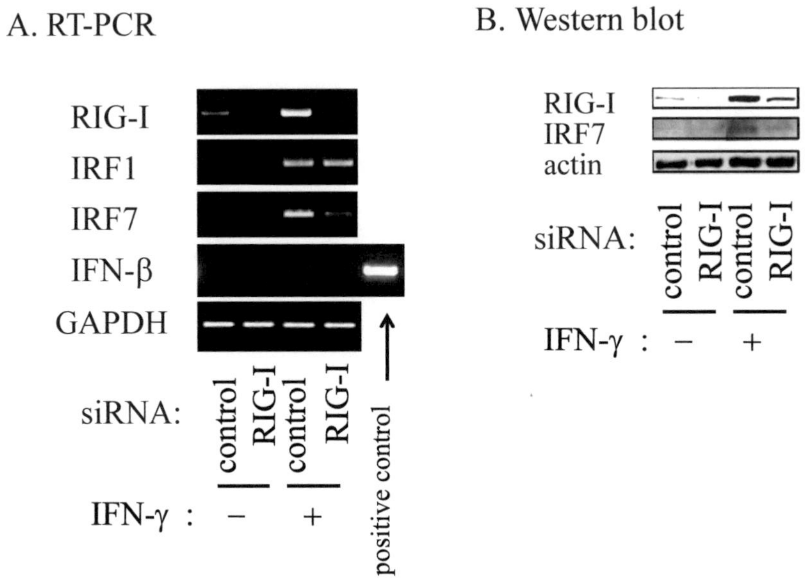

Figure 2. The cells were transfected with siRNA against RIG-I or a negative control non-silencing siRNA. At 24 h after the transfection, the cells were treated with 5 ng/ml IFN-γ for 24 h. (A) RNA was extracted from the cells and RT-PCR analyses for RIG-I, IRF1, IRF7, IFN-β and GAPDH were performed. (B) The cells were lysed and the lysates were subjected to western blot analysis for RIG-I, IRF7 and actin. (Imaizumi, et al. Lupus 2010)

Interestingly, the pretreatment of cells with dexamethasone inhibited the IFN- γ -induced expression of MCP-1 mRNA but did not affect the induction of mRNA for RIG-I or IRF7 in MCs. The induction of MCP-1 mRNA by IFN-γ was not inhibited by the knockdown of NF-κB p65, indicating that the NF−κB signaling pathway was not involved. Our results suggest selective regulation of the expression of IRFs by RIG-I in human MCs. The function of IRF7 has been well studied, mainly in dendritic cells and in mouse embryonic fibroblasts, and IRF7 is thought to be an important transcriptional factor that affects anti-viral responses by inducing the production of type I IFN [20]. However, neither IFN-γ treatment nor knockdown of RIG-I affected the expression of IFN-β in MCs. Although the functional significance of IRF7 expression in MCs remains to be elucidated, our recent observations suggest that the IFN-γ/RIG-I/IRF7 signaling pathways may be involved in the pathogenesis of lupus nephritis [15]. To date, it has been reported that TLR3, TLR4, TLR7 and TLR9 may play a role in the modulation of inflammatory processes in lupus nephritis [1, 3]. TLR7 and TLR9 recognize mammalian nucleic acids as well as bacterial DNA or viral single-stranded RNA (ssRNA), suggesting that the generation of some autoantibodies may be attributable to a possible role of TLR7 and TLR9 in selected patients with lupus nephritis [21]. Our previous clinical and experimental observations provide additional knowledge in the pathogenesis of lupus nephritis, although this remains preliminary. We believe that the involvement of the newly observed the IFN-γ/RIG-I/IRF7 pathway in MCs may contribute to mesangial inflammation, and the intervention of these signaling pathway may lead to the development of an optimal

http://dx.doi.org/10.5772/53026

future therapeutic strategies in lupus nephritis. Further clinical and experimental issues remain to be examined in future studies [22].

3. TLR3 and RIG-I in human MCs

Viral dsRNA is a potent inducer of type I IFNs and the downstream molecules of the innate immune pathway. Thus, in order to evaluate the potential role of RIG-I in response to viral dsRNA in human MC, we treated the cells with poly IC, an authentic dsRNA, in the next experiment. The cells were simply treated with poly IC, not transfected using poly/cationic lipid complex, in this experiment. Treatment with poly IC is a model of cells exposed to viral dsRNA released from dying cells. Stimulation with poly IC resulted in an increase in the expression of both RIG-I mRNA and protein in a concentration- and time-dependent manner, and this was accompanied with CCL5 expression [16]. Furthermore, treatment with RIG-I siRNA significantly lowered poly IC-induced CCL5 expression. In contrast, the poly IC-induced expression of CCL2 mRNA was not affected by RIG-I siRNA (Figure 3.). Interestingly, the poly IC-induced RIG-I expression was suppressed in response to treatment with siRNA against TLR3. Furthermore, TLR3 siRNA downregulated the poly IC-induced expressions of TLR3 and IFN-β, but RIG-I siRNA did not affect the expression of either TLR3 or IFN-β. In order to examine the role of IFN-β as a potential mediator of poly IC-induced RIG-I expression, IFN-β siRNA were used. The results showed that the poly IC-induced expressions of IFN-β and RIG-I were markedly inhibited in cells transfected with IFN-β siRNA. Pretreatment of the cells with a blocking antibody against the type I IFN receptor also reduced the poly IC-induced expression of RIG-I. Moreover, pretreatment of the cells with dexamethasone reduced the poly IC-induced expression of both RIG-I and IFN-β, but this treatment had no effect on IFN-β-induced RIG-I expression [16]. Our results suggest that the expression of CCL5 was selectively regulated by RIG-I expression in human MCs, because poly IC-induced CCL5 expression was inhibited in response to the knockdown of RIG-I, while the expression of CCL2 was not affected by treatment with RIG-I siRNA. A recent report suggested that RIG-I, and not TLR3, mediated the secretion of type I IFN in poly IC/ cationic lipid complex-treated glomerular endothelial cells [14]. Our findings reveal another aspect of glomerular inflammation, as the cross talk between glomerular endothelial cells and MCs may be an important factor of glomerular inflammation, and the RIG-I/CCL5 pathway in mesangial cells may contribute to glomerular inflammation, particularly after viral infection [16].

Both TLR3 and RIG-I are reported to serve as receptors for viral dsRNA. Our recent study showed that siRNA-mediated knockdown of TLR3 inhibited the poly IC-induced expression of both IFN-β and RIG-I. However, RIG-I knockdown had no effect on poly IC-induced IFN-β expression. Thus, RIG-I may function downstream to TLR3 in the signaling cascade activated by poly IC-induced expression of CCL5 in MCs [16]. In addition, the inhibitory effect of dexamethasone may depend on the suppression of IFN-β production, and not on the IFN-β-induced RIG-I expression. In this signaling pathway in MCs, TLR3 and newly synthesized IFN-β are involved in poly IC-induced RIG-I expression. Since dexamethasone had no effect on IFN-β-induced RIG-I expression, the inhibitory effect of dexamethasone may depend on the suppression of IFN-β production. On the basis of these results, we propose the TLR3/IFN-β/RIG-I/CCL5 pathway (Figure 4.). This pathway may play an important role in immune and inflammatory reactions against viral infection in MCs. Since a viral infection may sometimes trigger the development of an inflammatory renal disease or the worsening of pre-existing renal disease, we believe that our recent findings are informative enough for the field of nephrology. Interestingly, it has been reported that tacrolimus (Tac) reduces proteinuria and mesangial alterations due to suppression of glomerular IFN-γ mRNA expression in rat models [23]. Thus, an immunosuppressant, Tac, may be a possible candidate for the intervention of these signaling pathways, although this remains to be elucidated in future studies.

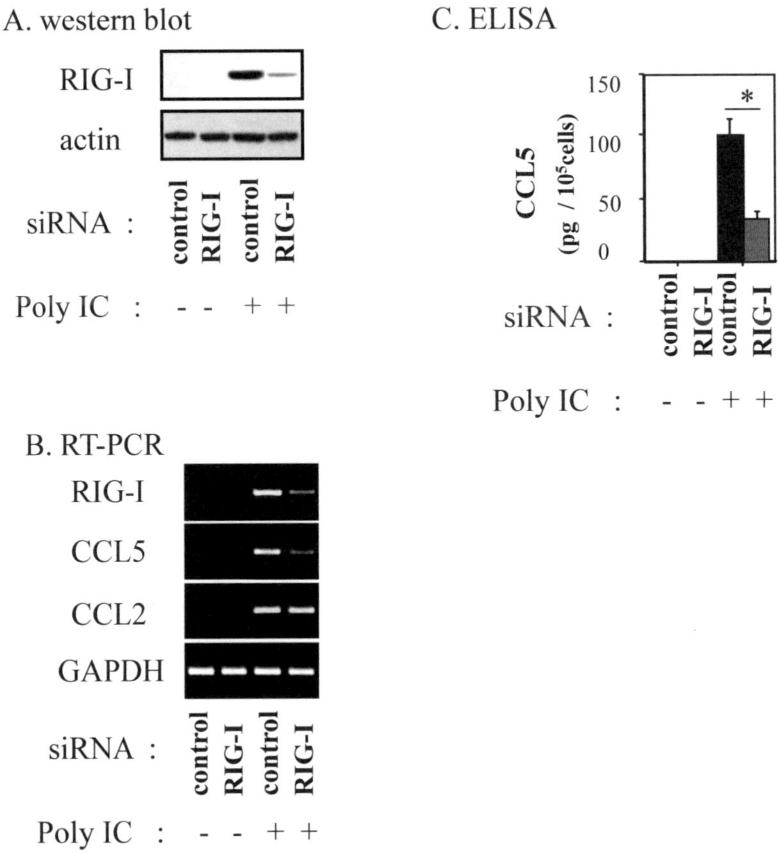

Figure 3. Knockdown of RIG-I reduces the poly IC-induced expression of CCL5 in human mesangial cells. The cells were transfected with siRNA against RIG-I or control siRNA and then stimulated with 20 mg/ml of poly IC. (A) After 24 h of poly IC treatment, the cells were lysed and western blotting for CCL5 was performed. (B) The cells were incubated for 16 h with poly IC, RNA was extracted, and RT-PCR was performed for RIG-I, CCL5, and CCL2. (C) The culture medium was collected after 24 h, and the concentration of CCL5 was determined by ELISA (n=3, *p<0.01). (Imaizumi, et al. NDT 2010)

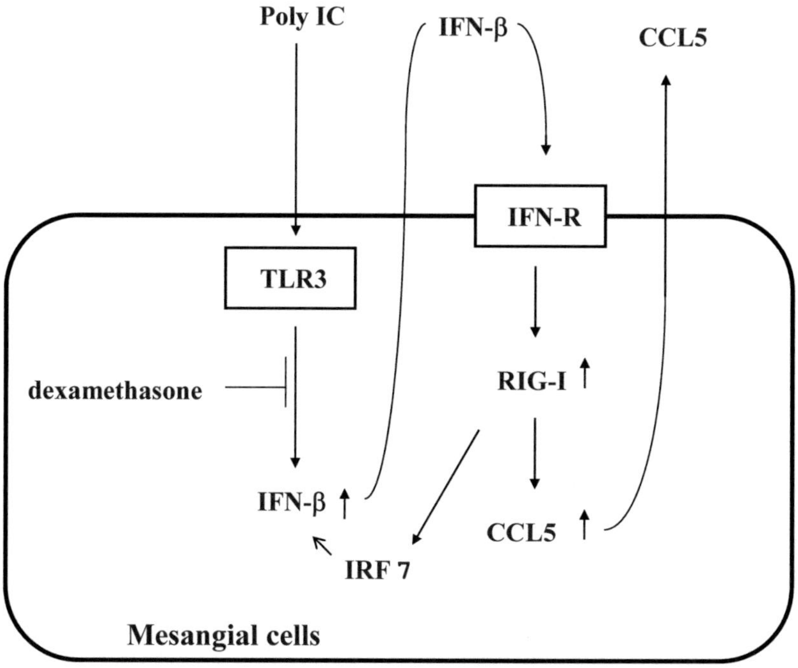

Figure 4. Proposed TLR3/IFN-β/RIG-I/CCL5 and IFN-γ/RIG-I/IRF7 signaling pathways in human mesangial cells (See the main document and Ref. no. 15 and 16).

4. TLR3 and IFN-stimulated gene (ISG) 20 in MCs

Interferon (IFN)-stimulated gene 20 (ISG20) is a 3′ - to - 5′ exonuclease specific for ssRNA and is involved in host defense reactions against RNA viruses [24, 25]. IFNs are key cytokines that regulate antiviral reactions and ISGs are class of major effector molecules for IFNs. Apart from antiviral reaction, ISGs may be involved in the pathogeneisis of a lupus model in mice [26]. We addressed the effect of poly IC on the expression of ISG20 in cultured MCs [17]. Poly IC treatment of MCs induced the expression of ISG20 in concentration- and time-dependent manners. Also, treatment of cells with poly IC induced the expression of IFN-β mRNA, but this was not the case with IFN-α. Transfection of the cells with siRNA against TLR3 or IRF3 suppressed the poly IC-induced expression of ISG20 mRNA and protein, while non-silencing control siRNA had no effect. On the other hand, siRNA against RIG-I, MDA5 or p65 did not affect the ISG20 expression (Figure 5.) [17]. Although siRNA may induce the expression of ISG20 nonspecifically, non-silencing control siRNA did not induce the expression of ISG20 under the condition we examined. Moreover, RNA interference against NF-κB p65 failed to inhibit poly IC-induced ISG20 expression.

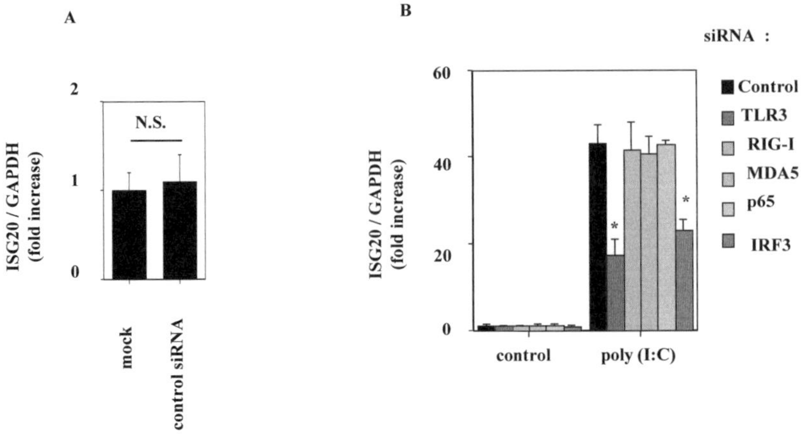

Figure 5. TLR3 and IRF3 are involved in poly IC-induced ISG20 expression. A. MCs were transfected with non-silencing control siRNA. After incubating for 24 h, RNA was extracted from cells. Expression of ISG20 mRNA was examined by real-time PCR. B. MCs were transfected with siRNA against TLR3, RIG-I, MDA5, p65, IRFr or a non-silencing control siRNA. 24 h after trasfections, the cells were treated for 16 h with 50 μg/ml poly IC and analyzed by real-time PCR for ISG20 mRNA (*p<0.01, n=3) (Imaizumi et al. Nephron Exp Nephrol 2011).

Transfection of the cells with IFN-β siRNA markedly inhibited the poly IC-induced expression of ISG20. Pretreatment of the cells with blocking antibody against type I IFN receptor also reduced the poly IC-induced expression of ISG20. Alternatively, transfection of the cells with an expression plasmid for IFN-β resulted in the over expression of ISG20 (Figure 6.) [17]. These observations suggest that *de novo* synthesized IFN-β is involved in poly IC-induced ISG20 expression.

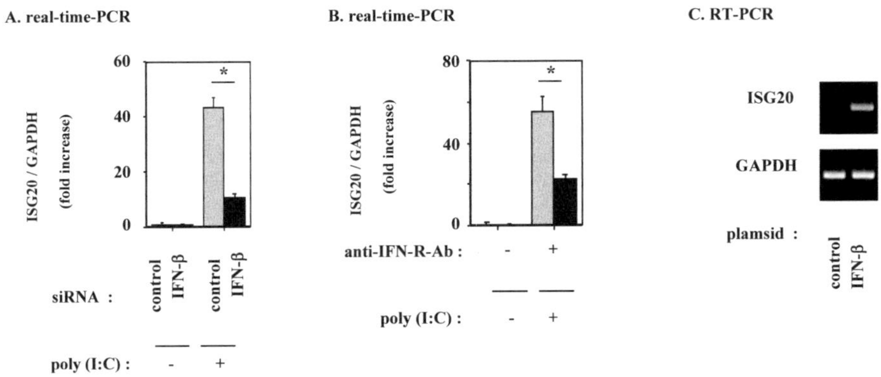

Figure 6. MCs were transfected with siRNA against IFN-β or a non-silencing control siRNA. A. After 24 h of transfection, the cells were treated with 50 μg/ml poly IC, RNA was extracted from cells after 16 h treatment with poly IC, and real-time PCR analysis for ISG20 was performed (*p<0.01, n=3). B. The cells were pretreated with a blocking antibody against type I IFN receptor (anti-IFN-ab) for 1 h, and subsequently treated with 50 μg/ml poly IC for 24 h (*p<0.01, n=3). C. The cells were transfected with an expression plasmid for IFN-β and incubated for 24 h (Imaizumi, et al. Nephron Exp Nephrol 2011).

Dexamethasone inhibits the induction of IFN-β and ISG20 by poly IC, but it did not affect the expression of ISG20 by IFN-β. Thus, the inhibitory effect of dexamethasone may depend on the suppression of IFN-β production, which is consistent with our previous report on the proposed TLR3/IFN-β/RIG-I/CCL5 pathway [16]. Transfection of MCs with a poly IC/cationic lipid complex induced the expression of ISG20 mRNA and protein. Knockdown of RIG-I, but not of TLR3 or MDA5, inhibited the induction of ISG20 by poly IC/cationic lipid complex.

On the basis of these results, TLR3, IFR3 and *de novo* synthesized IFN-β may mediate the expression of ISG20 induced by the simply treatment of poly IC, while RIG-I, but not MDA5, may be involved in the expression of ISG20 induced by poly IC/cationic lipid complex in this setting using cultured normal human MCs [17]. A previous study showed the recognition of a poly IC/cationic lipid complex by MDA5, not by RIG-I, in murine MCs [6]. The molecular mechanisms of pathogen recognition may vary between species. Although clinical impact of ISG20 expression in MCs except for antiviral responses remains to be elucidated in future studies [26], we found the novel TLR3/IRF3/IFN-β/ISG20 pathway in poly IC signaling in MCs, and this pathway may play an important role in immune and inflammatory reactions against viral infection in MCs.

5. TLR3, MDA5 and RIG-I in MCs

Recently, it was shown that MDA5 and RIG-I function as pathogen recognition receptor against viral dsRNA in the cytosome, and both the receptor may play an important role in innate immune reactions [4, 5]. Although the expression of MDA has been documented in murine MCs [6], and human MCs [17], detailed implications for the expression of MDA5 in human MCs have not been clarified. Thus, we next examined the effect of poly IC and the role of MDA5 in C-X-C motif chemokine 10 (CXCL10) (or IFN-γ-induced protein 10, IP-10) expression in cultured human MCs [8]. Poly IC, either simply applied to the cells or transfected as a complex with a cationic lipid, induced MDA5 expression in concentration- and time-dependent manners. Transfection of the cells with siRNA against TLR3 suppressed the poly IC-induced expression of MDA5 mRNA and protein, while siRNA against TLR3 did not suppress the poly IC/cationic lipid complex-induced expression of MDA5. On the other hand, siRNA against RIG-I significantly inhibited the MDA5 expression induced by poly IC/cationic lipid complex (Figure 7.) Knockdown of MDA5 had no effects on the expression of RIG-I induced by poly IC or poly IC/cationic lipid complex (Figure 8.). Thus, MDA5 may be located in the downstream of RIG-I in this signaling pathway in cultured human MCs [8]. These results are inconsistent with a previous report dealing with MDA5 expression in murine MCs [6]. The molecular mechanisms of pathogen recognition may vary between species, although this issue remains to be elucidated in future studies [17].

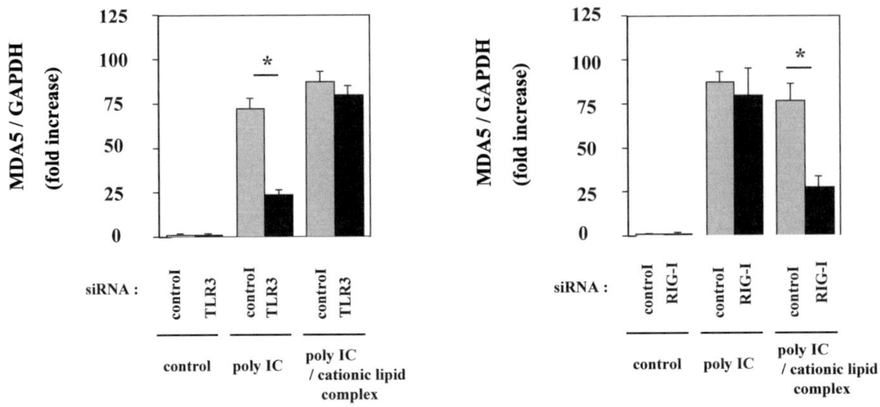

Figure 7. MCs were transfected with siRNA against TLR3, RIG-I, MDA5 or a non-silencing control siRNA. 24 h after transfection, the cells were treated with 30 μg/ml poly IC or were transfected with the complex of 1 ng/ml poly IC/ cationic lipid. After 16 h or 24 h incubation, the cells were subjected to real-time PCR analysis (Imaizumi et al. Tohoku J Exp Med 2012).

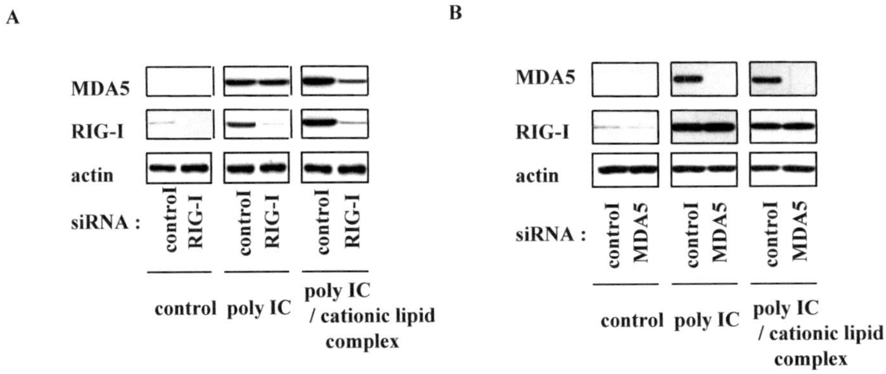

Figure 8. MCs were transfected with siRNA against RIG-I, MDA5, or non-silencing control siRNA. 24 h after transfection, the cells were treated with 30 μg/ml poly IC or were transfected with the complex of 1 ng/ml poly IC/cationic lipid. After 16 h or 24 h incubation, the cells were subjected to western blot analysis (Imaizumi et al. Tohoku J Exp Med 2012).

Induction of IFN-β mRNA was observed in the cells treated with poly IC or those transfected with a poly IC/cationic lipid complex. In this experiment, TLR3 knockdown suppressed IFN-β induction in the poly IC-treated cells, while RIG-I knockdown suppressed the induction in the cells transfected with poly IC/cationic lipid. Transfection of the cells with IFN-β siRNA markedly inhibited production of MDA5 and CXCL10 induced by poly IC treatment or poly IC/cationic lipid transfection. On the other hand, MDA5 was markedly induced by the transfection with an IFN-β expression plasmid. Thus, it is considered that newly synthesized IFN-β mediates poly IC-induced MDA5 expression (Figure 9.). Apart from anti-viral property, IFN-β has been reported to be involved in the pathogenesis of autoimmune diseases. IFN-β is an important mediator in virus-associated glomerulonephritis and immune complex-mediated glomerulonephritis exacerbated by viral infections [27]. In our previous studies, poly IC treatment of MCs induced the expression of IFN-β and de novo synthesized IFN-β mediated the expressions of RIG-I and ISG20 [16, 17]. In the present study, we observed that IFN-β is induced either by poly IC or a poly IC/cationic lipid complex, and *de novo* synthesized IFN-β may mediate the expression of MDA5 [8]. RIG-I is involved in IFN-β expression induced by poly IC/cationic lipid complex, but not in the MDA expression by IFN-β. CXCL10, a chemokine with chemotactic activity for the leukocytes with CXCR3, is involved in the pathogenesis of glomerular diseases. MDA5 is known to mediate CXCL10 induction in human bronchial epithelial cells infected with Rhinovirus [28]. We observed that MDA5 is involved in the poly IC-mediated expression of CXCL10 in MCs. Further, we found that the TLR3/IFN-β/MDA5/CXCL10 pathway activates by poly IC treatment, while RIG-I/IFN-β/MDA5/CXCL10 pathway activates by poly IC/cationic lipid complex treatment in anti-viral and inflammatory reactions in MCs.

Stored kidney specimens in good condition obtained from 6 cases (diffuse proliferative lupus nephritis, 2; proteinuric IgA nephropathy, 2; minimal change nephrotic syndrome, 1; nutcracker syndrome, 1) were used for immunefluorescent study of MDA5 and RIG-I expression. After blocking by incubation with 1% goat serum, the slides were incubated with an anti-MDA5 antibody (1:100) or an anti-RIG-I antibody (1:1000). Intense MDA5 immunoreactivity was detected in MCs of the specimens from diffuse proliferative lupus nephritis and proteinuric IgA nephropathy, while the expression in non-immune complex mediated renal diseases was undetectable. Interestingly, RIG-I immunoreactivity was only in diffuse proriferative lupus nephritis (Figure 10.) [8].

In human subjects, mesangial expressions of TLR3 and RIG-I have been reported in patients with lupus nephritis [13, 18]. In addition, we observed mesangial MDA5 immunoreactivity in biopsy specimens from patients with severe lupus nephritis and proteinuric IgA nephropathy while no MDA5 expression in patients with non-inflammatory renal diseases [8]. Interestingly, there was no mesangial expression of RIG-I in the specimens from patients with IgA nephropathy, despite of positive staining of MDA5. These observations suggest the expression of MDA5 in severe lupus nephritis is associated with the activation of signaling pathway via RIG-I, but MDA expression in IgA nephropathy is independent on RIG-I, although this theory remains speculative. Differential roles of MDA5 and RIG-I in severe lupus nephritis and protenuric IgA nephropathy may predict specific molecular mechanisms for these glomerulonephritis. This should be further investigated in future studies.

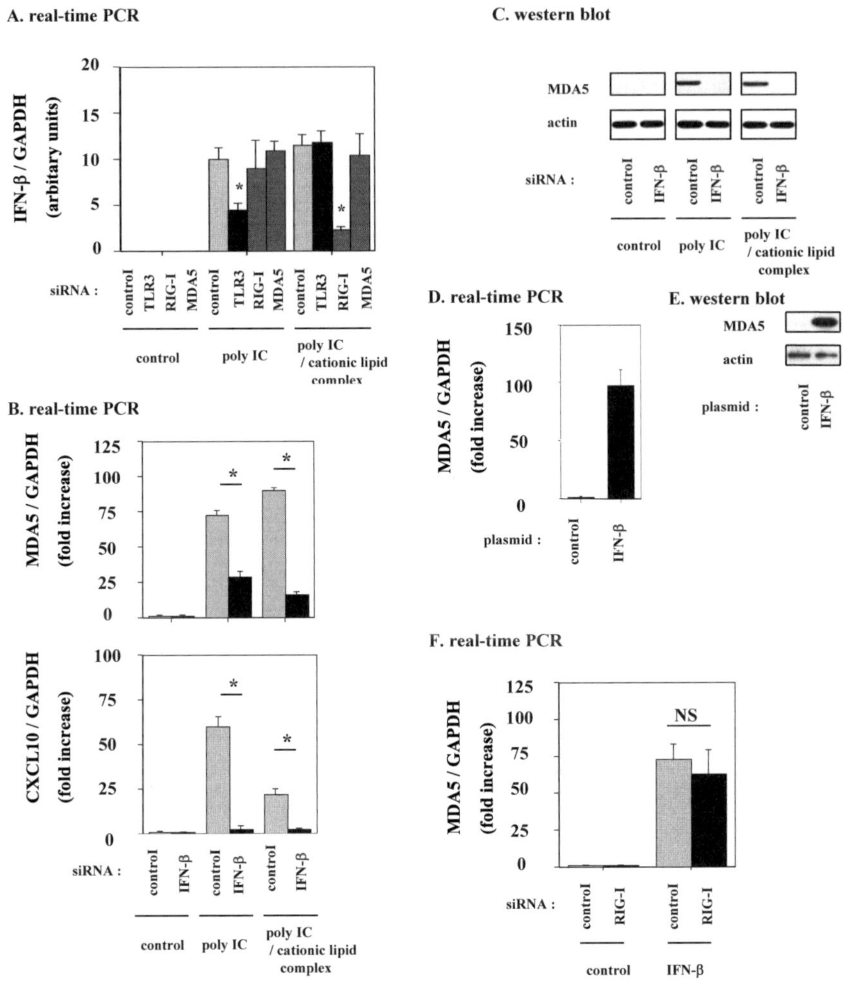

Figure 9. A. The cells were transfected with a non-silencing control siRNA, siRNA against TLR3, RIG-I or MDA5. After 24 h of transfection, the cells were treated or transfected with poly IC. RNA was extracted from cells after additional 4 h incubation, and the expression of IFN-β mRNA was examined using real-time PCR analysis (*p<0.01 vs. control, n=3). B and C. The cells were transfected with siRNA against IFN-β, and subsequently treated or transfected with poly IC. RNA was extracted after additional 16 h incubation, and real-time PCR analysis for MDA5 or CXCL10 was performed (*p<0.01, n=3). The cells were lysed after additional 24 h incubation, and lysates were subjected to western blot analysis for MDA5. The conditioned medium was collected, and the concentration of IFN-β was measured using an ELISA (*p<0.01, n=3). D and E. The cells were trenafected wit an expression plasmid for IFN-β and incubated for 24 h. Real-time PCR and western blot analysis for MDA5 were performed. F. The cells were transfected with siRNA aginst RIG-I.After 24 h incubation, the cells were treated with 10 ng/ml r(h) IFN-β for 8h. RNA was extracted from the cells and real-time PCR analysis for MDA5 was performed (Imaizumi et al. Tohoku J Exp Med 2012).

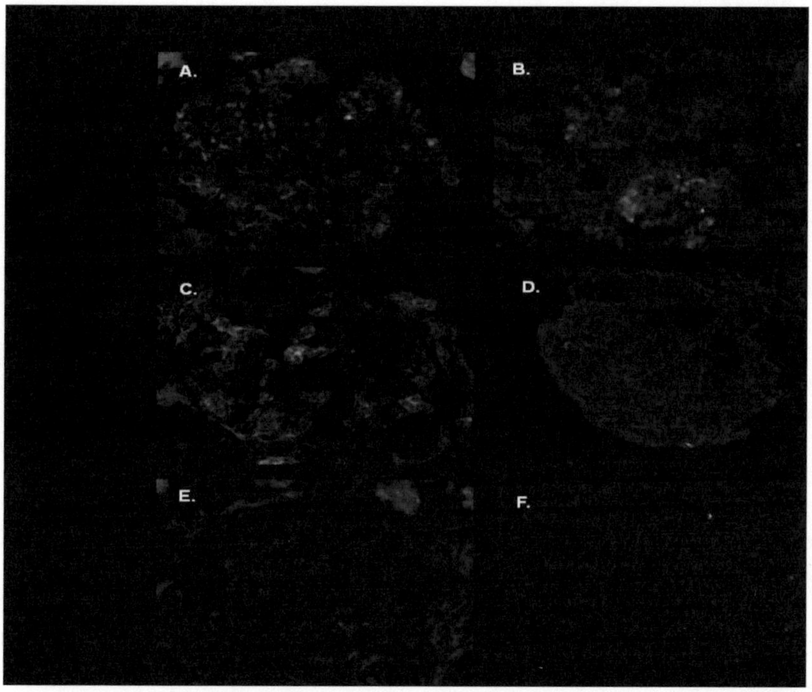

Figure 10. Intense MDA immunereactivity was detected in mesangial area of diffuse proliferative lupus nephritis (A) and proteinuric IgA nephropathty (C), but not in nutcracker syndrome (E). On the other hand, significant increase in the immunestaining intensity for RIG-I was observed only in severe lupus nephritis (B) (Imaizumi et al. Tohoku J Exp Med 2012).

6. Conclusion

We believe that involvement of the novel signaling pathways in MCs: the RIG-I-mediated IFN-γ/RIG-I/IRF7, TLR3/IFN-β/RIG-I/CCL5, RIG-I/IFN-β/MDA5/CXCL10 pathways, and the RIG-I-independent TLR3/IRF3/IFN-β/ISG20, and TLR3/IFN-β/MDA5/CXCL10 pathways may contribute to mesangial inflammation. Cross-talk of these signaling pathways may be involved in pathogenesis of human glomerulonephritis, and in the aggravation of glomerulonephritis due to viral infections. Although our findings remain preliminary, the intervention of these signaling pathways may lead to the development of future therapeutic strategies in the glomerular diseases. We found the involvement of novel RIG-I-mediated signaling pathways in mesangial inflammation in human MCs and there differences from TLR3 triggering, which addressed clinical significance.

Acknowledgements

These works were supported by grants-in-aid for Science from the Ministry of Education, Culture, Sports, Science and Technology of Japan, a grant from The Mother and Child Health Foundation (Osaka), and a grant from the Karoji Memorial Fund for Medical Research in Hirosaki University (Hirosaki). The Authors have no conflict of interest to declare.

Author details

Hiroshi Tanaka[1,2] and Tadaatsu Imaizumi[3]

*Address all correspondence to: hirotana@cc.hirosaki-u.ac.jp

1 Department of Pediatrics, Hirosaki University Hospital, Japan

2 Department of School Health Science, Faculty of Education Hirosaki University, Japan

3 Department of Vascular Biology, Graduate School of Medicine, Hirosaki University, Hirosaki, Japan

References

[1] Robson MG. Toll-like receptors and renal disease. Nephron Exp Nephrol 2009;113: e1-e7.

[2] Coppo R, Amore A, Peruzzi L, Vergano L, Camilla R. Innate immunity and IgA nephropathy. J Nephrol 2010; 23: 626-632.

[3] Patole PS, Pawar RD, Lech M, Zecher D, Schmidt H, Segerer S, Ellwart A, Henger A, Kretzler M, Anders HJ. Expression and regulation of Toll-like receptors in lupus-like immune complex glomerulomephritis of MRL-Fas (lpr) mice. Nephrol Dial Transplant 2006; 21: 3062-3073.

[4] Takeuchi O, Akira S. MDA5/RIG-I and virus recognition. Curr Opin Immunol 2008; 20: 17-22.

[5] Yoneyama M, Kikuchi M, Natsukawa T, Shinobu N, Imaizumi T, Miyagishi M, Taira K, Akira S, Fujita T. The RNA helicase RIG-I has an essential function in double-stranded RNA-induced innate antiviral responses. Nat Immunol 2004; 5: 730-737.

[6] Flur K, Allam R, Zecher D, et al. Viral RNA induces type I Interferon-dependent cytokine release and cell death in mesangial cells via melanoma-differentiation-associated gene-5. Implications for viral infection-associated glomerulonephritis. Am J Pathol 2009; 175: 2014-2022.

[7] Imaizumi T, Tanaka H, Uesato R, Tsugawa K, Matsumiya T, Yoshida H, Ishibashi Y, Satoh K. Involvement of retinoic acid-inducible gene-I (RIG-I) in rheumatoid arthritis and lupus nephritis. Hirosaki Med J 2011; 62 (Suppl.): S46-S49.

[8] Imaizumi T, Aizawa-Yashiro T, Tsuruga K, Tanaka H, Matsumiya T, Yoshida H, Tatsuta T, Xing F, Hayakari R, Satoh K. Melanoma differentiation-associated gene 5 regulates the expression of a chemokine CXCL10 in human mesangial cells: implications for chronic inflammatory renal diseases. Tohoku J Exp Med 2012; 228: 17-26.

[9] Wörnle M, Schmid H, Banas B, Merkle M, Henger A, Roeder M, Blattner S, Bock E, Kretzler M, Gröne HJ, Schlöndorff D. Novel role of Toll-like receptor 3 in hepatitis C-associated glomerulonephritis. Am J Pathol 2006; 168: 370-385.

[10] Lai AS, Lai KN. Viral nephropathy. Nat Clin Pract Nephrol 2006; 2: 254-262.

[11] Wörnle M, Roeder M, Sauter M, Riberio. Role of matrix metalloproteinases in viral-associated glomerulonephritis. Nephrol Dial Transplant 2009; 24: 1113-1121.

[12] Wörnle M, Roeder M, Sauter M, Merkle M, Ribeiro A. Effect of dsRNA on mesangial cell synthesis of plasminnogen activator inhibitor type 1 and tissue plasminogen activator. Nephron Exp Nephrol 2009; 113: e57-e65.

[13] Patole PS, Grone HJ, Segerer S, Ciubar R, Belemezova E, Henger A, Kretzier M, Schlöndorff D, Anders HJ. Viral double-stranded RNA aggravates lupus nephritis through Toll-like receptor 3 on glomerular mesangial cells and antigen-presenting cells. J Am Soc Nephrol 2005; 16: 1326-233.

[14] Hagele H, Allam R, Pawar RD, Anders HJ. Double-stranded RNA activates type I interferon secretion in glomerular endothelial cells via retinoic acid-inducible gene (RIG)- I. Nephrol Dial Transplant 2009; 24: 3312-3318.

[15] Imaizumi T, Tanaka H, Tajima A, Tsuruga K, Oki E, Sashinami H, Matsumiya T, Yoshida H, Inoue I, Ito E. Retinoic acid-inducible gene-I (RIG-I) is induced by IFN-γ in human mesangial cells in culture: possible involvement of RIG-I in the inflammation in lupus nephritis. Lupus 2010; 19: 830-836.

[16] Imaizumi T, Tanaka H, Matsumiya T, Yoshida H, Tanji K, Tsuruga K, Oki E, Aizawa-Yashiro T, Ito E, Satoh K. Retinoic acid-inducible gene-I is induced by double-stranded RNA and regulates the expression of CC chemokine ligand (CCL) 5 in human mesangial cells. Nephrol Dial Transplant 2010; 25: 3534-3539.

[17] Imaizumi T, Tanaka H, Mechti N, Matsumiya T, Yoshida H, Aizawa-Yashiro T, Tsuruga K, Hayakari R, Satoh K. Polyinosinic-polycytidylic acid induces the expression of interferon-stimulated gene 20 in mesangial cells. Nephron Exp Nephrol 2011; 119: e40-e48.

[18] Suzuki K, Imaizumi T, Tsugawa K, Ito E, Tanaka H. Expression of retinoic acid-inducible gene-I in lupus nephritis. Nephrol Dial Transplant 2007; 22: 2407-2409.

[19] Tsugawa K, Suzuki K, Oki E, Imaizumi T, Ito E, Tanaka H. Expression of mRNA for functional molecules in urinary sediment in glomerulonephritis. Pediatr Nephrol 2008; 23: 395-401.

[20] Honda K, Yanai H, Negishi H, Asagiri M, Sato M, Mizutani T, Shimada N, Oba Y, Takaoka A, Yoshida N, Taniguchi T. IRF-7 is the master regulator of type-I interferon-dependent immune responses. Nature 2005; 434: 772-777.

[21] Papadimitraki ED, Tzardi M, Bertsias G, Sotsiou E, Boumpas DT. Glomerular expression of toll-like receptor-9 in lupus nephritis but not in normal kidney: implications for the amplification of the inflammatory response. Lupus 2009; 18: 831-835.

[22] Tanaka H, Imaizumi T. Treatment of pediatric-onset lupus nephritis: New option of less cytotoxic immunosuppressive therapy. In: Hung FP. (ed.) Autoimmune Disorders: Current concepts & advances from bedside to mechanistic insights. Rijeka: InTech; 2011. p275- 288.

[23] Ikezumi Y, Kanno K, Koike H, Tomita M, Uchiyama M, Shimizu F, Kawachi H. FK506 ameliorate proteinuria and glomerular lesions induced by anti-Thy 1.1 monoclonal antibody 1-22-3. Kidney Int 2001; 61: 1339-1350.

[24] Allam R, Lichnekert J, Moll AG, Taubiz A, Vielhauer V, Anders HJ. Viral RNA and DNA trigger common antiviral responses in mesangial cells. J Am Soc Nephrol 2009; 20: 1986-1996.

[25] Degols G, Eldin P, Mechti N. ISG20, an actor of the innate immune response. Biochimie 2007; 89: 831-835.

[26] Nacionales DC, Kelly-Scumpia KM, Lee PY, Weinstein JS, Lyons R, Sobel E, Satoh M, Reeves WH. Deficiency of the type I interferon receptor protects mice from experimental lupus. Arthritis Rheum 2007; 56: 3770-3783.

[27] Anders HJ, Lichnekert J, Allam R. Interferon-α and $-\beta$ in kidney inflammation. Kidney Int 2010; 77: 848-854.

[28] Wang Q, Nagarkar DR, Bowman ER, Schneider D, Gosangi, Lei J, Zhao Y, McHenry CL, Burgens RV, Miller DJ, Sajjan U, Hershenson MB. Role of double stranded RNA pattern recognition receptors in Rhinovirus-induced airway epithelial cell responses. J Immunol 2009; 183: 6989-6997.

Chapter 4

Gene Expression Pattern Characterises Development of Multiple Sclerosis

Lotti Tajouri, Ekua W. Brenu, Kevin Ashton,
Donald R. Staines and Sonya M. Marshall-Gradisnik

Additional information is available at the end of the chapter

http://dx.doi.org/10.5772/53316

1. Introduction

Multiple sclerosis (MS) is a serious neurological disorder affecting young Caucasian individuals, usually with an age of onset at 18 to 40 years old. Females account for approximately 60% of MS cases and the manifestation and course of the disease is highly variable from patient to patient. The disorder is characterised by the development of plaques within the central nervous system (CNS). MS remains the most frequent cause of neurological disability, with the exception of trauma, for young adults. Investigations on twins show higher concordance rates of MS in monozygotic compared to dizygotic twins. In addition, familial susceptibility studies show that around 15% of MS patients have an affected relative. Familial risk for MS is thus very high compared to the lifetime prevalence in the general population of approximately 0.2%. Genome wide screens for MS have provided potential data for finding specific chromosomal loci involved in MS susceptibility. A series of whole genome screens for linkage to MS have been undertaken and resulted in the discovery of significant chromosomal susceptibility loci in the genome. These data have triggered a lot of interest in the regions found associated with MS and interestingly there are a number of genes that may plausibly be involved in the aetiology and pathophysiology of MS. These candidate genes have been implicated in a variety of approaches but usually involve immunological and/or genetic studies. One of the most consistent findings has been an association of specific major histocompatibility molecules which genes are located in the chromosome 6p21. However, other significant Non HLA regions pinpoint the involvement of several candidate genes that are currently under investigation at the sequencing and proteomic levels. Many gene expression studies have been undertaken to look at the specific patterns of gene transcript levels in MS. Human tissues and experimental mice were used in these gene-profiling studies and a very valuable and interesting set of data has resulted from these various expression studies. In general, genes showing variable expression include mainly immunological and inflammatory genes, stress and antioxidant genes, as well as metabolic and central nervous system markers. Of particular interest are a number of genes localised to susceptible loci previously shown to be in linkage with MS. However due to the clinical complexity of the disease, the heterogeneity of the tissues used in expression studies, as well as the variable DNA chips/membranes used for the gene profiling, it is difficult to interpret the available information. Although this information is essential for the understanding of the pathogenesis of MS, it is difficult to decipher and define the gene pathways involved in the disorder. Experiments in gene expression profiling in MS have been numerous and lists of candidates are now available for analysis. Researchers have investigated gene expression in peripheral mononuclear white blood cells (PBMCs), in MS animal models (EAE) and post mortem MS brain tissues. The genetic hallmarks of MS genetics, found to date, will be discussed in this chapter and particular conclusion on gene pathways and interactions proposed to possibly unravel the unknown aetiology of MS. Discussions on the effect of some MS medication and their effect in both cellular and molecular levels will be discussed.

2. MS genetics and overview

MS is a complex disease affecting the central CNS showing demyelinating nervous events due to an active autoimmune activity. Several patches of white matter degeneration are observed and are the results of multifocal entry of inflammatory immune cells in the CNS. These lesions scattered in the CNS vary in diameter and are most prominent within the periventricular myelin but can be present in various other parts of the CNS (Lumsden, 1970). The sclerotic appearance follows a classification where plaques are categorised as acute or chronic active, chronic silent plaques and importantly poor correlation is observed with the clinical classification of the disease. Clinical pathology is characterised by varying severity with MS being variable in onset and progression. These include Relapsing Remitting MS (RR-MS), Secondary Progressive MS (SP-MS) and Primary Progressive MS (PP-MS). While the lesions and symptoms are disseminated in time and space, the clinical classification of MS is mainly based on the occurrence of attacks, recovery states, and neurological deficits (Lumsden, 1970). Several concordance rate studies undertaken in twins showed a higher MS concordance in monozygotic, compared to dizygotic twins (Sadovnick et al., 1993) showing a clear involvement of genetics in MS. In addition, fifteen precents of MS patients have an affected relative that strengthen the genetic of MS. Interestingly, MS is more prevalent in women and accounts for more than two thirds of all MS sufferers (Weinshenker et al.,1994). Current and exponential knowledge in MS genetics enhances the clinical diagnosis for MS sufferers with the findings of genetic susceptibility loci and molecular markers. Some approaches have been and are currently investigated to generate new avenues to better diagnose MS, comprehend its pathophysiological cascades and importantly identify possible curative methods. Molecular genetic is one the scientific research area of choice to potentially unravel the yet unknown idiopathic disease. MS research investigations have concentrated efforts on gene expression profiling, determining DNA blue print, and comprehending the epigenetic in MS. All these efforts have provided an exciting opening of incoming transcriptomic, interactomic, epigenetic and proteomic discoveries all in relation to MS. Gene expression microarrays, Genome wide association studies, DNA methylation and miRNA profiling, copy number variation in MS that start to unravel specific loci in the genome, expression signatures and modulators of MS patho-physiology. Pro-inflammatory and anti-inflammatory take place in the pathophysiology of MS and include several cells of the immune system including the very important T regulatory T cells.

3. Immune tolerance disturbance in MS

Along with this immunosuppressive function, an important immune tolerance is known to take place. Immuno-tolerance characteristics, that directly have effects on pro-inflammatory cells, do rely on particular cells called T regulatory cells or Tregs (Kuniyasu et al., 2000). Tregs can be T4 lymphocytes or T8 lymphocytes, these cells are mostly immune-modulator actors particularly in inflamed regions. Such modulatory action is mediated interestingly by contact inhibition towards non Treg cells such as subsets of T4 and T8 lymphocytic cells. Specific markers are responsible are expressed to differentiate these subsets with regulatory or non-regulatory effective T-cell functionality (Teffs). Tregs CD25 markers denote CD4+ CD25+ and CD8+CD25+ cells as well as FoxP3+ marker, a repressor activator of activated T-cells found in CD4+CD25+FoxP3+ Treg cells or Cd8+ CD25+ CDFoxP3+ Treg cells. Other Treg marker can be encountered and include CXCR3+, a molecule present in CD8+ CXCR3+ Treg cells. The Treg functional role in restoring tolerance can be developed through different mechanisms. Tolerance could be undertaken by contact interaction such as Fas- Fas ligand interaction dictating an apoptotic faith to the Teff cells (Watanabe et al., 2002). In addition, Tregs installs tolerance on Teff cells by inhibiting Teff cytokine synthesis and subsequently Teff cytolytic activation is halted as well as Teff proliferation reduced (Duthoit et al., 2005). Teff cells can be either CD8+ or CD4+ cells with CD4+ classified as TH1 and TH2 types with both differing in action as pro-inflammatory and anti-inflammatory actions respectively. Briefly, the Th1 activation pathway is mediated by interferon γ on binding to interferon γ surface receptor on T cells with subsequent intracellular cascade activation. Such cascade leads to the activation of the transcription factor T-bet that ultimately binds DNA responsive elements of genes within the nucleus. The main responsive elements controlled and activated by T-bet are the interferon γ and IL-12 receptor $\beta 2$ chain genes. Upon activation, IL-12 receptor expression becomes widely available at higher amounts and the proteins co-locate in the cellular T-cell membrane surface. This receptor on the membrane becomes available for activation in the presence of local IL-12 cytokine. IL-12 receptor activation and expression induces an intracellular Stat 4 dependent cascade that enhances further the expression of the T-bet transcription factor. Relation between Tregs and pro-inflammatory TH1 and CD8+ T-cells demonstrate an interesting phenomenon that is built around the competition for Interleukin 2 binding. In sites of inflammation, binding of IL-2 by Tregs diminishes the availability of IL-2 to Teffs and therefore would limit their growth, function and even at early stage turning Teffs to become anergic towards antigens. Briefly, T-cells are activated through the physical contact of antigens with their T-cell receptor. The antigen is presented by antigen presenting cells under the restriction of MHC class molecules. Such binding activates p56lck tyrosine kinase with activation of downstream phosphorylation of proteins and activation of phospholipase C. Such phospholipase generates turns phosphatidyl inositol diphosphate into two compounds; the diacyl glycerol and inositol tri-phosphate, IP3. The endoplasmic reticulum IP3 receptor is therefore activated by IP3 and enables the release of calcium in the cytosol. Such Ca2++ induces a membrane activation of the cell membrane calcium release activated calcium channel named CRAC to subsequently increase highly the intracellular pool Ca2++ concentration. High levels of Ca2++ activate caclineurin, a phosphatase that dephosphorylates the transcriptional factor NFAT (nuclear factor of activated T-cells). Such dephosphorylated form of NFAT can translocate consequently into the nucleus to reach and bind responsive elements of Il-2, AP1 and NFKB genes. Beside the roles of Tregs as pro-apoptotic inducers of cytolytic Teff cells and inhibitors of Teff cells expansion, Tregs are also capable to modulate inflammation and modulate the pattern observed in inflammation sites. Inflammation modulation of Tregs is mediated by their capacities to synthesize and secrete both anti-inflammatory TGFβ and interleukin 10 molecules. In addition, Teffs in presence of TGFβ expresses an additional pool of Interleukin 10 which maintains a positive feedback as Il-10 action dictates Teffs to respond with much higher affinity to TGFβ. Interestingly, expression of the transcription factor Foxp3 in Tregs is also subject to TGFβ action (Pyzic et al., 2007. In multiple sclerosis, both Foxp3 and TGFβ have been found to be down regulated in expression (Huan et al., 2005 and Mirshafley et al., 2009)

4. Which gene expression microarrays started to enlighten gene expression in MS

4.1. Major post mortem brain tissue microarrays undertaken in MS

In 1999, the work of Whitney (Whitney et al., 1999) described the analysis of MS acute lesions from a single female MS patient with PP-MS. Patient's plaques and white matter were compared for gene expression and results showed 62 differentially expressed genes. The genes with increased expression in acute plaques included leukotriene A-4 hydroxylase, TNF α receptor, the auto-antigen annexin XI, interferon regulatory factor 2 (IRF-2), activin Type II receptor (ACVR2), protein kinase C type β-1 (PRKCB1), myelin transcription factor-1 (MYT1) and many several candidates. Two years later, Withney (Whitney et al., 2001) undertook microarray experiments using 2 MS patients. One patient's 16 chronic inactive (silent) plaques and the second patient's acute and chronic active plaque were used in the investigation. Gene expression analysis compared the levels of mRNA plaques and compared with control normal white matter RNA. Several gene candidates were found dysregulated in expression in these human tissues and validated in animal MS models. It included thrombin receptor, proteinase activated receptor 3 (PAR3) which is a gene previously found up-regulated in macrophages while in presence of granulocyte-macrophage colony-stimulating factor (GM-CSF) (Colognato et al., 2003). Jun-D and the putative ligand for the IL-1 receptor- related molecule (T1/ST2) were also found to be overexpressed in their animal studies. Interestingly, the arachidonate 5-lipoxygenase gene (5-LO) was found up-regulated in expression in MS. 5-LO is a gene coding for a key enzyme in the leucotriene pathway and responsible for the conversion of arachidonic acid to leukotriene A4 (LTA4). Interestingly their previous microarray study using human MS brain tissue (Whitney et al., 1999) showed an over-expression of leukotriene A4 hydrolase (LTA4H). The gene LTA4H is responsible for the conversion of LTA4 to LTB4. LTBA4 that acts on leukotriene B4 receptor 1 (BLTR), is a potent chemotaxic factor for neutrophils and induces leucocyte adhesion to endothelial cells (Yokomizo et al., 1997). These findings show clearly the importance of the leukotriene cascade in MS pathology. Genes involved in both the chemoattraction events and genes involved in the formation of the LTB4 chemoattractor molecule such as LTB4 omega hydroxylase or Cytochrome P450 family 4 subfamily F polypeptide 3 (LTBAH or CYP4F3) have also previously been studied. LTBA4H is a gene encoding two possible isoforms, CYP4F3A and CYP4F3B that aim at catabolising the effect of LTB4 action (Shak et al., 1984). Interestingly a study in 2009 (Parkinson et al., 2009) has shown that LTA4h is a marker in inflammatory perivascular cuffs and actively demyelinating plaques in relapsing-remitting and progressive human MS.

4.2. Discussion on key hallmark: Arachidonic pathway in MS

The over expression of prostaglandin D synthase interrogates once again about the important role that may play arachidonic acid related metabolites in MS neuroinflammation. Whitney et al. (Whitney et al., 1999 and 2001), showed the enzymatic involvement of the 5-lipoxygenase and leukotriene A4 hydrolase gene in the production of leucotriene pro-inflammatory molecules in MS disorder. In addition, Chabas (Chabas et al., 2001) showed that the second enzymatic pathway that metabolises acid arachidonic might also be playing a significant role in MS pathology. The cyclo-oxygenase pathway, with prostaglandin- endoperoxide synthase 1 and 2 (COX 1 and COX2), transforms arachidonic acid (AA) into prostaglandins (PGG2 series and PGH2 series). PGH2 is turned into PPD2 by prostaglandin D synthase, the enzyme that Chabas et al. found in high amounts in MS cDNA libraries (Chabas et al., 2001). The prostaglandins and leucotrienes are both pro-inflammatory molecules and might play a significant role in MS pathology. Ligand of the peroxisome proliferator activated receptor (PPAR gamma). PPAR gamma acts as an anti-inflammatory element and inhibits the pro-inflammatory IL12 cytokine. IL12p40 production correlates with disease activity and is found increased in expression in SP-MS individuals (Balashove et al, 1999; Soldan et al, 2004). However, research demonstrated that IL23 rather than IL12 plays a higher role in brain autoimmune inflammation (Cua et al., 2003). PPAR gamma was found with higher gene expression levels in EAE mice treated with Lovastatin drugs (Paintlia et al., 2004). Further evidence was implicating the cycloxygenase enzymatic pathway in which Lovastatin treated EAE mice showed reduced expression of the COX2 enzyme. Taken together, this suggests that the transformation of PGD2 into PGJ2 might play a potential role in MS. Enzymatically, PGD2 can be either transformed into PGJ2 or PGF2. Of note, the product of prostaglandin synthase (PFS), PGF2, was reported to be involved in acute demyelination of peripheral nerves (Hu et al., 2003).

The first MS gene expression study was investigated in 1997 by Becker (Becker et al., 1997). To undertake such investigating, a normalized cDNA library from CNS lesions of a PP-MS sufferer was studied. The most important finding was a set of 16 genes all involved in autoimmunity. Three of these genes coded for proteins previously implicated in MS and include MBP, PLP and α-β crystallin. Of note, seven of these 16 genes are autoantigens associated with systemic lupus erythematosus (SLE) and two are associated with insulin dependent diabetes mellitus (IDDM).

In 2001, Chabas's study (Chabas et al., 2001) was performed involving a high throughput sequencing of expressed sequence tags. The authors used non-normalised cDNA brain libraries from MS brain lesions and normal control brains. They identified 330 gene transcripts common for all libraries with several of these involved in inflammatory response. Genes that were found highly expressed included Prostaglandin D synthase (PTGDS), prostatic binding protein (PBP), ribosomal protein L17 (RPL17), osteopontin (SPP1), heat shock protein 70 (HSP70), myelin basic protein (MBP) and glial fibrillary acidic protein (GFAP). In Tajouri et al., 2003, over expression of HSP 70 within chronic active plaques was found. The inducible form of HSP 70 has been shown to promote myelin autoantigen presentation in APCs (Mycko et al., 2003). Of note, HSP 70 was though found to be down-regulated in other studies (Bomprezzi et al., 2003 and Lock et al., 2002).

Additionally, in Chabas (Chabas et al., 2001) decreased transcription levels were observed for synaptobrevin (VAMP3), amyloid beta precursor protein-binding, family B, member 1 (APBB1), LDL-receptor related protein (LRP1), glycogen synthase kinase 3 alpha (GSK3A), brain specific sodium-dependent inorganic phosphate co-transporter or solute carrier family 17 (SLC17A7). Chabas's team placed their attention on the increase of osteopontin transcripts in MS. A closer analysis of this candidate was performed on EAE mice. Interestingly, a knock out mouse for osteopontin showed in their study a decrease in EAE severity when compared to control mice. However, a comment made on Chabas's work has been raised (Blom et al., 2003) with the publication of an independent study using a knockout mouse for the osteopontin gene (OPN-/- 129/C57/BL10 with q haplotype: B10.Q usually susceptible to EAE). In Blom's study the gene OPN was solely and completely inactivated with the use of fully backcrossed mice. EAE mice were induced by injections of recombinant rat MOG myelin proteins emulsified in complete Freund adjuvant. The results from Blom et al. showed no decrease in severity of these EAE OPN-/- mice and such data were in direct contradiction with Chabas's findings. Blom hypothesized that the knock out mouse model used in Chabas's work could have knockout OPN-linked polymorphic genes and explain the decrease in EAE severity. The genes closely linked to OPN that have potential inflammatory functions were cited and accounted for 14 genes. This would include the IFN-gamma-inducible protein 10 (IP-10 or CXCL10) a chemo-attractant factor localised on chromosome 4q21.

4.3. Discussion on key hallmark: Chemokine IP-10 in MS

CXCL10 or IP-10 is a chemokine that preferentially attracts Th1 cells through its receptor CXCR3, expressed at high levels on these cells (Loetscher et al., 1996). IP-10 is induced in a variety of cells in response to the Th1 cytokine IFN-gamma (Luster et al., 1985). IP-10 expression is most often associated with Th1-type inflammatory diseases, where it is thought to play an important role in the recruitment of Th1 lymphocytes into tissues. Of note, Tajouri's work (Tajouri et al., 2003) showed that CXCL10 was over-expressed in chronic active plaques by a fold increase of 2.5 whereas this increase was more prominent in acute plaques in secondary progressive MS brains. Relapses in MS often are preceded by increased TH1 cytokine levels and decreased levels of TH2 cytokines. Remissions, on the other hand, exhibit a rise in the anti-inflammatory TH2 cytokines (Wingerchuk, et al., 1997 and Young et al., 1998). CXCL10 levels are related to clinical relapses in EAE (Fife et al., 2001 and Camody et al., 2002) and the source of production of CXCL10 is from astrocytes in EAE mice (Tani et al., 1996). Immuno-reactivity to CXCL10 was shown in demyelinating plaques (Huang et al., 2000). Also, this protein is found in higher levels within the CSF of MS patients compared to healthy controls (Franciotta et al., 2001) and such levels of expression correlate with the count of leucocytes in the CSF (Sorensen et al., 2002). Anti- CXCL10 reduces disease activity in common EAE (Fife et al., 2001). In viral model of MS (chronic demyelinating phase of mouse hepatitis virus infection of the CNS), mice showed a decrease severity of their pathology (Liu et al., 1997). CXCL10 acts on a receptor, the CXC chemokines Receptor 3 (CXCR3) that is localised genetically on chromosome X (Xq13). The gene for CXCR3 was localised on human chromosome Xq13 which is in clear contrast to all other chemokine receptor genes, suggesting unique function(s) for this receptor and its ligands that may lie beyond their established role in T cell-dependent immunity (Loetscheret al., 1996). CXCR3 is found over-expressed in macrophages, T cells and reactive astrocytes in MS plaques (Simpson et al., 2000). Perivascular cuffs in post mortem MS lesions showed CXCR3+ cells presence correlating with an increase of interferon gamma production (Balashov et al., 1999). Additional findings of elevated chemokine receptors CXCR3 has been reported in peripheral blood of progressive forms of MS (Vacknin- Dembinski et al, 2006). In 2002, Sorensen et al showed a continuous accumulation of CXCR3 +cells in lesion formation of MS patients (Sorensen et al., 2002). Targeting the CXCR3 receptor via antagonists could alter T-cell diapedesis through the CNS in MS (Ransohoff et al., 2000). Hong's study (Hong et al., 2004) demonstrated that treatment with Glatiramer acetate was significantly reducing the expression of CXCR3. In Tajouri's study (Tajouri et al., 2003), the author used RNA from MS chronic active and MS acute lesions. RNA was extracted, and compared with patient matched normal white matter by fluorescent cDNA microarray hybridisation analysis. This resulted in the identification of 139 genes that were differentially regulated in MS plaque tissue compared to normal tissue. Of these, 69 genes showed a common pattern of expression in the chronic active and acute plaque tissues investigated; while 70 transcripts were uniquely differentially expressed (>1.5-fold) in either acute or chronic active tissues. These results included known markers of MS such as the myelin basic protein (MBP) and glutathione S-transferase (GST) M1, nerve growth factors, such as nerve injury-induced protein 1 (NINJ1), X-ray and excision DNA repair factors (XRCC9 & ERCC5) and X-linked genes such as the ribosomal protein, RPS4X. Several genes were involved in inflammation including a number of leucocyte markers that are present in MS plaques. As an example, the gene granulin has been found to be slightly up-regulated compared to normal controls. Granulin is a novel class of growth regulators expressed by leucocytes (Bateman et al., 1993). This gene is normally not expressed in normal brains but in brain glial tumour cells (Liau et al., 2000) and located at 17q21.32, a region of suggestive linkage in MS pathology (GAMES and the Transatlantic Multiple Sclerosis Genetics Cooperative., 2003). In addition complement molecules or acute phase proteins such as Complement component 1, q subcomponent, beta polypeptide (C1QB) were found to be up-regulated in expression in the most inflammatory forms of plaque types, the acute plaques.

The expression of C1QB may originally come from blood vessel endothelial cells and could act detrimentally on the CNS with this complement inflammatory molecule (Klegeris et al., 2000). Interestingly, this inflammatory gene is involved in sporadic amyotrophic lateral sclerosis neuro-degeneration in which high levels of gene expression are found in post mortem tissues (Grewal et al., 1999). In parallel, anti-inflammatory proteins such as endothelial protein C receptor (PROCR) were found, in Tajouri et al., 2003 to be dramatically down-expressed in acute inflammatory plaques but this effect was less pronounced in chronic active plaques.

Lock's study (Lock et al., 2002) investigated the differences in gene expression between acute and chronic silent plaques from 4 MS individuals and found 1080 genes with a fold change of >2 in at least 2 out of 4 MS samples. Genes expressed in 4/4 MS samples were classified according to the type of lesion studied. Over-expressed genes included T- B and macrophage cell related genes, growth and endocrine factors, granulocyte and mast cell related genes as well as neurogenic and remyelinating factors. As an example, interleukin 17 (IL-17), transforming growth factor 3 (TGF- β 3), adrenocorticotropic hormone receptor (ACTHR), tryptase-III and immunoglobulin E receptor and matrix metalloproteinase 19 (MMP-19) were up-regulated in expression only in chronic silent plaques. In acute plaques, melanocortin- 4 receptor (MC4R), signal transducer and activator of transcription 5B (STAT5B), insulin like growth factor 1 or somatomedin C (IGF1), granulocyte colony stimulating hormone (G-CSF) and interferon, alpha-inducible protein (G1P2) transcripts were over represented. Of note, G-CSF was also found over-expressed in the acute phase of EAE animals (Camody et al., 2002). Of interest as well, some pregnancy related genes were differentially expressed such as an increased of expression of pregnancy-specific β1 glycoprotein (PSG3) in acute plaques, a decreased expression for PSG11 in chronic silent. In Tajouri study (Tajouri et al., 2003), the author experimented a dramatic increase of PSG3 occurs in acute plaques and interestingly this gene is genetically localised on 19q13.2, a promising MS linked susceptibility locus (Pericak-Vance et al., 2004). Of note, PSG molecules are actually co-expressed in the late stage of placenta formation with gut-enriched Kruppel-like zinc finger protein gene (GKLF4) (Blanchon et al., 2001). Of interest, GKLF4 is found prominently decreased in expression with interferon β therapy (Sturzebecher et al., 2003), a treatment of high efficacy in treating relapsing remitting MS (RR-MS) affecting mostly women.

The author Mycko (Mycko et al., 2003) established arrays to compare MS chronic active plaques and chronic inactive plaques. They investigated as well the differential gene expression in between the centre and the margin of such plaques. This resulted in the identification of very interesting features such as an increased level of expression of adenosine A1 receptor (ADORA1) in the marginal zone of the chronic active plaques. Studies on EAE animals depleted of the ADORA1 gene showed an increased severity of the disease course [66]. Consequently, ADORA1 may be involved in reducing the ongoing worsening effect of inflammation in MS lesions. The purine nucleoside adenosine inhibits IL-12 and this effect results in the increase of the Th2 type IL 10 mediator [19]. Additionally in Mycko's study (Mycko et al., 2003), an up regulation of expression was observed for the myelin transcription factor (MyT1) in the margins of chronic active lesions. Such MyT1 factor, precluding of ongoing attempts of remyelination in MS plaques, was previously identified as over-expressed in acute plaques in Whitney's study (Whitney et al., 1999). DNA repair related genes such as the X-ray repair complementing defective repair in Chinese hamster cells 9 (XRCC9) were also found up-regulated in the margins of chronic active and silent plaques. In our array data of this current thesis, XRCC9 gene was down regulated in MS acute and chronic active plaques.

The author Lindberg (Lindberg et al., 2004) used oligonucleotide DNA chips that included a total of 12 633 probes. Lindberg investigated the gene expression of MS lesions and NAWM (surrounding these lesions) that were extracted from SP-MS brain patients. Common immune responsive and neural homeostatic related genes were altered in expression. As an example, the neural development factor Ephrin receptor (EPBR), the cytoskeletal genes tubulin A and B and the pro-inflammatory interleukin 6 receptor were all increased in expression. The gene lysosome–associated membrane protein 2 (LAMP2), a neuro-lysosomal protector was down-expressed as well as synaptojanin 2b (SYNJ2), a gene involved in vesicle recycling.

5. Major peripheral blood mononuclear cell gene expression microarrays undertaken in MS

Peripheral blood cells (PBMC) from MS individuals have been used to extract mRNA and to investigate gene expression levels by microarray experiments. Bomprezzi et al., 2003 used a set of PBMC from fresh blood obtained from 14 MS patients and 7 controls but also frozen blood from 3 MS patients and 2 controls. A second set of cells was investigated and obtained from frozen blood of 10 MS patients and 10 controls. All of these patients were chosen under the condition of non-previous therapy. The differential gene expression from this study revealed 303 differentially expressed candidate genes. Among these, the platelet activating factor acetyl hydrolase (PAFAH1B1), a gene involved in brain development and chemo-attraction during inflammation and allergy, was found with an increased transcript expression in MS peripheral blood cells when compared to controls. Tumour necrosis factor receptor (TNFR or CD27) is found also highly regulated in these MS cells. This gene is a co-stimulator for T cell activation and is crucial for immune response development. The T cell receptor (TCR) gene was also found increased in expression as well as the zeta chain associated protein kinase (ZAP70). TCR is essential for T cell mediated immune response and has been implicated in MS susceptibility (Beall et al., 1993). ZAP70 is directly implicated in TCR induced T cell activation (Chan et al., 1992). Other candidates such as zinc protein 128 (ZNF128) and transcription factor 7 (TCF7) play a role in T cells and both were found at higher expression levels in MS blood cells. Cytokines are numerous and act on cytokine receptors during inflammation. The interleukin 7 receptor (IL7 R) is up-regulated in in Bomprezzi's study (Bomprezzi et al., 2003) as well as the myelin and lymphocyte protein (MAL). This receptor plays roles in B cells and T cells activation and particularly is involved in γδ T cells. γδ T cells are present in MS lesions and their inhibition decrease the severity of EAE mice and induced the reduction of pro-inflammatory cytokines and iNOS expression (Rajan et al,. 1996). The main down-regulated genes under expressed were tissue inhibitor of metalloproteinase 1 (TIMP1), plasminogen activator inhibitor 1 (SERPINE 1), the histone coding genes, and the heat shock protein 70 (HSP70), an auto-antigen implicated in the ubiquitin proteasome pathway for the degradation of cytokines.

A second study (Ramanathan et al., 2001) investigated RR-MS patients within their clinical remission to investigate around 15 thousand genes. The results have shown common differential gene expression implicated in TCR activation such as the cAMP responsive element modulator and lymphocyte specific protein tyrosine kinase (LCK), both found at a high level of expression. Interleukin receptor gene was also found up-regulated in MS blood compared to controls. Detoxification genes were increased in expression such as haemoglobin scavenger receptor (M130 or CD 163 antigen), as well as high expression levels of auto-antigens such as auto-antigen PM-SCL. Interestingly, a high level of gene transcripts was found for the melanocyte specific transporter protein gene (P protein) a gene involved in the oculocutaneous albinism disorder (Lee et al., 1994).

6. Treatment regimen and consequences in gene expression of MS patients

6.1. Common treatment available in MS

The existence of spontaneous remissions makes treatment difficult to evaluate. Several accepted regimes exist with indication being dependent upon the stage of the disease. Acute stages are treatable with oral prednisone, or dexamethasone until manifestation remit. Interferon β in high doses given every other day (subcutaneously) may reduce the frequency of neurological exacerbations in patients with RR-MS. The processes of demyelination and relapse are currently being treated with the drugs Avonex (interferon β-1a), Betaferon (interferon beta-1β), Copaxone (Glatiramer acetate, Co-polymer-1 or COP-1), Rebif (interferon β-1a), and Novantrone (chemotherapeutic agent) in the United States and United Kingdom. Of particular interest is the drug Copaxone. This drug is an oligopeptide (L-glutamic acid, L-alanine, L-tyrosine and L-lysine) leading to a diminution of exacerbation rates in RR-MS (Johnson et al., 1998) inhibiting the migration of lymphocytes (Prat et al., 1999) and inhibition of T cell activation (Miller et al., 1998). Copaxone was shown as well to act on T cells by increasing their secretion of neurotrophic factors such as the brain derived neurotrophic factor (BDNF) (Chen et al., 2003) with relevance to new research investigations for therapeutics (Ziemssen et al., 2003). Recent advances in the discovery of new treatments are encouraging. The classical immuno-modulator, β-interferon decreases the level of inflammation and has been shown to decrease the blood brain barrier monocyte infiltration within the CNS of MS animal models (Floris et al., 2002). However, patients on β-interferon therapy tend to produce neutralising antibodies against the drug, reducing overall beneficial effects of this type of therapy (Bertolotto et al., 2003). Furthermore, discontinuation of β-interferon treatment further increases antibody production and as a result leads to further reduction of interferon efficiency (Reske et al., 2004). Steroids are usually used in an attempt to reduce neutralising antibody production (Bagnato et al., 2003), however benefits of interferon therapy are now debatable following a recent study that showed no effect of interferon β in PP-MS (Leary et al., 2003). New therapeutic attempts are under investigation with the example of the use of pluripotent cells. Haematopoietic stem cell implantation in humans offers new hopes to patients with MS (Burt et al., 2003) and studies using neural precursor cells in EAE rat models published promising results with a decrease of disease severity and reduced CNS inflammation (Ben-Hur et al., 2003). Additionally, some other studies have also been carried out with the use of statins (3-hydroxy-3-methylglutaryl conenzyme A reductase inhibitors). As an example, results of a recent study showed a 43 % decrease in the mean number of MRI lesions using Simvastatin (Zocor drug) in 30 patients investigated with relapsing remitting MS (Vollmer et al., 2004). Patients with RR-MS currently follow the ABC therapy (Avonex, Betaseron and Copaxone) to minimise the neuro-inflammation course of the disease but presently, there is no curative therapy for MS. New drug discoveries show preliminary promising data and researchers are attempting to find new strategies to cure MS. With new trials under way and increasing research undertaken in MS, sufferers may hope for a normal life with newly developed drugs.

6.2. Major peripheral blood mononuclear cell gene expression microarrays undertaken in therapeutic treated MS patients

Other studies on PBMCs were undertaken but differential expression studies have focused on MS patients treated with particular therapeutics and comparison of their response was made against non treated controls. Interferon β therapy (Betaferon and Avonex drugs) in MS is effective due to its immunosuppression activity and was investigated in a few studies. The action of interferon beta is thought to play a role in decreasing the MHC class II molecules on the surface of glial cells (thus diminishing their capacity as antigen presenting cells) (Satoh et al., 1995. Also, interferon β is thought to decrease the disruption of the blood brain barrier (Young et al., 1998) and to shift a pro-inflammatory Th1 mediated immunity to Th2 immunity (Karp et al., 2000).

Koike et al., 2003 performed microarray experiments on T cells using 13 MS patients, before and after interferon β therapy. Data showed 21 differentially expressed genes after treatment with beta interferon and nine of these genes possess interferon responsive elements. Of particular interest, this study upon interferon beta treatment showed the down regulation of gene expression of tumour necrosis factor alpha induced protein 6 (TNFAIP6 or TSG-6). TSG-6 is a gene previously found implicated with murine experimental arthritis, another form of autoimmune disease (Bardos et al., 2001). An interesting conclusion held by the author is the exclusion of the hypothesis that interferon β treatment in MS actually shifts immunity from a Th1 to Th2 shift. This is in concordance with the work of Wandinger (Wandinger et al., 2001 and Sturzebecher et al., 2003). Sturzebecher investigated the gene expression profile of PBMCs ex vivo and in vitro from 10 RRMS patients with interferon therapy. The authors noted altered gene expression for interferon related genes such as an up-regulation of STAT1. Interestingly, they found the down regulation of IL 8 gene, a known chemo-attractant for neutrophils, but as well a down-regulation of a fair number of proliferative effectors. This anti-proliferative effect was evident especially via the down regulation of gene expression of FBJ murine osteosarcoma viral [v-fos] oncogene homolog (cFos), proto-oncogene cJun (c-Jun) and FMS-related tyrosine kinase 3 (Flt-3). The gut-enriched Kruppel-like zinc finger protein (GKLF4) was found prominently decreased in expression with interferon β therapy. This gene is thought to play a role in pregnancy specific glycoproteins (PSG) gene expression control since both GKLF4 and PSG molecules are co-expressed in the late stage of placenta formation (Blanchon et al., 2001). Of interest, studies on Pregnancy in Multiple Sclerosis (PRIMS) show that the third trimester of pregnancy is the subject of a marked reduction in relapse rate (Vukusic et al., 2004). Surprisingly, Sturzebecker reports an up-regulation of pro-inflammatory chemokines such as interferon-gamma-inducible protein 10 (IP-10 or CXCL10), monocyte chemo-attractant protein 1 (MCP1 or SCYA2 or CCL2) and karyopherin beta-2 (Mip1). Previous gene profiling studies by the same research team by Wandinger et al., 2001, has shown that pro-inflammatory factors such as interleukin 12 receptor β2 (IL12Rβ2) chain as well as chemokine, CC motif, receptor 5 (CCR5) were also up-regulated in expression in MS peripheral blood cells after interferon beta treatment. IL12 Rβ2 is also found by Hong et al. (Hong et al., 2004), to be significantly over-expressed with interferon β. Although, the inhibition of IL12R has been reported to be mediated by interleukin β induced interleukin 10 dependant activation pathway (Wang et al., 2000), such various findings show the eventual reason why some MS patients do fail to respond to interferon β treatment. The cytokine gene profiling results from Wandinger et al. [68] also rules out partially the hypothesis that interferon β therapy induces a Th1-Th2 shift in PBMC of MS patients. Such an idea is further supported by additional findings showing increased expression, after interferon β therapy, of other Th1 mediators such as Chemokine (C-C) receptor 5 (CCR5). CCR5 being the chemokine receptor for normal T-cell expressed and secreted (RANTES) and the two isoforms of the chemoattractor macrophage inflammatory protein 1 cited above (MIP1α and MIP1β). The gene CCR5 has already been found at high level of expression in acute phase of EAE animals and low in expression during the recovery phase of these animals Camody et al., 2002). CCR5 is found increased in expression on T cells in peripheral blood with this receptor only found up regulated in Progressive forms of MS and not in relapsing-remitting MS (Vaknin-Dembinsky et al, 2007) Interestingly, CCR5 is significantly down-expressed in MS with Glatiramer acetate drug treatment (Hong et al., 2004) and such a treatment could compensate for the interferon β inability to decrease CCR5. Of note, CCR5 is also down-regulated in expression with Lovastatin drug treatment in EAE mice (Paintlia et al., 2004) and seems to be a key factor in remission in EAE mice (Camody et al., 2002). Also, the up-regulation of some pro-inflammatory markers after interferon β therapy has been noted.

An interesting study by Der et al., 1998 performed oligonucleotide array experiments with untreated HT1080 cells and cells treated with interferon α-β or γ. The results attempted to identify levels of gene expression of interferon regulated and non-regulated genes. The interferon regulated genes such as interferon induced protein P78 (MxA) (MxA is homolog to Myxovirus influenza resistance 1: MX1) and the interferon-inducible protein p78, second locus (MxB, homolog MX2) showed an up-regulation of gene expression following interferon β treatment but were not differentially expressed with interferon β. Consequently, MxA and MxB over-expression with interferon β are in favour and support the findings of Wandinger et al [68]. Significant increase of expression of MxA was also found in MS peripheral blood cells after interferon β therapy [20]. However, in Wandinger et al., 2001 large multifunctional protease 2 (LMP2), with a role in antigen presentation and IL-15R α chain were found with high levels of transcripts after interferon β therapy. Additional microarray experiments examining interferon β-responsive transcripts in PBMC of MS patients, have shown that in Avonex-treated MS patients (with interferon β treatment), the gene LMP2 is inversely modulated compared to Avonex non treated MS patients [(Igelsias et al., 2004). Such high levels of LMP2 in both studies may not be due to the interferon β therapy by itself but simply due to the increase of interferon γ concentration along with interferon β therapy. Der's (Der et al., 1998) research has also shown that over representation of transcripts from LMP2 is dependent on interferon γ exclusively but not dependent on interferon β treatment. Interestingly, Wandinger et al., 2001 reports that IFN-γ gene expression is actually increasing transiently after two months of interferon β therapy during the course of MS pathology.

Hong et al., 2004, investigated PBMC from 18 MS patients treated with interferon β-1a and a group of 12 MS patients treated with Glatiramer acetate. Interferon related genes were differentially expressed with interferon β but also Th1 type molecules were increased in expression. Additionally, Glatiramer acetate treatment shows that some of these pro-inflammatory molecules were indeed down-expressed with this drug. Iglesisas et al., 2004 undertook a study investigating Avonex treatment. The methodology consisted in comparing peripheral blood cells from 5 RR-MS, treated with the drug, to 5 RR-MS without Avonex free. A second comparison was made against healthy blood donors. A set of 6800 genes was screened in this microarray experiment and data were focused mainly on the E2F pathway, a pathway of high interest in autoimmunity (Murga et al., 2001). This pathway is triggered by interleukin 2, a potent interleukin involved in maturation and activation of T cells. Briefly, IL2 acts on IL2 receptor leading to a phosphatidyl 3-kinase dependant intracellular cascade inducing subtypes of E2F proteins (E2F 1-3 are downstream activators; E2f 4-5 are repressors). E2F transcription factors bind to DNA and induce immune cell proliferation and S phase entry in the cell cycle. The listing of genes resulting from the microarray experiments in Iglesias et al., 2004 showed a common up-regulation of expression of histone genes in MS. Interestingly, the histone genes and Fas1, that are normally increased in MS pathology, and decreased in expression in the presence of the Avonex drug. Additionally, the gene GM-CSF receptor β chain (CSF2RB), E2F3 and histone H4/D (HIST1H4A), were increased in MS but were inversely modulated in PBMCs from Avonex-treated patients when compared to untreated MS patients. Of interest, the H4/D gene is localised at 6p21, a strong MS linked chromosomal locus. On the other hand the gene E2F2, found up-regulated in PBMC of MS patients, was not inversely modulated by the action of Avonex. Avonex appears to be inhibiting the E2F3 pathway and has a strong negative effect on the monocyte activation factor GM-CSF but no effect on the differentiation of thymocytes from precursor cells [absence of inverse modulation found for the gene thymopoeitin (TMPO)]. The author also found the down-regulation of expression in MS PBMC of the gene O-6-methylguanine-DNA methyltransferase (MGMT), a gene involved in DNA repair. DNA repair mechanism may interact directly with the E2F pathway (Ren et al., 2002). Of note, data from our array experiments showed two differentially genes expressed that relate to DNA repair mechanism, the base excision repair gene (UNG) and BRCA1-associated RING domain protein 1 (BARD1). These two genes are involved in the E2F pathway (Ren et al., 2002) and both were down-regulated with the UNG gene being down-regulated only in chronic active plaques and the BARD1 gene being down-expressed in both chronic active and acute plaques. Of note, BARD1 showed lower down expression in chronic active plaques than within acute plaques. Satoh et al., 2006 established the gene expression pattern using T cells and non T cells of Japanese MS individuals. Their result showed a down regulation of genes involved in DNA repair but as well a very abundant number of apoptotic genes. Such genes included the down regulation in MS of BCL2, TRAIL and DAXX and E2F5. In addition, they confirmed the up regulation of genes associated with inflammation such as IL1 receptor type 2, CXCL2 and ICAM1. In 2006, the same author Satoh (Satoh et al., 2006b) demonstrated the influence of interferon β therapy in MS. A particular gene CXCL9 was suppressed in long term treatment of interferon β in RRMS patients. Besides the findings of the common genes known to be differentially expressed in MS such as CXCl10 expression, Satoh demonstrated (Satoh et al., 2006b) again that pro-inflammatory chemokines are up-regulated following interferon β therapy. Such pro-inflammatory chemokines include CCR2 (monocytic) and CXCR3 (thymocytic).

7. Conclusions

Large power Microarray studies for gene expression in MS are undertaken with subcellular isolated immune cells and post-mortem brain tissues. This area of research is still revealing altered expression of candidate genes. A series of gene expression were studied to assess specific patterns of gene expression in MS patients and animal models. Data demonstrated a strong immunological and inflammatory gene involvement along with a number of stress and antioxidant related genes, metabolic and CNS markers. Particular interest is drawn on genes that are genetically located at MS susceptible loci, loci that were previously revealed by linkage and genome wide screen studies. Present research tends to replicate similar high throughput gene expression investigation but importantly the present investigations are using starting tissue material that presents both with higher quality & integrity. In addition, the research in MS gene expression is undertaken using homogenous cellular material where researchers carefully purify and isolate subpopulation of cells to undertake the gene expression profiling in post mortem brains and blood cells. Promising results are ahead of us; results that need to be replicated and emanating from large power studies with, in this case, the potential and probability to find new gene candidates and their pathways. Genome wide association studies are enhancing the findings but MS remains still unknown at this stage with a complex pathological mechanism that needs to be unravelled. Combination of GWAS data and Microarrays is with no doubt narrowing the list of key genes that are possibly part of the aetiology of MS and represents therefore an interesting and exciting time for MS research. Clustering analysis should aid in providing a means to classify candidates into global functional groups in the disease course. The large amount of data arising from all these studies is daunting but enhanced statistical analysis and storage of data is promising and would be fast rewarding to find new therapeutics. However, the gene expression experiments in MS brains should be carried out in more accessible and other types of tissue to gain a better picture of MS. Pharmacologically, gene profiling analysis has indicated that some pro-inflammatory molecules are drug resistant to interferon β therapy and seem indeed to be repressed by Lovastatin drug. Intensive investigation of each candidate gene and implicated pathways is the next step in MS research and will require further research at the proteomic level and increased new pharmaceutical trials. Of particular interest are a number of specific genes genetically localised at susceptible loci found to be in linkage with MS (largely reported in genome wide screen studies). However due to clinical complexity of the disease, the heterogeneity of the tissues used as well as the DNA chips/membranes used for the gene profiling, one is faced with a phenomenal load of differentially expressed genes. Although this information is essential for the understanding of the pathogenesis of MS, one must now depict and comprehend the gene pathways and interactome involved in the MS disorder.

Author details

Lotti Tajouri[1,2], Ekua W. Brenu[1,2], Kevin Ashton[1,2], Donald R. Staines[1,3] and Sonya M. Marshall-Gradisnik[4]

1 Faculty of Health Science and Medicine, Population Health and Neuroimmunology Unit, Bond University, Robina, Queensland, Australia

2 Faculty of Health Science and Medicine, Bond University, Robina, Queensland, Australia

3 Queensland Health, Gold Coast Population Health Unit, Southport, Queensland, Australia

4 Griffith University, Griffith Institute of Health and Medical Research, Southport, Queensland, Australia

References

[1] Bagnato F, Pozzilli C. Pharmacological methods to overcome IFN-beta antibody formation in the treatment of multiple sclerosis. Expert Opin Investig Drugs. 2003;12(7): 1153-63.

[2] Balashov, K.E., Rottman, J.B., Weiner, H.L., Hancock, W.W. CCR5(+) and CXCR3(+) T cells are increased in multiple sclerosis and their ligands MIP-1alpha and IP-10 are expressed in demyelinating brain lesions. Proc. Natl. Acad. Sci. U S A. 1999, 96(12) : 6873-8.

[3] Bardos, T., Kamath, R.V., Mikecz, K., Glant, T.T. Anti-inflammatory and chondroprotective effect of TSG-6 (tumour necrosis factor-alpha-stimulated gene-6) in murine models of experimental arthritis. Am. J. Pathol. 2001, 159(5): 1711-21.

[4] Bateman, A., Belcourt, D., Bennett, H., Lazure, C., Solomon, S. Granulins, a novel class of peptide from leukocytes. Biochem. Biophys. Res. Commun. 1990, 173(3) : 1161-8.

[5] Beall, S.S., Biddison, W.E., McFarlin, D.E., McFarland, H.F., Hood, L.E. Susceptibility for multiple sclerosis is determined, in part, by inheritance of a 175-kb region of the TcR V beta chain locus and HLA class II genes. J. Neuroimmunol. 1993, (1-2): 53-60.

[6] Becker, K.G., Mattson, D.H., Powers, J.M., Gado, A.M., Biddison, W.E. Analysis of a sequenced cDNA library from multiple sclerosis lesions. J. Neuroimmunol. 1997, 77(1): 27-38.

[7] Ben-Hur T, Einstein O, Mizrachi-Kol R, Ben-Menachem O, Reinhartz E, Karussis D, Abramsky O. Transplanted multipotential neural precursor cells migrate into the inflamed white matter in response to experimental autoimmune encephalomyelitis. Glia. 2003;41(1):73-80.

[8] Bertolotto A, Gilli F, Sala A, Capobianco M, Malucchi S, Milano E, Melis F, Marnetto F, Lindberg RL, Bottero R, A Di Sapio, MT Giordana, Persistent neutralizing antibodies abolish the interferon beta bioavailability in MS patients. Neurology. 2003;60(4): 634-9.

[9] Blanchon, L., Bocco, J.L., Gallot, D., Gachon, A.M., Lemery, D., Dechelotte, P., Dastugue, B., Sapin, V. Co-localization of KLF6 and KLF4 with pregnancy-specific glycoproteins during human placenta development. Mech. Dev. 2001, 105(1-2): 185-9.

[10] Blom, T., Franzen, A., Heinegard, D., Holmdahl, R. Comment on "The influence of the pro-inflammatory cytokine, osteopontin, on autoimmune demyelinating disease". Science 2003, 299(5614): 1845.

[11] Bomprezzi, R., Ringner, M., Kim, S, Bittner, M.L., Khan, J., Chen, Y., Elkahloun, A., Yu, A., Bielekova, B., Meltzer, P.S., Martin, R., McFarland, H.F., Trent, J.M. Gene expression profile in multiple sclerosis patients and healthy controls: identifying pathways relevant to disease. Hum. Mol. Genet. 2003, 12(17) : 2191-9.

[12] Bomprezzi, R., Ringner, M., Kim, S., Bittner, M.L., Khan, J., Chen, Y., Elkahloun, A., Yu, A., Bielekova, B., Meltzer, P.S., Martin, R., McFarland, H.F., Trent, J.M. Gene expression profile in multiple sclerosis patients and healthy controls: identifying pathways relevant to disease. Hum. Mol. Genet. 2003, 12(17): 2191-9.

[13] Burt RK, Cohen BA, Russell E, Spero K, Joshi A, Oyama Y, Karpus WJ, Luo K, Jovanovic B, Traynor A, Karlin K, Stefoski D, Burns WH. Hematopoietic stem cell transplantation for progressive multiple sclerosis: failure of a total body irradiation-based conditioning regimen to prevent disease progression in patients with high disability scores. Blood. 2003;102(7):2373-8.

[14] Carmody, R.J., Hilliard, B., Maguschak, K., Chodosh, L.A., Chen, Y.H. Genomic scale profiling of autoimmune inflammation in the central nervous system: the nervous response to inflammation. J. Neuroimmunol. 2002, 133(1-2): 95-107.

[15] Chabas, D., Baranzini, S.E., Mitchell, D., Bernard, C.C., Rittling, S.R., Denhardt, D.T., Sobel, R.A., Lock, C., Karpuj, M., Pedotti, R., Heller, R., Oksenberg, J.R., Steinman, L. The influence of the pro-inflammatory cytokine, osteopontin, on autoimmune demyelinating disease. Science 2001, 294(5547): 1731-5.

[16] Chan, A.C., Iwashima, M., Turck, C.W., Weiss, A. ZAP-70: a 70 kd protein-tyrosine kinase that associates with the TCR zeta chain. Cell. 1992, 71(4): 649-62.

[17] Chen M, Valenzuela RM, Dhib-Jalbut S. Glatiramer acetate-reactive T cells produce brain-derived neurotrophic factor. J Neurol Sci. 2003;215(1-2):37-44.

[18] Colognato, R., Slupsky, J.R., Jendrach, M., Burysek, L., Syrovets, T., Simmet, T. Differential expression and regulation of protease activated receptors in human peripheral monocytes and monocytederived antigen-presenting cells. Blood. 2003, 102(7): 2645-52.

[19] Cua DJ, Sherlock J, Chen Y, Murphy CA, Joyce B, Seymour B, et al. Interleukin-23 rather than interleukin-12 is the critical cytokine for autoimmune inflammation of the brain. Nature 2003;421:744.

[20] Der, S.D., Zhou, A., Williams, B.R.G., Silverman, R.H. Identification of genes differentially regulated by interferon , or using the oligonucleotide arrays. PNAS. 1998, 95: 15623-15628.

[21] Duthoit CT, Mekala DJ, Alli RS, Geiger TL. Uncoupling of IL-2 signaling from cell cycle progression in naïve CD4+ T cells by regulatory CD4+CD25+ T lymphocytes. J Immunol. 2005 Jan 1;174(1):155-63.

[22] Fife, B.T., Kennedy, K.J., Paniagua, M.C., Lukacs, N.W., Kunkel, S.L., Luster, A.D., Karpus, W.J. CXCL10 (IFN-gamma-inducible protein-10) control of encephalitogenic CD4+ T cell accumulation in the central nervous system during experimental autoimmune encephalomyelitis. J. Immunol. 2001, 166: 7617– 7624.

[23] Floris S, Ruuls SR, Wierinckx A, van der Pol SMA, Döpp E, van der Meide PH, Dijkstra CD, De Vries HE. Interferon-beta directly influences monocyte infiltration into the central nervous system. Journal of Neuroimmunology. 2002;127(1-2):69-79.

[24] Franciotta, D., Martino, G., Zardini, E., Furlan, R., Bergamaschi, R., Andreoni, L., Cosi, V. Serum and CSF levels of MCP-1 and IP- 10 in multiple sclerosis patients with

acute and stable disease and undergoing immunomodulatory therapies. J. Neuroimmunol. 2001, 115(1-2): 192–198.

[25] GAMES and the Transatlantic Multiple Sclerosis Genetics Cooperative. A meta-analysis of whole genome linkage screens in multiple sclerosis. J. Neuroimmunol. 2003, 143: 39– 46

[26] Grewal, R.P., Morgan, T.E., Finch, C.E. C1qB and clusterin mRNA increase in association with neurodegeneration in sporadic amyotrophic lateral sclerosis. Neurosci. Lett. 1999, 271(1): 65-7.

[27] Hong, J., Zang, Y.C., Hutton, G., Rivera, V.M., Zhang, J.Z. Gene expression profiling of relevant biomarkers for treatment evaluation in multiple sclerosis. J. Neuroimmunol. 2004, 152(1-2): 126- 39.

[28] Hu, W., Mathey, E., Hartung, H.P., Kieseier, B.C. Cyclooxygenases and prostaglandins in acute inflammatory demyelination of the peripheral nerve. Neurology 2003, 61(12): 1774-9.

[29] Huan J, Culbertson N, Spencer L, et al. Decreased FOXP3 levels in multiple sclerosis patients. J Neurosci Res 2005;81:45–52.

[30] Huang, D., Han, Y., Rani, M.R., Glabinski, A., Trebst, C., Sørensen, T., Tani, M., Wang, J., Chien, P., O'Bryan, S., Bielecki, B., Zhou, Z.L., Majumder, S., Ransohoff, R.M. Chemokines and chemokine receptors in inflammation of the nervous system: manifold roles and exquisite regulation. Immunol. Rev. 2000, 177: 52– 67.

[31] Iglesias, A.H., Camelo, S., Hwang, D., Villanueva, R., Stephanopoulos, G., Dangond, F. Microarray detection of E2F pathway activation and other targets in multiple sclerosis peripheral blood mononuclear cells. J. Neuroimmunol. 2004, 150(1-2): 163-77.

[32] Johnson KP, Brooks BR, Cohen JA, Ford CC, Goldstein J, Lisak RP, Myers LW, Panitch HS, Rose JW, Schiffer RB, Vollmer T, Weiner LP, Wolinsky JS. Extended use of glatiramer acetate (Copaxone) is well tolerated and maintains its clinical effect on multiple sclerosis relapse rate and degree of disability. Copolymer 1 Multiple Sclerosis Study Group. Neurology. 1998;50(3):701-8.

[33] Karp, C.L., Biron, C.A., Irani, D.N. Interferon beta in multiple sclerosis: is IL-12 suppression the key? Immunol. Today. 2000, 21(1): 24-8.

[34] Klegeris, A., Bissonnette, C.J., Dorovini-Zis, K., McGee,r P.L. Expression of complement messenger RNAs by human endothelial cells. Brain Res. 2000, 871(1): 1-6.

[35] Koike, F., Satoh, J., Miyake, S., Yamamoto, T., Kawai, M., Kikuchi, S., Nomura K., Yokoyama, K., Ota, K., Kanda, T., Fukazawa, T., Yamamura, T. Microarray analysis identifies interferon betaregulated genes in multiple sclerosis. J. Neuroimmunol. 2003, 139(1-2): 109 18.

[36] Kuniyasu Y, Takahashi T, Itoh M, Shimizu J, Toda G, Sakaguchi S. Naturally anergic and suppressive CD25(+)CD4(+) T cells as a functionally and phenotypically distinct immunoregulatory T cell subpopulation. Int Immunol. 2000;12(8):1145-55.

[37] Leary SM, Miller DH, Stevenson VL, Brex PA, Chard DT, Thompson AJ. Interferon beta-1a in primary progressive MS: an exploratory, randomized, controlled trial. Neurology. 2003;60(1):44-51.

[38] Lee, S.T., Nicholls, R.D., Schnur, R.E., Guida, L.C., Lu-Kuo, J., Spinner, N.B., Zackai, E.H., Spritz, R.A. Diverse mutations of the P gene among African-Americans with type II (tyrosinase-positive) oculocutaneous albinism (OCA2). Hum. Mol. Genet. 1994, 3(11) : 2047-51.

[39] Liau, L.M., Lallone, R.L., Seitz, R.S., Buznikov, A., Gregg, J.P., Kornblum, H.I., Nelson, S.F., Bronstein, J.M. Identification of a human glioma-associated growth factor gene, granulin, using differential immuno-absorption. Cancer Res. 2000, 60(5): 1353-60.

[40] Lindberg, R.L., De Groot, C.J., Certa, U., Ravid, R., Hoffmann, F., Kappos, L., Leppert, D. Multiple sclerosis as a generalized CNS disease comparative microarray analysis of normal appearing white matter and lesions in secondary progressive MS. J. Neuroimmunol. 2004, 152(1 2): 154-67.

[41] Liu, N., Lamerdin, J.E., Tucker, J.D., Zhou, Z.Q., Walter, C.A., Albala, J.S., Busch, D.B., Thompson, L.H. The human XRCC9 gene corrects chromosomal instability and mutagen sensitivities in CHO UV40 cells. Proc. Natl. Acad. Sci. USA 1997, 94(17): 9232- 7.

[42] Lock, C., Hermans, G., Pedotti, R., Brendolan, A., Schadt, E., Garren, H., Langer-Gould, A., Strober, S., Cannella, B., Allard, J., Klonowski, P., Austin, A., Lad, N., Kaminski, N., Galli, S.J., Oksenberg, J.R., Raine, C.S., Heller, R., Steinman, L. Genemicroarray analysis of multiple sclerosis lesions yields new targets validated in autoimmune encephalomyelitis. Nat. Med. 2002, 8(5): 500-8.

[43] Loetscher, M., Gerber, B., Loetscher, P., Jones, S.A., Piali, L., Clark-Lewis, I., Baggiolini, M., Moser, B. Chemokine receptor specific for IP10 and mig: structure, function, and expression in activated T-lymphocytes. J. Exp. Med. 1996, 184(3): 963-9.

[44] Loetscher, M., Loetscher, P., Brass, N., Meese, E., Moser, B. Lymphocyte- specific chemokine receptor CXCR3: regulation, chemokine binding and gene localization. Eur. J. Immunol. 1998, 28(11): 3696-705.

[45] Lumsden, C.E. The neropathology of multiple sclerosis. Handb. Clin. Neurol. 1970, 9: 217

[46] Luster, A.D., Unkeless, J.C., Ravetch, J.V. Gamma-interferon transcriptionally regulates an early-response gene containing homology to platelet proteins. Nature 1985, 315(6021): 672-6..

[47] Miller A, Shapiro S, Gershtein R, Kinarty A, Rawashdeh H, Honigman S, Lahat N. Treatment of multiple sclerosis with copolymer-1 (Copaxone): implicating mechanisms of Th1 to Th2/Th3 immune-deviation. J Neuroimmunol. 1998;92(1-2):113-21.

[48] Mirshafiey A, Mohsenzadegan M.TGF-β as a promising option in the treatment of multiple sclerosis Neuropharmacology. 2009;56(6–7):929–936

[49] Murga, M., Fernandez-Capetillo, O., Field, S.J., Moreno, B., Borlado, L.R., Fujiwara, Y., Balomenos, D., Vicario, A., Carrera, A.C., Orkin, S.H., Greenberg, M.E., Zubiaga, A.M. Mutation of E2F2 in mice causes enhanced T lymphocyte proliferation, leading to the development of autoimmunity. Immunity 2001, 15(6): 959-70.

[50] Mycko, M.P., Cwiklinska, H., Szymanski, J., Szymanska, B., Kudla, G., Kilianek, L., Odyniec, A., Brosnan, C.F., Selmaj, K.W. Inducible heat shock protein 70 promotes myelin autoantigen presentation by the HLA class II. J. Immunol. 2004, 172(1):202-13.

[51] Mycko, M.P., Papoian, R., Boschert, U., Raine, C.S., Selmaj, K.W. cDNA microarray analysis in multiple sclerosis lesions: detection of genes associated with disease activity. Brain 2003, 126(Pt 5): 1048-57.

[52] Paintlia, A.S., Paintlia, M.K., Singh, A.K., Stanislaus, R., Gilg, A.G., Barbosa, E., Singh, I. Regulation of gene expression associated with acute experimental autoimmune encephalomyelitis by Lovastatin. J. Neurosci. Res. 2004, 77(1): 63-81.

[53] Parkinson JF, Guilford WJ, Mendoza LM, Rosser M, Post J, Schaefe C, Halks-Miller M, Kirkland T, Cleve A, Lassmann H and Reder AT. New Roles for LTA4 Hydrolase, LTB4 and BLT1 in Multiple Sclerosis and Experimental Allergic Encephalomyelitis. The Journal of Immunology, 2009, 182, 48.9

[54] Pericak-Vance, M.A., Rimmler, J.B., Haines, J.L., Garcia, M.E., Oksenberg, J.R., Barcellos, L.F., Lincoln, R., Hauser, S.L., Cournu-Rebeix, I., Azoulay-Cayla, A., Lyon-Caen, O., Fontaine, B., Duhamel, E., Coppin, H., Brassat, D., Roth, M.P., Clanet, M., Alizadeh, M., Yaouanq, J., Quelvennec, E., Semana, G., Edan, G., Babron, M.C., Genin, E., Clerget-Darpoux, F. Investigation of seven proposed regions of linkage in multiple sclerosis: an American and French collaborative study. Neurogenetics 2004, 5(1): 45-8.

[55] Prat A, Al-Asmi A, Duquette P, Antel JP. Lymphocyte migration and multiple sclerosis: relation with disease course and therapy. Ann Neurol. 1999;46(2):253-6.

[56] Pyzik M, Piccirillo CA. TGF-beta1 modulates Foxp3 expression and regulatory activity in distinct CD4+ T cell subsets. J Leukoc Biol. 2007; 82(2):335-46.

[57] Rajan, A.J., Gao, Y.L., Raine, C.S., Brosnan, C.F. A pathogenic role for gamma delta T cells in relapsing-remitting experimental allergic encephalomyelitis in the SJL mouse. J. Immunol. 1996, 157(2): 941-9.

[58] Ramanathan, M., Weinstock-Guttman, B., Nguyen, L.T., Badgett, D., Miller, C., Patrick, K., Brownscheidle, C., Jacobs, L. In vivo gene expression revealed by cDNA ar-

rays: the pattern in relapsingremitting multiple sclerosis patients compared with normal subjects. J. Neuroimmunol. 2001, 116(2): 213-9.

[59] Ransohoff, R.M., Bacon, K.B. Chemokine receptor antagonism as a new therapy for multiple sclerosis. Expert Opin. Investig. Drugs. 2000, 9: 1079– 1097.

[60] Ren, B., Cam, H., Takahashi, Y., Volkert, T., Terragni, J., Young, R.A., Dynlacht, B.D. E2F integrates cell cycle progression with DNA repair, replication, and G(2)/M checkpoints. Genes Dev. 2002, 16(2): 245-56.

[61] Reske D, Walser A, Haupt WF, Petereit HF. Long-term persisting interferon beta-1b neutralizing antibodies after discontinuation of treatment. Acta Neurol Scand. 2004;109(1):66-70.

[62] Sadovnick, A.D., Armstrong, H., Rice, G.P., Bulman, D., Hashimoto, L., Paty, D.W., Hashimoto, S.A., Warren, S., Hader, W., Murray, T.J. A population-based study of multiple sclerosis in twins: update. Ann. Neurol. 1993 , 33: 281-285.

[63] Satoh, J., Nakanishi, M., Koike, F., Miyake, S., Yamamoto, T., Kawai, M., Kikuchi, S., Nomura, K., Yokoyama, K., Ota, K., Kanda, T., Fukazawa, T., Yamamura, T. Microarray analysis identifies an aberrant expression of apoptosis and DNA damageregulatory genes in multiple sclerosis. Neurobiol. Dis. 2005, 18(3): 537-50.

[64] Satoh, J., Nakanishi, M., Koike, F., Onoue, H., Aranami, T., Yamamoto, T., Kawai, M., Kikuchi, S., Nomura, K., Yokoyama, K., Ota, K., Saito, T., Ohta, M., Miyake, S., Kanda, T., Fukazawa, T., Yamamura, T. T cell gene expression profiling identifies distinct subgroups of Japanese multiple sclerosis patients. J. Neuroimmunol. 2006, 174(1-2): 108-18.

[65] Satoh, J., Paty, D.W., Kim, S.U. Differential effects of beta and gamma interferons on expression of major histocompatibility complex antigens and intercellular adhesion molecule-1 in cultured fetal human astrocytes. Neurology 1995, 45(2): 367-73.

[66] Satoh, J., Nanri, Y., Tabunoki, H., Yamamura, T. Microarray analysis identifies a set of CXCR3 and CCR2 ligand chemokines as early IFNbeta-responsive genes in peripheral blood lymphocytes in vitro: an implication for IFNbeta-related adverse effects in multiple sclerosis. BMC Neurol. 2006b, 6: 18.

[67] Shak, S., Goldstein, I.M. Omega-oxidation is the major pathway for the catabolism of leucotriene B4 in human polymorphonuclear leukocytes. J. Biol. Chem. 1984, 259(16): 10181-7.

[68] Simpson, J.E., Newcombe, J., Cuzner, M.L., Woodroofe, M.N. Expression of the interferon-gamma-inducible chemokines IP-10 and Mig and their receptor, CXCR3, in multiple sclerosis lesions. Neuropathol. Appl. Neurobiol. 2000, 26(2): 133-42.

[69] Soldan SS, Alvarez Retuerto AI, Sicotte NL, Voskuhl RR. Dysregulation of IL-10 and IL-12p40 in secondary progressive multiple sclerosis. J Neuroimmunol 2004;146:209.

[70] Sorensen, T.L., Trebst, C., Kivisakk, P., Klaege, K.L., Majmudar, A., Ravid. Multiple sclerosis: a study of CXCL10 and CXCR3 colocalization in the inflamed central nervous system. J. Neuroimmunol. 2002, 127: 59-68.

[71] Sturzebecher, S., Wandinger, K.P., Rosenwald, A., Sathyamoorthy, M., Tzou, A., Mattar, P., Frank, J.A., Staudt, L., Martin, R., McFarland, H.F. Expression profiling identifies responder and nonresponder phenotypes to interferon-beta in multiple sclerosis. Brain 2003, 126(Pt 6): 1419-29.

[72] Tajouri, L., Mellick, A.S., Ashton, K.J., Tannenberg, A.E., Nagra, R.M., Tourtellotte, W.W., Griffiths, L.R. Quantitative and qualitative changes in gene expression patterns characterize the activity of plaques in multiple sclerosis. Brain Res. Mol. Brain Res. 2003, 119(2): 170-83.

[73] Tani, M., Glabinski, A.R., Tuohy, V.K., Stoler, M.H., Estes, M.L., Ransohoff, R.M. In situ hybridization analysis of glial fibrillary acidic protein mRNA reveals evidence of biphasic astrocyte activation during acute experimental autoimmune encephalomyelitis. Am. J. Pathol. 1996, 148: 889– 896

[74] Vaknin-Dembinsky A, Balashov K, Weiner HL. IL-23 is increased in dendritic cells in multiple sclerosis and down-regulation of IL-23 by antisense oligos increases dendritic cell IL-10 production. J Immunol 2006;176:7768.

[75] Vollmer T, Key L, Durkalski V, Tyor W, Corboy J, Markovic-Plese S, Preiningerova J, Rizzo M, Singh I. Oral simvastatin treatment in relapsing-remitting multiple sclerosis. Lancet. 2004;363(9421):1607-8.

[76] Vukusic, S., Hutchinson, M., Hours, M., Moreau, T., Cortinovis- Tourniaire, P., Adeleine, P., Confavreux, C. The Pregnancy In Multiple Sclerosis Group; Pregnancy In Multiple Sclerosis Group. Pregnancy and multiple sclerosis (the PRIMS study): clinical predictors of post partum relapse. Brain 2004, 127(Pt 6): 1353-60.

[77] Wandinger, K.P., Sturzebecher, C.S., Bielekova, B., Detore, G., Rosenwald, A., Staudt, L.M., McFarland, H.F., Martin, R. Complex immunomodulatory effects of interferon-beta in multiple sclerosis include the upregulation of T helper 1-associated marker genes. Ann.Neurol. 2001, 50(3): 349-57.

[78] Wang, X., Chen, M., Wandinger, K.P., Williams, G., Dhib-Jalbut, S. IFN-beta-1b inhibits IL-12 production in peripheral blood mononuclear cells in an IL-10-dependent mechanism: relevance to IFN-beta-1b therapeutic effects in multiple sclerosis. J. Immunol. 2000, 165(1): 548-57.

[79] Watanabe T, Yoshida M, Shirai Y, Yamori M, Yagita H, Itoh T, Chiba T, Kita T, Wakatsuki Y. Administration of an antigen at a high dose generates regulatory CD4+ T cells expressing CD95 ligand and secreting IL-4 in the liver. J Immunol. 2002;168(5): 2188-99.

[80] Weinshenker, B.G. Natural history of multiple sclerosis. Ann. Neurol. 1994, 36: S6-11.

[81] Whitney, L.W., Becker, K.G., Tresser, N.J., Caballero-Ramos, C.I., Munson, P.J., Prabhu, V.V., Trent, J.M., McFarland, H.F., Biddison, W.E. Analysis of gene expression in mutiple sclerosis lesions using cDNA microarrays. Ann. Neurol. 1999, 46(3): 425-8.

[82] Whitney, L.W., Ludwin, S.K., McFarland, H.F., Biddison, W.E. Microarray analysis of gene expression in multiple sclerosis and EAE identifies 5-lipoxygenase as a component of inflammatory lesions. J. Neuroimmunol. 2001, 121(1-2):40-8.

[83] Wingerchuk, D., Liu, Q., Sobell, J., Sommer, S., Weinshenker, B.G. A population-based case-control study of the tumour necrosis factor alpha-308 polymorphism in multiple sclerosis. Neurology 1997, 49(2): 626-8.

[84] Yokomizo, T., Izumi, T., Chang, K., Takuwa, Y., Shimizu, T. A Gprotein- coupled receptor for leucotriene B4 that mediates chemotaxis. Nature 1997, 387(6633): 620-4.

[85] Young, V.W., Chabot, S., Stuve, O., Williams, G. Interferon beta in the treatment of multiple sclerosis: mechanisms of action.Neurology 1998 , 51: 682-689.

[86] Ziemssen T, Kumpfel T, Klinkert WE, Neuhaus O, Hohlfeld R. Glatiramer acetate-specific T-helper 1- and 2-type cell lines produce BDNF: implications for multiple sclerosis therapy. Brain-derived neurotrophic factor. Brain. 2002;125(Pt 11):2381-91.

Chapter 5

Costimulatory Molecules in Rheumatic Diseases Revisited with an Emphasis on Their Roles in Autoimmune Sjögren's Syndrome

Adrienne E. Gauna and Seunghee Cha

Additional information is available at the end of the chapter

http://dx.doi.org/10.5772/54480

1. Introduction

Sjögren's syndrome (SjS) is a chronic, inflammatory autoimmune disorder characterized by dry mouth and dry eyes, in which lymphocytic infiltration (primarily CD4 T-cells) of the salivary and lacrimal glands destroy their secretion abilities. Since abnormal activation of T-cells are a key feature of SjS, as well as for other autoimmune conditions, defining the processes for T-cell activation and inhibition are important for understanding SjS autoimmune pathogenesis.

The molecules CD80 (B7.1) and CD86 (B7.2), here forth collectively referred to as B7, are critical costimulatory ligands during the process of antigen presentation because of their abilities to support T-cell receptor (TCR)-mediated responses through their binding to and activation of CD28 receptors on T-cells. Binding of either of these B7 ligands to cytotoxic T-Lymphocyte Antigen 4 (CTLA-4, CD152) counter receptor are crucial for attenuating T-cell responses. Additionally, these processes of activation and inhibition have been shown to be modulated in part by regulatory T (Treg) cells, which are a naturally occurring cell population capable of directly suppressing effector T (Teff) cells activation and proliferation, especially to self-antigens.

In autoimmune diseases, dysfunction of Treg cells is a potential contributor to disease development, where costimulatory requirements for Treg cell proliferation and suppression capabilities may not be met. It is possible that the relative contribution of CD86/CD80 and CD28/CTLA-4 signals to Treg and Teff cells could dictate the potency of suppression and phenotypes of cells. This is important in understanding autoimmune diseases where abnormal expression of CD86 and CD80 is seen in the target tissue sites and dysregulation of specific Treg populations may contribute to development of autoimmune disorders.

Elucidating biological function and mechanisms of action of the CD86/CD80:CD28/CTLA-4 molecules have been the focus of much research over the past several decades since their seminal discoveries in the early 1990s. However, there are still many questions as to how these molecules interact to form specific immune responses in vivo, especially in the field of autoimmunity. In this book chapter, we will describe potential processes for T-cell activation and inhibition and investigate the contribution of abnormal costimulatory/inhibitory signals from CD80/CD86 to the establishment of autoimmune disorders, such as SjS.

2. Overview of costimulatory molecules for T-cell activation and inhibition

Much of the difficulties in achieving a cohesive understanding of the CD86/CD80:CD28/CTLA-4 system stem from various complexities, such as, cell type-specific expression (including varying protein levels and kinetics of expression) and assorted ligand:receptor interactions that contribute to the overall immune phenotype. In this section, we will focus on the expression, interactions, and overall function of these receptors and ligands, especially related to Treg cell activation and suppression function.

2.1. Expression of CD86/CD80:CD28/CTLA-4

The CD28 and CTLA-4 receptors are members of the CD28 family of immunoglobulin-like glycoproteins that are genetically linked on human chromosome 2 and mouse chromosome 1, although they each have distinct patterns of cell surface expression. CD28 is well known to be constitutively present at the surface of all T-cells (CD4 and CD8), where its surface levels are further increased to maximal by 24 hours following TCR activation. CTLA-4 on the other hand is found predominantly located in intracellular vesicles. CTLA-4 is well known to be rapidly removed from the cell surface by clatherin adaptor complex AP-2-mediated endocytosis, such that only a small fraction of CTLA-4 is present on the cell surface under steady-state conditions [1-5]. Following TCR activation CTLA-4 still retains its endocytosis capabilities [6] and yet, its surface concentration is quickly increased by 48 hours after T-cell activation. Delivery of CTLA-4 receptor to the immune synapse has also been shown to be associated with the strength of TCR signaling [7]; indicating that T-cells with higher affinity TCRs are potentially more likely to be attenuated by CTLA-4 receptor activation.

The two known CD28 and CTLA-4 ligands, CD86 and CD80, are members of the B7 family of immunoglobulin-like proteins expressed on a variety of antigen presenting cell (APC) types including dendritic cells (DCs), macrophages, and B-cells [8, 9]. Similar to the CD28 family, the B7 family of ligands appears to derive from gene duplication events, where they are genetically linked on human chromosome 3 and mouse chromosome 16, although, they too have very distinct patterns of expression from each other. CD86 is most commonly constitutively expressed on the surface of professional antigen presenting cells (APCs) or cells such as monocytes [8-10]. On these cell types CD86 is generally more abundantly expressed than CD80. CD86 is rapidly upregulated and maximally expressed by 48 hours in response to its interaction with CD28 receptor or other inflammatory stimuli [9, 11, 12]. Typically, CD80 is not constitutively present on unactivated cells. Following initiation of CD28 or inflammatory stimulation the expression of CD80 is produced at a much slower rate [9]. Interestingly, immature DCs (and Langerhans cells) show evidence that CD80 is the predominantly expressed ligand compared to CD86 [13-15]. These findings are indicative of a predominant role for CD80 in immature or regulatory cells [16-18].

2.2. Relative interaction properties of CD86/CD80:CD28/CTLA-4

The CD28/CTLA-4 receptors and the CD86/CD80 ligands function as multi-subunit proteins comprising of identical protein subunits that provide unique ligand:receptor interactions. CD28 is well known as a homodimer. However, this homodimer configuration only possesses a single ligand binding site, in stark contrast to CTLA-4 homodimer, which is shown to possess two ligand binding sites [19, 20]. Regarding the ligands themselves, CD80 exists as a weak noncovalently bound homodimer based on analytical ultracentrifugation and crystal structure of CD80 [21]. This same dimeric conformation was also observed following crystallization of CD80 complexed with CTLA-4 [20, 21] and photo-bleaching FRET confirmed that CD80 exists predominantly as a dimer on the surface of APCs [22]. On the other hand, CD86 primarily exists as a monomer as detected by analytical ultracentrifugation and gel filtration studies [23]. The crystal structure analysis of CD86 also revealed poor dimer interface [21], but interestingly, crystallization of CD86 complex with CTLA-4 indicates that it can potentially form a dimer as well as crosslink CTLA-4 receptors [24]. Again, crystallization of CD86 without CTLA-4 or in solution indicates that CD86 is unlikely to form stable dimers [19, 23]. Findings based on photo-bleaching FRET also confirmed that CD86 exists as a monomer on the cell surface [22], where CD86 tends to have a faster association and dissociation rate than CD80 to either receptors [25]. The issue for potential receptor mediated dimerization of CD86 is currently unresolved. These findings altogether suggest that CD28 is restricted to having one ligand binding partner, whereas, CTLA-4 is potentially capable of crosslinking linking a single ligand, probably CD80, and forming complex network of interactions receptor:ligand interactions.

Along these similar lines, actual affinity of CTLA-4 for the B7 ligands is much higher than with CD28. However, the differences between CD80 and CD86 binding to T-cell receptors are less remarkable. Relative interaction properties of these molecules indicate preferential interaction between CD80 and CTLA-4, whereas CD86 more biased towards CD28 [19, 20]. CD80 binds CTLA-4 with a modest 10-fold higher affinity than does CD86 ligand [19]. As such, all other things being equal, when CD86 is expressed on APCs, then CD28 is more favored interaction than CTLA-4 at the T-cell:APC interface. Thus, the activation signals elicited by CD86:CD28 are less likely to be attenuated by coincident CTLA-4 ligation and enhancing the costimulatory effects [19]. Actual preferences of each B7 molecule with CD28 and CTLA-4 were tested in APCs deficient in either CD86 or CD80, where relative sequestration of CD28 and CTLA-4 in the immunological synapse was evaluated. Results from this study do indicate that CD80 does preferentially bind to CTLA-4 and CD86 shows better interaction with CD28 on the cell surface [26].

2.3. Functions of CD86/CD80:CD28/CTLA-4

As mentioned previously, the receptors CD28 and CTLA-4 are members of the CD28 family of immunoglobulin-like glycoproteins expressed on both CD4+ and CD8+ T-cells. These receptors share the same B7 ligands; however, they have opposing functions on T-cells. CD28 receptor activation supplies additional signals to support TCR-mediated responses, such as, T-cell proliferation, cytokine production, cell survival, and promotes T-cell help to B cells [1, 27-29]. As expected, CD28 deficient mice have impaired T-cell activation in response to antigen [30], as well as, defective B cell responses [29, 31]. These additional costimulatory signals provided by CD28 have been suggested to function to decrease the threshold for T-cell activation, thereby, reducing the contact time with APC required for T-cell activation [32, 33]. CTLA-4 receptor activation provides signals to effectively attenuate T-cell responses. The inhibitory function of CTLA-4 was first described from CTLA-4 deficient mice that exhibit a fatal CD4+ T-cell hyperproliferation and multi-organ infiltration [34-36]. These abnormally activated T-cells are potentially reactive to multiple self-antigens despite apparently normal thymic selection [37]. These T-cells are primarily mediated through activation of CD28, since mice deficient in both CTLA-4 and B7 do not develop disease [38, 39] and where a specific mutation in CD28 prevents disease induction [40]. CTLA-4 has now been better established in its role in the suppressive function of Treg cells [41-44]. The mechanisms by which CTLA-4 in Treg cells directly suppresses immune responses includes the delivery of negative signal towards inhibition of Teff cell proliferation and activation [45, 46], as well as, through the removal of B7 molecules from the surface of the APCs [47]. However, there is also the potential for CTLA-4 competition with CD28 for ligands that could contribute to suppression functions as well. Altogether, CTLA-4 has a major role in modulating CD28-mediated activation.

The differences in CD80 and CD86 function in regards to T-cell activation and inhibition are not so well appreciated. There is still a general perception that CD80 and CD86 are interchangeable costimulators with differences only in kinetics of expression and cell type distribution. Despite the obvious overlapping functions, these B7 molecules do show evidence of distinct biological effects, predominantly with CD80 having more inhibitory roles and effects on Treg cells. A classic example of this phenomenon is in the non-obese diabetic (NOD) mouse model. In this model, blockade of CD80 by monoclonal antibodies (MAbs) exacerbates disease, while blockade of CD86 prevents disease [48]. It is possible that with blocking of CD86, the available CD80 could have enhanced interactions and would thus be free to interact with CTLA-4, thus attenuating T-cell activation. Blocking of CD80 would potentially free CD86 to interact with CD28 making it more likely to provide help activate self-reactive T-cells. Since NOD Tregs appear more dependent on CD80 for their maintenance, these self-reactive T-cells may not be attenuated as well [49].

A more recent regulatory function has also been found for CD80, where CD80 acts as an alternate ligand for programmed death ligand 1 (PD-L1, B7H1, CD274) [50]. PD-L1 is well known to induce inhibitory signals in T-cells and to inhibit T cell proliferation. The affinity of CD80 for PD-L1 is intermediate between its affinity for CD28 and CTLA-4, yet still three-fold less than the affinity of PD-L1 for PD-1 [50]. The function of this CD80:PD-L1 interaction in immune responses was shown in vivo where this pathway was shown to prevent alloimmune responses and where these tolerogenic effects were mediated by the interactions of PD-L1 on APCs eliciting an inhibitory signal through CD80 expressed on T-cells [51]. Specific blockade of this CD80/PD-L1 interaction indicates that the inhibitory signal from CD80 but not PD-L1 is responsible for attenuation of T-cell expansion and enhancement of T-cell anergy. Blocking of this interaction specifically led to enhanced expansion and restored antigen responsiveness in previously anergized T-cells [52].

2.3.1. *Regulatory T cells*

There are several lines of evidence suggesting that the expression of CD80 and CD86 ligands by APCs are important in maintaining Treg cell homeostasis and suppressive function in the periphery. B7 blockade experiments have indicated that continual expression of B7 in the periphery is necessary to maintain the Treg compartment as indicated by the reduced CD25 expression following blockade [53]. Additionally, blocking antibodies to B7 also was capable of inhibiting the natural turnover of adoptively transferred Treg cells in vivo [54].

The relative contribution of CD86 and CD80 to Treg cell responses is more difficult to describe because of their overlapping functions, however, definite differences have been indicated. The relative expression levels of CD86 and CD80 on DCs are well known to be modulated during the progression from immature to mature state. For example, DCs expressing high levels of CD86, makes them particularly proficient at driving Treg cell proliferation [55], where CD86 was shown to be more important than CD80 in this regard [56]. These findings are all consistent with CD86 being a better ligand for CD28 in the face of CTLA-4 expression and potentially better at stimulating Treg proliferation in these settings. CD80 appears to contribute more to the inhibitory functions of Treg cells through its involvement with CTLA-4. For example, in the presence of antibodies to either CD80 or CTLA-4, Treg suppression abilities were impaired when the CD25- responder T cells are not exposed to the blocking antibodies [56]. Evidence also suggests that Teff cells from B7-deficient mice are resistant to suppression by wild type Tregs, where CD80 on Teff cells was largely shown to be the dominant ligand for mediating suppression capabilities of Treg cells [57]. This effect is potentially mediated by a CD80 cell-intrinsic negative signal into Teff cells that helps facilitate suppression. The receptor for B7 that mediated this effect was not identified, but due to the requirement for Treg cells it appears to be mediated by CTLA-4 [57].The transfection of either CD80 or CD86 into Chinese hamster ovary cells (CHO), indicate CD80 could direct CTLA-4-mediated inhibition of resting human T cells through the activities of CD25+CTLA-4+ Treg cells [43]. Additional to the effects of CD80 through CTLA-4, suppressive functions of CD80 have shown that the PD-L1/CD80 pathway also leads to promotion of the in vivo expansion of donor natural Tregs in allogeneic recipients [58]. The proposed mechanism of action is that IFN-gamma upregulates tissue expression of the PD-L1 on APCs and parenchymal cells. Expression of PD-L1 on those cells in normal tissues is thought to be capable of interacting with CD80 expressed on Treg cells, promoting development and maintenance of Treg cells [58].

Therefore, it is possible that under a steady state condition, low CD80 and PD-L1 expressed by immature DCs preferentially interacts with CTLA-4 and CD80 predominantly expressed by Treg cells, thus, promoting Treg function and maintenance. However, specific mechanisms of controlling Treg cell maintenance and suppression functions through these signaling molecules are still areas requiring exploring. Following inflammatory stimuli and DC maturation, where there is a relative upregulation of CD86 compared to CD80 along with higher levels of antigenic stimulation, Treg suppressive capacity should become reduced. This is supported by the finding that CD28 and TCR stimulation could antagonize suppressive function of Treg cells [43, 59]. Therefore, CD80 and CD86 may have somewhat opposing roles in aiding suppressive capacity through CTLA-4 vs. activation of T-cells cells through CD28, where their relative expression could influence this balance (Figure 1).

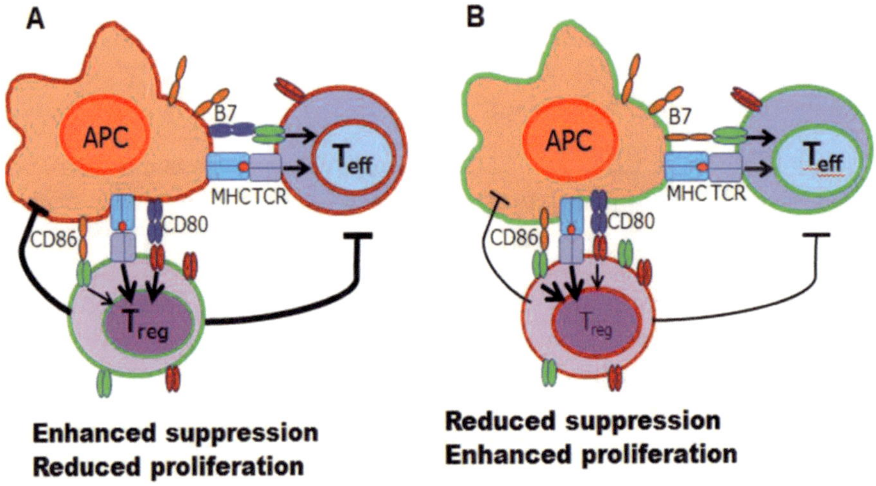

Figure 1. Mechanism by which Treg cells balance responses to B7 ligand stimulation. (A) Relatively high expression of CD80 on APC favours enhancing suppressive function of Treg cell and inhibits T-cell proliferation. (B) Increase in CD86 following activation of APC favours inhibition of Treg cells and enhances T-cell proliferation. Specific signalling requirements of Treg activation and inactivation are still to be determined.

3. Impact of CD86/CD80 molecules in autoimmune disease

The relative contribution of CD86 and CD80 to the development of autoimmunity is difficult to evaluate because of the diverse cells and interactions involved in disease pathogenesis. However, interesting trends have appeared where alterations in relative expression of CD86 and CD80 in the target tissues and alterations in Treg numbers and function may contribute to the onset of autoimmune diseases. In this section we will review some information on the rheumatic autoimmune diseases systemic lupus erythematosus and rheumatoid arthritis as well as cover important findings regarding autoimmune diabetes. The major focus of this section will be on elucidating the pathogenesis of Sjögren's syndrome as it is related to target tissue expression of B7 molecules and role of Treg cells in these tissues.

3.1. Systemic lupus erythematosus

Systemic lupus erythematosus (SLE) is a chronic multi-organ autoimmune disease distinguish by imbalanced T-cell homeostasis towards activated Teff cell subsets Th1 and Th2 and can affect multiple organs and systems of the body. It is well characterized by the number and variety of autoantibodies produced and is well marked by anti-nuclear antibody production. Many of the symptoms are caused by impaired antigen-antibody complex clearance and thus triggering inflammatory responses in multiple sites. Because of the difficulty in evaluating patient disease progression several mouse models have been used to evaluate how abnormal costimulation and Treg cells contribute to disease. The autoimmune BXD2 mice indicates that type I IFN can promote autoimmune responses through the upregulation of CD86high expression on marginal zone precursor B-cells, which were shown to be located at the T-B-cell border of the spleen germinal centers [60]. In regards to Treg maintenance, the (NZB x NZW)F1 and (SWR/NZB)F1 lupus-prone mice had reduced numbers of CD4+CD25+ cells [61]. There was no intrinsic defect in the suppressive function of the (NZB x NZW) F1 mice [62]. Additionally, only marginal defects in Treg suppression were observed in MRL/Mp mice [63]. MRL/lpr mice with strong lupus disease were found to have normal percentages of peripheral CD4+CD25high T-cells and that Foxp3 expression was unaltered. However, they do display a reduced capacity to suppress and effector CD4+CD25- T-cells were significantly less susceptible to suppression. Importantly they also found that CD80/CD86 were under-expressed on Teff, APCs, and on Treg cells, suggesting that the reduction in these molecules could be contributing to the reduced abilities of Treg cells to suppress [64].

3.2. Rheumatoid arthritis

Rheumatoid Arthritis (RA) is a chronic inflammatory disease characterized by inflammation of the joints and surrounding tissue including mononuclear cell infiltration of synovial tissue. Predominant lymphocytes present in rheumatoid synovium focal infiltrates are lymphocytes (predominantly CD4+ T-cells with relatively few positive for CD25), macrophages, and plasma B cells. The expression of CD86 was readily detectable in the synovium compared to osteoarthritis synovial [65]. In contrast, CD80 expression was not significantly expressed in the synovium [65]. Overall, the expression of CD80 on APCs in the synovium is generally low, while expression of CD86 is relatively high and is expressed on several APCs including DCs, B-cells, and macrophages [66-70]. Blocking of CD28 signaling pathway has also been shown to prevent or even treat autoimmune disease [71], indicating that CD28 is probably a regulator in the induction of autoimmune diseases. For instance, CD28 deficient mice are resistant to collagen induced arthritis [72] and inhibition of both CD80 and CD86 during the induction phase of collagen induced arthritis prevents the development of disease [71, 73, 74]. Arthritis is also abolished and autoantibody production is suppressed in MLR/lpr mice lacking CD28, however, the accumulation of abnormal T cells is almost unchanged [75]. Indicating CD28 may have a better role in aiding B cell responses in this model. Most importantly, treatment with blocking CTLA-4-Ig also significantly improved signs and symptoms and Treg function of RA patients in clinical trials [76]. In general, Treg cells with diminished suppressive capacity were obtained from synovial fluid of patients with RA [77, 78]. Functional studies of Treg cell defects in mice related to RA indicate that defects in CD4+Foxp3+ Treg cells in K/BxNsf mice exhibited earlier onset and more aggressive progression of arthritis than K/BxN littermates [79]. This was accompanied by plasmacytoid dendritic cells expressing high levels of CD86 and CD40, but not CD80, in synovia and increase memory CD4+ T-cells in the spleen and draining lymph nodes [79]. These mice also exhibit an abnormal accumulation of mature plasma cells in spleen and associated loss of bone marrow plasma cells. These plasma cells were also less susceptible to cell death [80]. Overall, it appears the function of CD28 to the pathogenesis of RA, potentially mediated through over expression of CD86 appears to have a major function in disease pathogenesis.

3.3. Autoimmune diabetes

B7 molecules have potential influence on autoreactive T cells in animals genetically predisposed to autoimmune disease. Adoptive transfer of NOD B-cells previously blocked with B7 MAbs along with diabetogenic T-cells into NOD.scid mice protected associated type 1 diabetes [81].Again, as mentioned previously NOD mice treated with blocking CD86 MAbs prevents the spontaneous development of diabetes, whereas blocking CD80 accelerates and worsened disease [48]. Treatment of NOD mice older than 10 weeks of age with blocking CD86 MAbs did not alter the course of disease [48]. These results indicate that in the NOD background, the influence of CD86 to promotion and CD80 to suppression of disease occurs early on in disease pathogenesis. Breeding of CD86 deficiency onto NOD background prevented the development of diabetes, as expected from previous studies. However, aging mice around age 20 weeks would develop a peripheral neuropathy characterized by demyelization and defective nerve function due to mononuclear cell infiltration of peripheral nerves [82]. This was accompanied by a high level of CD80 expression on the APCs in the spleen as well as on the nerves of affected animals [82]. This is similar to reports seen in Experimental Autoimmune Epithelitis (EAE) and Multiple Sclerosis (MS) patients [83, 84], where downregulation of CD86 and upregulation of CD80 is observed on CNS-infiltrating cells and splenocytes. These somewhat conflicting findings for autoimmune diseases can potentially be explained by differences in interplay of local cellular interactions, cytokines and chemokines that may alter B7 expression. In this case, high expression of CD80 could potentially allow activation of CD28 signaling and autoimmune activation rather than suppression.

There is still some debate on whether Treg cells contribute to autoimmunity with regards to their deficits and functionality in autoimmune diabetes. Treg depletion or B7-deficiency (significant loss in CD4+CD25+ cell population) in NOD mice leads to accelerated disease onset

[53, 54]. The importance of Treg number to quality of suppression was shown with polyclonal Treg adoptive transfer to NOD.scid at a 2:1 ratio (Treg:Th1) was unable to suppress, while 5:1 ratio was able to provide protection in approximately half of the recipients. Therefore, with sufficiently large populations of Tregs, there may be adequate numbers of antigen-specific Tregs capable of suppressing diabetes [85]. It is interesting to note that Treg cells developed in vitro from induced GAD-IgG transduced splenocytes were capable of suppressing diabetes in NOD mice. This was accompanied by a higher ratio of CD80 compared to CD86 expression in splenocytes, which was sufficient to allow development of functional Treg cells (Foxp3+) in this model [86-88]. Depletion of CD4+CD25+ cells from transduced splenocytes transferred into NOD mice showed increased ratio of CD86 to CD80 in splenocytes. Blocking of CD80, but not CD86, reduced the relative quantity of Foxp3 [87]. Along these lines, a progressive decrease was observed in the Treg cell:Teff cell ratio in inflamed islets but not in pancreatic lymph nodes in NOD mice. Intra-islet Treg cells expressed reduced amounts of CD25 and Bcl-2, where the administration of low-dose interleukin-2 (IL-2) promoted Treg cell survival and protected mice from developing diabetes. Together, these results suggest intra-islet Treg cell dysfunction is a root cause of the progressive breakdown of self-tolerance and the development of diabetes in nonobese diabetic mice [89]. However, there is still some debate on whether NOD mouse Treg cells are sufficient in regulating Teff, since Tregs from NOD and B6g7 mice were equally effective but NOD T conventional cells were hyper-responsive to stimulation [90].

3.4. Sjögren's syndrome

Recently in SjS, as with some of the other autoimmune diseases previously mentioned, the emphasis of pathogenicity has been placed on CD86 expression in the salivary gland environment. Expression of CD86 and CD80 in SjS patient salivary gland tissue compared to patients with nonspecific sialadenitis was first described in 1999, where expression of both ligands were found in ductal and acinar regions of immunohistochemically stained tissue sections [91]. It was recently shown that the functional expression of CD86 on salivary gland epithelial cells derived from SjS patients are capable of interacting with CD28, but its binding to CTLA-4 was reduced [92]. Therefore, salivary epithelial cells are possibly functioning to promote production of IL-2 and T-cell proliferation. This paper also indicates that expression of CD80, contrary to other immunohistochemistry results suggesting that CD80 is expressed [93],[94], could not be established in their salivary gland epithelial cells. It is difficult to establish the relative expression of these molecules in vivo, since several other studies were conducted on cell lines derived from patient biopsies under cytokine stimulating conditions or from immunohistochemistry of tissue sections using BB1 antibody, which potentially shares reactivity with non-B7 proteins such as MHC class II invariant chain [92, 95]. Further studies may be required to verify the production of CD80 as well as the relative expression of each of these ligands in the salivary glands of patients and healthy controls.

However, in C57BL/6 (B6) mice the overall expression of B7 is relatively low (CD86 greater than CD80) in normal mouse submandibular salivary glands compared to lymphoid tissues and is located predominantly along the ducts and among acini as previously indicated in human patients (data unpublished, [96]). Presumably, these cells are salivary gland epithelial cells, where the expression of low level costimulatory ligands is presumed normal and possibly protective. As for mouse models for SjS, retinoblastoma-associated protein 48 (RbAp48) transgenic mice, using a salivary gland specific promoter [97], resulted in the development of SjS-like symptoms. In salivary gland tissues of these mice the protein expression of MHC class II, CD86, CD80, and ICAM-1 were all upregulated in affected mice salivary glands. Where the expression levels of CD86 is higher than CD80 in the SMX, indicating a potential pathogenic role of CD86 to disease initiation [96]. Another mouse model of SjS, the C57BL/6.NOD-*Aec1Aec2* is a double congenic mouse model of primary SjS syndrome that contains two genetic regions (Idd3 and Idd5) derived from the NOD mouse model [98]. These genetic regions confer spontaneous development of SjS-like syndrome on the B6 background. A recent study using this model highlighted the importance of local B7 molecules and signaling through CD28 to disease progression [99]. In this report AAV transduced expression of the CTLA-4-Ig (blocks B7 molecules interactions) in the salivary glands of SjS-prone mouse model. Delivery of this gene construct via AAV prior to disease onset prevented glandular damage and lymphocytic cell infiltration commonly associated with disease, as well as, prevented loss of saliva secretion in the treated mice [99]. This was also accompanied by a significant increase in transforming growth factor beta-1 (TGF-B1) in the salivary glands and draining lymph nodes of these mice [99]. These results suggest a potential regulatory role (either Treg or epithelial cells) involved with treatment of CTLA-4-Ig. Authors of this paper did not explore the mechanisms of action of this molecule. Along similar lines, another study involving treatment of blocking CD86 MAbs to another mouse model of primary SjS, the NFS/sld 3-day thymectomized mutant, was shown to prevent the autoimmune lesions and autoantibody production to a-fodrin [100]. Along with previous lines of research indicating a negative regulatory role of CD80, no significant effects were seen in mice treated with anti-CD80 MAbs [100]. These results together outline the importance of costimulation to disease onset and severity and highlight the influence of CD86-CD28 as a potential mediator of disease initiation in salivary and lacrimal glands.

Results regarding Treg involvement in the pathogenesis of SjS have been contradictory. However, increasing evidence details defects in Treg contributing to disease. Recently it has also been shown that in situ patrolling Tregs are essential for protection against autoimmune exocrinopathy. In this system, CCR7 deficient mice were unable to allow Treg egress from lymph nodes into peripheral tissues such as salivary and lacrimal glands, and that this resulted in disease resembling SjS [101]. Interestingly, wild-type C57BL/6 mice evaluation showed approximately 30% lacrimal and 23% salivary expression of Foxp3+ cells under steady-state conditions, while CCR7-deficient mice had approximately 7% and 9% respectively [101]. The Foxp3-deficient scurfy mouse model (essentially deficient in Treg cells) adds more complexity to the issue of roles of Tregs, since these mice do not develop inflammation or inflammatory cell infiltration into their salivary or lacrimal glands, however, adoptive transfer to Rag-deficient mice induces multi-organ inflammation in salivary, lacrimal glands, stomach, small intestine, pancreas, colon, and even skeletal muscle. This included inflammation in the lacrimal and salivary glands as well as inhibited salivary function, where infiltration was located primarily in the acini and granular convoluted tubules [102].

SjS patients have also been shown to have decreased number of Tregs (CCR7+Foxp3+) in salivary glands compared to controls [101]. In line with this direct tissue evidence, there are also several other reports of fewer salivary Tregs present in patients with SjS [103, 104] and reports of Tregs with decreased suppression capabilities [105]. Reports of increased number of Foxp3+ Treg cells in the salivary glands of patients with SjS [105, 106], was positively correlated with the grade of infiltration as evaluated by Chisholm score [106]. The authors do not address potential mechanisms for this observation. The observed number of Foxp3+ cells in the peripheral blood was unchanging between SjS, RA, and healthy controls [106]. It is possible that the observations of increased numbers of Treg cells in the salivary glands of patients with SjS could be a result of proliferative enrichment due to increased costimulatory signaling (CD28 and CD86), and may have altered suppressive function as a result.

4. Conclusions

In autoimmune diseases, dysfunction of Treg cells is a potential contributor to disease development, where costimulatory requirements for Treg cell proliferation and suppression capabilities may not be met. Based on reviewed research on autoimmune diseases, it appears that contribution of CD86 to Teff cells via CD28 signaling are potentially one of the initiating factors of disease, at least in the cases RA, autoimmune diabetes, and SjS. The lack of CD80 regulatory effects on these diseases appears in general to be due to a lack of expression on certain cell types, such as resident epithelium as in RA and SjS. In the previously mentioned model where CD80 helps suppressive Treg function, this relative lack of CD80 earlier in disease onset could be contributing to the allowance of autoreactive T-cells to respond towards self-antigens. However, regulatory mechanisms of B7 ligand expression as well as the differential signaling mechanisms that control Treg maintenance and function with regards to CD80 and CTLA-4 signaling pathways have yet to be elucidated. Some of the previously mentioned contradictory findings as to abnormal expression of B7 molecules and their function in autoimmune diseases could be explained by multiple factors such as genetic background, relative expression of B7 ligands, immune microenvironment, and timing of critical immunological events. Better understanding costimulatory and inhibitory requirements of CD80 and CD86 are worth further looking into since clinical trials involving CTLA-4-Ig (Abatacept, Orencia) have shown promise in clinical improvement for RA [107] but not so well in controlling flares in patients with non-life threatening SLE [108]. Clinical trials are also underway for MS and Type I diabetes, where findings do show efficacy in controlling disease activity in MS [109] and delaying beta cell loss in diabetes patients [110]. There is no data available for use of CTLA-4-Ig in SjS patients. However, the previously mentioned findings with CTLA-4-Ig in SjS-prone mice do show promise for the use of costimulatory blockade in prevention of disease [99]. Mechanisms involving these observed protective effects of blocking B7 with regards to Treg maintenance and function should also be explored, since regulation of specific Treg populations may contribute to development of autoimmunity. Overall, there are still many questions as to how the CD86/CD80:CD28/CTLA-4 family interacts to form specific immune responses in vivo, especially in the areas of Treg development, homeostasis, and suppression function. It is well established that Treg cells are important to the prevention of autoimmunity. Whether targeting costimulatory molecules to drive desirable Treg development and function to a complete reversal of disease phenotype needs to be further clarified in autoimmune diseases, especially in SjS.

Author details

Adrienne E. Gauna and Seunghee Cha*

Oral and Maxillofacial Diagnostic Sciences, University of Florida, Gainesville, USA

References

[1] Linsley, P.S., et al., Binding of the B cell activation antigen B7 to CD28 costimulates T cell proliferation and interleukin 2 mRNA accumulation. J Exp Med, 1991. 173(3): p. 721-30.

[2] Chuang, E., et al., Interaction of CTLA-4 with the clathrin-associated protein AP50 results in ligand-independent endocytosis that limits cell surface expression. J Immunol, 1997. 159(1): p. 144-51.

[3] Zhang, Y. and J.P. Allison, Interaction of CTLA-4 with AP50, a clathrin-coated pit adaptor protein. Proc Natl Acad Sci U S A, 1997. 94(17): p. 9273-8.

[4] Schneider, H., et al., Cytolytic T lymphocyte-associated antigen-4 and the TCR zeta/CD3 complex, but not CD28, interact with clathrin adaptor complexes AP-1 and AP-2. J Immunol, 1999. 163(4): p. 1868-79.

[5] Shiratori, T., et al., Tyrosine phosphorylation controls internalization of CTLA-4 by regulating its interaction with clathrin-associated adaptor complex AP-2. Immunity, 1997. 6(5): p. 583-9.

[6] Mead, K.I., et al., Exocytosis of CTLA-4 is dependent on phospholipase D and ADP ribosylation factor-1 and stimulated during activation of regulatory T cells. J Immunol, 2005. 174(8): p. 4803-11.

[7] Egen, J.G. and J.P. Allison, Cytotoxic T lymphocyte antigen-4 accumulation in the immunological synapse is regulated by TCR signal strength. Immunity, 2002. 16(1): p. 23-35.

[8] Greenwald, R.J., G.J. Freeman, and A.H. Sharpe, The B7 family revisited. Annu Rev Immunol, 2005. 23: p. 515-48.

[9] Lenschow, D.J., T.L. Walunas, and J.A. Bluestone, CD28/B7 system of T cell costimulation. Annu Rev Immunol, 1996. 14: p. 233-58.

[10] Azuma, M., et al., CD28 interaction with B7 costimulates primary allogeneic proliferative responses and cytotoxicity mediated by small, resting T lymphocytes. J Exp Med, 1992. 175(2): p. 353-60.

[11] Hathcock, K.S., et al., Comparative analysis of B7-1 and B7-2 costimulatory ligands: expression and function. J Exp Med, 1994. 180(2): p. 631-40.

[12] Inaba, K., et al., The tissue distribution of the B7-2 costimulator in mice: abundant expression on dendritic cells in situ and during maturation in vitro. J Exp Med, 1994. 180(5): p. 1849-60.

[13] Geissmann, F., et al., TGF-beta 1 prevents the noncognate maturation of human dendritic Langerhans cells. J Immunol, 1999. 162(8): p. 4567-75.

[14] Kodaira, Y., et al., Phenotypic and functional maturation of dendritic cells mediated by heparan sulfate. J Immunol, 2000. 165(3): p. 1599-604.

[15] McGuirk, P., C. McCann, and K.H. Mills, Pathogen-specific T regulatory 1 cells induced in the respiratory tract by a bacterial molecule that stimulates interleukin 10 production by dendritic cells: a novel strategy for evasion of protective T helper type 1 responses by Bordetella pertussis. J Exp Med, 2002. 195(2): p. 221-31.

[16] Steinman, R.M. and M.C. Nussenzweig, Avoiding horror autotoxicus: the importance of dendritic cells in peripheral T cell tolerance. Proc Natl Acad Sci U S A, 2002. 99(1): p. 351-8.

[17] Shklovskaya, E., et al., Langerhans cells are precommitted to immune tolerance induction. Proc Natl Acad Sci U S A, 2011. 108(44): p. 18049-54.

[18] Wallet, M.A., P. Sen, and R. Tisch, Immunoregulation of dendritic cells. Clin Med Res, 2005. 3(3): p. 166-75.

[19] Collins, A.V., et al., The interaction properties of costimulatory molecules revisited. Immunity, 2002. 17(2): p. 201-10.

[20] Bhatia, S., et al., B7-1 and B7-2: similar costimulatory ligands with different biochemical, oligomeric and signaling properties. Immunol Lett, 2006. 104(1-2): p. 70-5.

[21] Stamper, C.C., et al., Crystal structure of the B7-1/CTLA-4 complex that inhibits human immune responses. Nature, 2001. 410(6828): p. 608-11.

[22] Bhatia, S., et al., Different cell surface oligomeric states of B7-1 and B7-2: implications for signaling. Proc Natl Acad Sci U S A, 2005. 102(43): p. 15569-74.

[23] Zhang, X., et al., Crystal structure of the receptor-binding domain of human B7-2: insights into organization and signaling. Proc Natl Acad Sci U S A, 2003. 100(5): p. 2586-91.

[24] Schwartz, J.C., et al., Structural basis for co-stimulation by the human CTLA-4/B7-2 complex. Nature, 2001. 410(6828): p. 604-8.

[25] Linsley, P.S., et al., Human B7-1 (CD80) and B7-2 (CD86) bind with similar avidities but distinct kinetics to CD28 and CTLA-4 receptors. Immunity, 1994. 1(9): p. 793-801.

[26] Pentcheva-Hoang, T., et al., B7-1 and B7-2 selectively recruit CTLA-4 and CD28 to the immunological synapse. Immunity, 2004. 21(3): p. 401-13.

[27] Boise, L.H., et al., CD28 costimulation can promote T cell survival by enhancing the expression of Bcl-XL. Immunity, 1995. 3(1): p. 87-98.

[28] McLeod, J.D., et al., Activation of human T cells with superantigen (staphylococcal enterotoxin B) and CD28 confers resistance to apoptosis via CD95. J Immunol, 1998. 160(5): p. 2072-9.

[29] Ferguson, S.E., et al., CD28 is required for germinal center formation. J Immunol, 1996. 156(12): p. 4576-81.

[30] Shahinian, A., et al., Differential T cell costimulatory requirements in CD28-deficient mice. Science, 1993. 261(5121): p. 609-12.

[31] Walker, L.S., et al., Co-stimulation and selection for T-cell help for germinal centres: the role of CD28 and OX40. Immunol Today, 2000. 21(7): p. 333-7.

[32] Iezzi, G., K. Karjalainen, and A. Lanzavecchia, The duration of antigenic stimulation determines the fate of naive and effector T cells. Immunity, 1998. 8(1): p. 89-95.

[33] Gett, A.V. and P.D. Hodgkin, A cellular calculus for signal integration by T cells. Nat Immunol, 2000. 1(3): p. 239-44.

[34] Waterhouse, P., et al., Lymphoproliferative disorders with early lethality in mice deficient in Ctla-4. Science, 1995. 270(5238): p. 985-8.

[35] Tivol, E.A., et al., Loss of CTLA-4 leads to massive lymphoproliferation and fatal multiorgan tissue destruction, revealing a critical negative regulatory role of CTLA-4. Immunity, 1995. 3(5): p. 541-7.

[36] Chambers, C.A., T.J. Sullivan, and J.P. Allison, Lymphoproliferation in CTLA-4-deficient mice is mediated by costimulation-dependent activation of CD4+ T cells. Immunity, 1997. 7(6): p. 885-95.

[37] Chambers, C.A., et al., Thymocyte development is normal in CTLA-4-deficient mice. Proc Natl Acad Sci U S A, 1997. 94(17): p. 9296-301.

[38] Tivol, E.A., et al., CTLA4Ig prevents lymphoproliferation and fatal multiorgan tissue destruction in CTLA-4-deficient mice. J Immunol, 1997. 158(11): p. 5091-4.

[39] Mandelbrot, D.A., A.J. McAdam, and A.H. Sharpe, B7-1 or B7-2 is required to produce the lymphoproliferative phenotype in mice lacking cytotoxic T lymphocyte-associated antigen 4 (CTLA-4). J Exp Med, 1999. 189(2): p. 435-40.

[40] Tai, X., et al., Induction of autoimmune disease in CTLA-4-/- mice depends on a specific CD28 motif that is required for in vivo costimulation. Proc Natl Acad Sci U S A, 2007. 104(34): p. 13756-61.

[41] Takahashi, T., et al., Immunologic self-tolerance maintained by CD25(+)CD4(+) regulatory T cells constitutively expressing cytotoxic T lymphocyte-associated antigen 4. J Exp Med, 2000. 192(2): p. 303-10.

[42] Read, S., V. Malmstrom, and F. Powrie, Cytotoxic T lymphocyte-associated antigen 4 plays an essential role in the function of CD25(+)CD4(+) regulatory cells that control intestinal inflammation. J Exp Med, 2000. 192(2): p. 295-302.

[43] Manzotti, C.N., et al., Inhibition of human T cell proliferation by CTLA-4 utilizes CD80 and requires CD25+ regulatory T cells. Eur J Immunol, 2002. 32(10): p. 2888-96.

[44] Taylor, P.A., R.J. Noelle, and B.R. Blazar, CD4(+)CD25(+) immune regulatory cells are required for induction of tolerance to alloantigen via costimulatory blockade. J Exp Med, 2001. 193(11): p. 1311-8.

[45] Krummel, M.F. and J.P. Allison, CTLA-4 engagement inhibits IL-2 accumulation and cell cycle progression upon activation of resting T cells. J Exp Med, 1996. 183(6): p. 2533-40.

[46] Walunas, T.L., C.Y. Bakker, and J.A. Bluestone, CTLA-4 ligation blocks CD28-dependent T cell activation. J Exp Med, 1996. 183(6): p. 2541-50.

[47] Qureshi, O.S., et al., Trans-endocytosis of CD80 and CD86: a molecular basis for the cell-extrinsic function of CTLA-4. Science, 2011. 332(6029): p. 600-3.

[48] Lenschow, D.J., et al., Differential effects of anti-B7-1 and anti-B7-2 monoclonal antibody treatment on the development of diabetes in the nonobese diabetic mouse. J Exp Med, 1995. 181(3): p. 1145-55.

[49] Bour-Jordan, H., et al., Costimulation controls diabetes by altering the balance of pathogenic and regulatory T cells. J Clin Invest, 2004. 114(7): p. 979-87.

[50] Butte, M.J., et al., Programmed death-1 ligand 1 interacts specifically with the B7-1 costimulatory molecule to inhibit T cell responses. Immunity, 2007. 27(1): p. 111-22.

[51] Yang, J., et al., The novel costimulatory programmed death ligand 1/B7.1 pathway is functional in inhibiting alloimmune responses in vivo. J Immunol, 2011. 187(3): p. 1113-9.

[52] Park, J.J., et al., B7-H1/CD80 interaction is required for the induction and maintenance of peripheral T-cell tolerance. Blood, 2010. 116(8): p. 1291-8.

[53] Salomon, B., et al., B7/CD28 costimulation is essential for the homeostasis of the CD4+CD25+ immunoregulatory T cells that control autoimmune diabetes. Immunity, 2000. 12(4): p. 431-40.

[54] Tang, Q., et al., Cutting edge: CD28 controls peripheral homeostasis of CD4+CD25+ regulatory T cells. J Immunol, 2003. 171(7): p. 3348-52.

[55] Yamazaki, S., et al., Direct expansion of functional CD25+ CD4+ regulatory T cells by antigen-processing dendritic cells. J Exp Med, 2003. 198(2): p. 235-47.

[56] Zheng, Y., et al., CD86 and CD80 differentially modulate the suppressive function of human regulatory T cells. J Immunol, 2004. 172(5): p. 2778-84.

[57] Paust, S., et al., Engagement of B7 on effector T cells by regulatory T cells prevents autoimmune disease. Proc Natl Acad Sci U S A, 2004. 101(28): p. 10398-403.

[58] Yi, T., et al., Host APCs augment in vivo expansion of donor natural regulatory T cells via B7H1/B7.1 in allogeneic recipients. J Immunol, 2011. 186(5): p. 2739-49.

[59] Takahashi, T., et al., Immunologic self-tolerance maintained by CD25+CD4+ naturally anergic and suppressive T cells: induction of autoimmune disease by breaking their anergic/suppressive state. Int Immunol, 1998. 10(12): p. 1969-80.

[60] Wang, J.H., et al., Type I interferon-dependent CD86(high) marginal zone precursor B cells are potent T cell costimulators in mice. Arthritis Rheum, 2011. 63(4): p. 1054-64.

[61] Wu, H.Y. and N.A. Staines, A deficiency of CD4+CD25+ T cells permits the development of spontaneous lupus-like disease in mice, and can be reversed by induction of mucosal tolerance to histone peptide autoantigen. Lupus, 2004. 13(3): p. 192-200.

[62] Scalapino, K.J., et al., Suppression of disease in New Zealand Black/New Zealand White lupus-prone mice by adoptive transfer of ex vivo expanded regulatory T cells. J Immunol, 2006. 177(3): p. 1451-9.

[63] Monk, C.R., et al., MRL/Mp CD4+,CD25- T cells show reduced sensitivity to suppression by CD4+,CD25+ regulatory T cells in vitro: a novel defect of T cell regulation in systemic lupus erythematosus. Arthritis Rheum, 2005. 52(4): p. 1180-4.

[64] Parietti, V., et al., Function of CD4+,CD25+ Treg cells in MRL/lpr mice is compromised by intrinsic defects in antigen-presenting cells and effector T cells. Arthritis Rheum, 2008. 58(6): p. 1751-61.

[65] Balsa, A., et al., Differential expression of the costimulatory molecules B7.1 (CD80) and B7.2 (CD86) in rheumatoid synovial tissue. Br J Rheumatol, 1996. 35(1): p. 33-7.

[66] Summers, K.L., et al., Dendritic cells in synovial fluid of chronic inflammatory arthritis lack CD80 surface expression. Clin Exp Immunol, 1995. 100(1): p. 81-9.

[67] Ranheim, E.A. and T.J. Kipps, Elevated expression of CD80 (B7/BB1) and other accessory molecules on synovial fluid mononuclear cell subsets in rheumatoid arthritis. Arthritis Rheum, 1994. 37(11): p. 1637-46.

[68] Liu, M.F., et al., The presence of costimulatory molecules CD86 and CD28 in rheumatoid arthritis synovium. Arthritis Rheum, 1996. 39(1): p. 110-4.

[69] Thomas, R. and C. Quinn, Functional differentiation of dendritic cells in rheumatoid arthritis: role of CD86 in the synovium. J Immunol, 1996. 156(8): p. 3074-86.

[70] Verwilghen, J., et al., Expression of functional B7 and CTLA4 on rheumatoid synovial T cells. J Immunol, 1994. 153(3): p. 1378-85.

[71] Webb, L.M., M.J. Walmsley, and M. Feldmann, Prevention and amelioration of collagen-induced arthritis by blockade of the CD28 co-stimulatory pathway: requirement for both B7-1 and B7-2. Eur J Immunol, 1996. 26(10): p. 2320-8.

[72] Tada, Y., et al., CD28-deficient mice are highly resistant to collagen-induced arthritis. J Immunol, 1999. 162(1): p. 203-8.

[73] Tellander, A.C., et al., Interference with CD28, CD80, CD86 or CD152 in collagen-induced arthritis. Limited role of IFN-gamma in anti-B7-mediated suppression of disease. J Autoimmun, 2001. 17(1): p. 39-50.

[74] Knoerzer, D.B., et al., Collagen-induced arthritis in the BB rat. Prevention of disease by treatment with CTLA-4-Ig. J Clin Invest, 1995. 96(2): p. 987-93.

[75] Tada, Y., et al., Role of the costimulatory molecule CD28 in the development of lupus in MRL/lpr mice. J Immunol, 1999. 163(6): p. 3153-9.

[76] Alvarez-Quiroga, C., et al., CTLA-4-Ig therapy diminishes the frequency but enhances the function of Treg cells in patients with rheumatoid arthritis. J Clin Immunol, 2011. 31(4): p. 588-95.

[77] Mottonen, M., et al., CD4+ CD25+ T cells with the phenotypic and functional characteristics of regulatory T cells are enriched in the synovial fluid of patients with rheumatoid arthritis. Clin Exp Immunol, 2005. 140(2): p. 360-7.

[78] van Amelsfort, J.M., et al., Proinflammatory mediator-induced reversal of CD4+,CD25+ regulatory T cell-mediated suppression in rheumatoid arthritis. Arthritis Rheum, 2007. 56(3): p. 732-42.

[79] Jang, E., et al., Deficiency of foxp3 regulatory T cells exacerbates autoimmune arthritis by altering the synovial proportions of CD4 T cells and dendritic cells. Immune Netw, 2011. 11(5): p. 299-306.

[80] Jang, E., et al., Foxp3+ regulatory T cells control humoral autoimmunity by suppressing the development of long-lived plasma cells. J Immunol, 2011. 186(3): p. 1546-53.

[81] Hussain, S. and T.L. Delovitch, Dysregulated B7-1 and B7-2 expression on nonobese diabetic mouse B cells is associated with increased T cell costimulation and the development of insulitis. J Immunol, 2005. 174(2): p. 680-7.

[82] Salomon, B., et al., Development of spontaneous autoimmune peripheral polyneuropathy in B7-2-deficient NOD mice. J Exp Med, 2001. 194(5): p. 677-84.

[83] Karandikar, N.J., et al., Tissue-specific up-regulation of B7-1 expression and function during the course of murine relapsing experimental autoimmune encephalomyelitis. J Immunol, 1998. 161(1): p. 192-9.

[84] Miller, S.D., et al., Blockade of CD28/B7-1 interaction prevents epitope spreading and clinical relapses of murine EAE. Immunity, 1995. 3(6): p. 739-45.

[85] Tonkin, D.R., et al., Regulatory T cells prevent transfer of type 1 diabetes in NOD mice only when their antigen is present in vivo. J Immunol, 2008. 181(7): p. 4516-22.

[86] Wildenberg, M.E., et al., Lack of CCR5 on dendritic cells promotes a proinflammatory environment in submandibular glands of the NOD mouse. J Leukoc Biol, 2008. 83(5): p. 1194-200.

[87] Wang, R., et al., GAD-IgG-inducing CD4+Foxp3+Treg cells suppressing diabetes are involved in the increasing ratio of CD80+:CD86+ CELLS in NOD mice. Arch Med Res, 2008. 39(3): p. 299-305.

[88] Song, L., et al., Retroviral delivery of GAD-IgG fusion construct induces tolerance and modulates diabetes: a role for CD4+ regulatory T cells and TGF-beta? Gene Ther, 2004. 11(20): p. 1487-96.

[89] Tang, Q., et al., Central role of defective interleukin-2 production in the triggering of islet autoimmune destruction. Immunity, 2008. 28(5): p. 687-97.

[90] D'Alise, A.M., et al., The defect in T-cell regulation in NOD mice is an effect on the T-cell effectors. Proc Natl Acad Sci U S A, 2008. 105(50): p. 19857-62.

[91] Manoussakis, M.N., et al., Expression of B7 costimulatory molecules by salivary gland epithelial cells in patients with Sjogren's syndrome. Arthritis Rheum, 1999. 42(2): p. 229-39.

[92] Kapsogeorgou, E.K., H.M. Moutsopoulos, and M.N. Manoussakis, Functional expression of a costimulatory B7.2 (CD86) protein on human salivary gland epithelial cells that interacts with the CD28 receptor, but has reduced binding to CTLA4. J Immunol, 2001. 166(5): p. 3107-13.

[93] Matsumura, R., et al., Glandular and extraglandular expression of costimulatory molecules in patients with Sjogren's syndrome. Ann Rheum Dis, 2001. 60(5): p. 473-82.

[94] Tsunawaki, S., et al., Possible function of salivary gland epithelial cells as nonprofessional antigen-presenting cells in the development of Sjogren's syndrome. J Rheumatol, 2002. 29(9): p. 1884-96.

[95] Freeman, G.J., et al., The BB1 monoclonal antibody recognizes both cell surface CD74 (MHC class II-associated invariant chain) as well as B7-1 (CD80), resolving the question regarding a third CD28/CTLA-4 counterreceptor. J Immunol, 1998. 161(6): p. 2708-15.

[96] Ishimaru, N., et al., Expression of the retinoblastoma protein RbAp48 in exocrine glands leads to Sjogren's syndrome-like autoimmune exocrinopathy. J Exp Med, 2008. 205(12): p. 2915-27.

[97] Mikkelsen, T.R., et al., Tissue-specific expression in the salivary glands of transgenic mice. Nucleic Acids Res, 1992. 20(9): p. 2249-55.

[98] Cha, S., et al., Two NOD Idd-associated intervals contribute synergistically to the development of autoimmune exocrinopathy (Sjogren's syndrome) on a healthy murine background. Arthritis Rheum, 2002. 46(5): p. 1390-8.

[99] Yin, H., et al., Local delivery of AAV2-CTLA4IgG decreases sialadenitis and improves gland function in the C57BL/6.NOD-Aec1Aec2 mouse model of Sjogren's syndrome. Arthritis Res Ther, 2012. 14(1): p. R40.

[100] Saegusa, K., et al., Treatment with anti-CD86 costimulatory molecule prevents the autoimmune lesions in murine Sjogren's syndrome (SS) through up-regulated Th2 response. Clin Exp Immunol, 2000. 119(2): p. 354-60.

[101] Ishimaru, N., et al., In situ patrolling of regulatory T cells is essential for protecting autoimmune exocrinopathy. PLoS One, 2010. 5(1): p. e8588.

[102] Sharma, R., et al., Regulation of multi-organ inflammation in the regulatory T cell-deficient scurfy mice. J Biomed Sci, 2009. 16: p. 20.

[103] Li, X., et al., T regulatory cells are markedly diminished in diseased salivary glands of patients with primary Sjogren's syndrome. J Rheumatol, 2007. 34(12): p. 2438-45.

[104] Liu, M.F., et al., Decreased CD4+CD25+bright T cells in peripheral blood of patients with primary Sjogren's syndrome. Lupus, 2008. 17(1): p. 34-9.

[105] Szodoray, P., et al., Cells with regulatory function of the innate and adaptive immune system in primary Sjogren's syndrome. Clin Exp Immunol, 2009. 157(3): p. 343-9.

[106] Sarigul, M., et al., The numbers of Foxp3 + Treg cells are positively correlated with higher grade of infiltration at the salivary glands in primary Sjogren's syndrome. Lupus, 2010. 19(2): p. 138-45.

[107] Vital, E.M. and P. Emery, Abatacept in the treatment of rheumatoid arthritis. Ther Clin Risk Manag, 2006. 2(4): p. 365-75.

[108] Merrill, J.T., et al., The efficacy and safety of abatacept in patients with non-life-threatening manifestations of systemic lupus erythematosus: results of a twelve-month, multicenter, exploratory, phase IIb, randomized, double-blind, placebo-controlled trial. Arthritis Rheum, 2010. 62(10): p. 3077-87.

[109] Viglietta, V., et al., CTLA4Ig treatment in patients with multiple sclerosis: an open-label, phase 1 clinical trial. Neurology, 2008. 71(12): p. 917-24.

[110] Orban, T., et al., Co-stimulation modulation with abatacept in patients with recent-onset type 1 diabetes: a randomised, double-blind, placebo-controlled trial. Lancet, 2011. 378(9789): p. 412-9.

Chapter 6

Immune Synapses Between Lymphocytes and Target Cells in Autoimmune Thyroid Diseases

Iwona Ben-Skowronek and Roman Ciechanek

Additional information is available at the end of the chapter

http://dx.doi.org/10.5772/53009

1. Introduction

The immune synapse is the interface between an antigen-presenting cell and a lymphocyte [1-4] as well as the interface between different lymphocytes, Natural Killer cells, and target cells [5]. This intercellular connection serves as a focal point for exocytosis and endocytosis [6]. Numerous investigations have elucidated the structure of the immunological synapse. The synapse is composed of a central region: a central supramolecular activation complex SMAC [cSMAC], a T cell receptor (TCR) cluster and associated signaling proteins, and peripheral SMAC (pSMAC) of a ring of tight adhesion between the reacting cells [7]. The separated space of SMAC is the place of exocytic and endocytic events in this site but the precise site of signaling is not known [8]. The early signaling process occurs in peripheral microclusters in the pSMAC and the cSMAC in T and B cell synapses [9-12]. CD4 T cells form long-lived synapses with APCs – the synapses live few hours. CD8 T cells form transient synapses, lasting only minutes, because the target cells are killed [13,14]. In this cytotoxic synapse, activated Src kinases were detected in the cSMAC [13]. The cSMACs play an important role not only in signaling but also in receptor recycling because endosomal compartments polarize to the point immediately beneath the cSMAC of the immunological synapse [15]. The endosome comes to lie underneath the cSMAC as polarization of the microtubule skeletons occurs during synapse formation. This polarization is antigen-dependent. The receptor activation leads to accumulation of actin across the synapse and formation of an outer ring around the synapse [16,17]. The cytotoxic reaction of lymphocytes CD8 is connected with release of specialized lysosomes containing the lytic pore-forming protein perforin, which enables gransymes to lead to rapid apoptosis of the target cell [17]; the centrosome in the lymphocytes is polarized right up to the plasma membrane containing the synapse cSMAC [18]. The lytic granules are delivered to a specialized secretory domain within the synapse by moving along the microtubules toward the centrosome. Granule contents are then released into a small cleft between the two cells [17]. Since the overall levels of surface and endocytosed proteins remain the same regardless of ICAM-1, this suggests that ICAM-1–LFA-1 engagement in the pSMAC acts to restrict and focus endocytic and exocytic events to the center of the synapse. Griffiths suggests that the centrosome may play a role in identifying a specialized area of membrane for focal endocytosis and exocytosis [6]. An important role in formation of the immunological synapse is played by the localization of mitochondria – the mitochondria can activate and terminate the activity of immune synapses [19]. The *in vivo* image of T cell activation is slightly more complex. In an experimental system that uses subcutaneous injection of labeled LPS-activated dendritic cells followed by intravenous injection of naive transgenic CD8+ T cells, behavior of these cells and a three-phase model for T cell activation were observed: [20]. Phase 1 includes initial transient T cell–DC interactions characterized by continued rapid T cell migration that can last from 30 min to 8 h depending on the pMHC density. Signals in phase 1 are integrated through kinapses. Phase 2 is a period of stable T cell–DC interactions lasting ~12 h, during which cytokines such as IL-2 are produced. Signals in phase 2 are integrated through the immune synapse. Phase 3 is a return to transient T cell–DC interaction and rapid T cell migration during which the T cell divides multiple times and then exits the lymphoid tissue. The correct interpretation of these stop and go signals is critical for generation of effector and memory T cells [21,22].

The aim of the study is presentation of the ultrastructure of immune synapses between T- cells and plasma cells and target cells *in vivo* in autoimmune thyroid diseases.

2. Material and methods

2.1. Patients

A group of children and adolescents was chosen for the study to exclude the impact of aging processes and other diseases connected with age: circulatory disorders, arterial sclerosis, and drug use.

The study involved 90 children: 30 children affected with Graves' disease, 30 children with Hashimoto's thyroiditis and 30 children as a control group. The children were treated in the Department of Pediatric Endocrinology and Neurology in Lublin and in the Pediatric Department in Rzeszow in the years 1994 – 2007 and operated on in the Surgery Department of the Regional Hospital in Lublin and in the Regional Hospital in Rzeszow.

The investigation was accepted by the local Ethical Committee at the Medical University in Lublin.

2.1.1. Control group

The control group consisted of 30 children aged 6-19 who had died in accidents and of other non-autoimmune diseases; the thyroid specimens were taken during autopsy (n=25). Some specimens were taken during a surgical operation of thyroglossal cysts and during surgery of parathyroid glands (n=5). These were fragments of routinely sampled tissue specimens for

http://dx.doi.org/10.5772/53009

standard pathologic investigations. All the children were in euthyreosis [Tab.1]. All children's parents signed an informed consent before autopsy or surgical operation.

2.1.2. Patient qualification procedure

All patients' parents signed an informed consent before these investigations.

All the patients received physical examination to assess the goiter and clinical signs and symptoms of thyroid disorders. The TSH (Thyroid-stimulating hormone), fT4 (free thyroxin) and TT3 (total triiodothyronine) hormones were assayed by MEIA (Abbott Kit, Langford, Ireland). The levels of TSH receptor antibodies were measured by RIA (TRAK assay BRAHMS Diagnostica GmbH, Berlin, Germany). The thyroperoxidase (TPO) and thyroglobulin (TG) antibodies were assayed by LIA (Lumitest BRAHMS Diagnostica GmbH, Berlin, Germany).

In the patients with Graves' disease, symptoms of thyrotoxicosis: goiter, tachycardia, sleeplessness, anxiety, high diastolic/systolic blood pressure amplitude, an increase in fT4 (mean 3.8± 0.7 ng/dl) and TT3 (mean 363±175.3 ng/dl), and a decrease in TSH (mean 0.004±0.003 mU/l) were observed. The levels of antibodies against the TSH receptor (TRAB) (7-462U/ml) and the levels of TPO antibodies (21-6663U/ml) and TG antibodies (25-13351U/ml) were usually increased. The patients were treated with methimazole in initial doses 0.9-0.5 mg/kg b.w./day during 4-6 weeks and after that time, when in euthyreosis, they got maintenance doses c.a.0.1 mg/kg b.w./ day (mainly 5mg/day) in combination with a low dose of l-thyroxin (25μg/day) during 18-24 months. Children with Graves' disease, whose early relapses of hyperthyreosis necessitated surgery treatment – thyroidectomy after 18-36 months, were qualified for the investigation [Tab. 1].

Hashimoto's thyroiditis was recognized in patients with parenchymal or nodular large size goiter accompanied by pressure to other neck structures in the phase of euthyreosis or hypothyreosis, rarely in hyperthyreosis (Hashitoxicosis). In ultrasonography, a non-homogenous structure of the thyroid was observed. The levels of TPO Ab and TG Ab were increased, but the levels of the TRAb were in normal ranges. In histopathological examination, mononuclear lymphatic infiltrations in the thyroid parenchyma were detected, and Hashimoto's thyroiditis was diagnosed. Before surgery, the patients were usually treated with l-thyroxin 25-100 μg/day. [Tab. 1].

	Patients number	Age [years]	TSH mIU/L	fT4 ng/dl	TPO Ab IU/L	TG Ab IU/L	TSI IU/L
Graves' disease	30	5-19	0,001-0,005	3,3-5,1	21-6663	25-13351	7-462
Hashimoto's thyroiditis	30	8-19	0,600-98,800	0,1—2,3	132-9856	128-14567	0-0,99
Control group	30	6-19	0,270-4,200	x	x	x	x
Normal ranges			0,270-4,200	0,8-2,3	<34	<115	<1

Table 1. Characteristics of the patients examined before treatment

3. Ultrastructural investigations

Specimens for ultrastructural investigations were obtained during thyroidectomy. Small segments of thyroid were cut into 0,5mm^3 pieces and fixed in 4% glutaraldehyde in 0,1 M cacodylate buffer, pH 7.4 for 24 h in 4ºC, post fixed in 2% OsO4 in the same buffer for 1h in room temperature, dehydrated in a graded series (up to 100%) of ethanol and embedded in 812 Epon. They were then polymerized at 60ºC. Five specimens were taken from every thyroid from each patient with Graves' disease, Hashimoto's thyroiditis, and from the control group. Epon blocks were cut with an RMC MT-7 ultramicrotome, USA. From every specimen were analyzed serial 10 slides. Ultrathin sections were contrasted with uranyl acetate and lead citrate and examined under the EM 900 Zeiss Germany Electron Microscope.

4. Results

In the control group of children without a thyroid disease, lymphocytes in the interstitium of the thyroid gland were observed sporadically. The lymphatic cells did not cross the basal membrane of thyroid follicles, were not in contact with thyrocytes and did not form groups. In Graves' disease, T cells that crossed the basal membrane of the vesicles were observed to be in contact with thyrocytes. The lymphocytes migrated to thyroid follicles from capillary vessels or from lymphatic follicles. The migrating T-cells had numerous projections – lamellipodia on their surface. Polarization of cell organelles was already visible in narrow capillaries. The lamellipodia, mitochondria, and the Golgi system were located in the same part of the lymphocyte [Fig.1]. T cells, which penetrated across the basal membrane between thyrocytes, looked similar [Fig. 2]. The T- cells formed numerous junctions with thyrocytes. The structure of these connections was similar to zonula occludens with an area of cell membrane fusion and area of free spaces between cells, in which protein substances were secreted [Fig.2]. The T-cells were not polarized in those connections with thyrocytes. The thyrocytes were not damaged, but were active and had numerous mitochondria, secretory vesicles and a big amount of euchromatin in the nuclei [Fig. 2].

In Hashimoto's thyroiditis, the sites of contact between T-cells and lymphocytes had the character of an immune synapse, too. The synapse, however, looked different. The T-cells were polarized – the centrioles, mitochondria, Golgi system, and secretory vesicles were present in the part connected with the thyrocytes. The synapse was composed of a distal part – an adhesion zone, and a central part – a space in which electron dense substances were secreted [Fig.3]. The thyrocytes staying in contact with T-cells exhibited the features of apoptosis: dark, concentrated heterochromatin in the nucleus, swollen mitochondria, and enlarged cisterns of endoplasmic reticulum.

In AITD, synapses between plasma cells and thyrocytes were observed. In Graves' disease, synapses were formed in the distal part – zonula adherens - without fusion of thyrocyte and plasmocyte cell membranes and in the central part - the space between membrane of plasma cells and thyrocytes. Electron dense substances from the rough endoplasmic reticulum of the

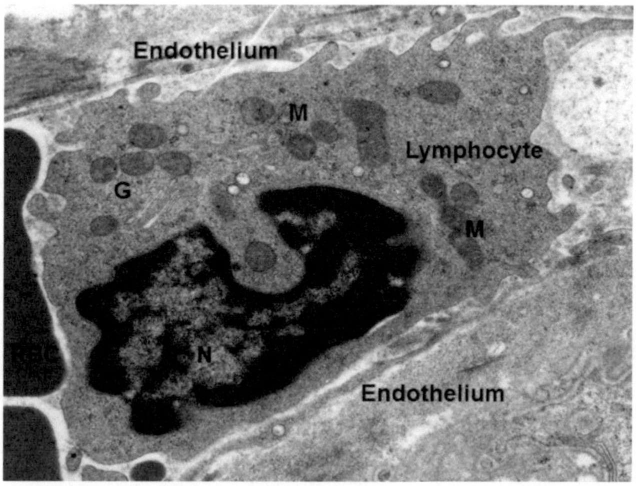

Figure 1. The lymphocyte migrating in the capillary vessel. Polarization of the lymphatic cell is visible: lamellipodia, mitochondria, and Golgi complex are present on the same side. N- nucleus, M- mitochondria, G-Golgi system, RBC- red blood cell. TEM magn. 15 000x

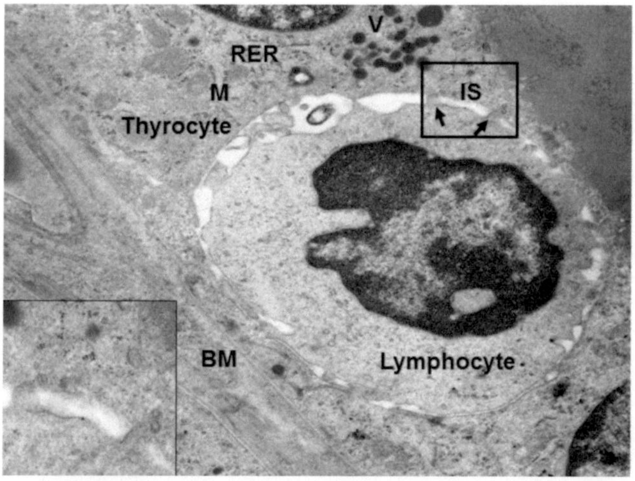

Figure 2. The lymphocyte between thyrocytes in the thyroid follicle in Graves' disease. The lymphocyte formed numerous immune synapses with the thyrocyte. The immune synapses are limited by zonula occludens (pSMAC with fusion of cell membranes). The space (cSMAC) is visible in the center of the immune synapse. The thyrocytes are active without signs of damage. RER – rough endoplasmic reticulum, M-mitochondria, V-secretory vesicle, MB- basal membrane, IS- immune synapse. TEM magn. 15 000x.

plasma cells – most probably immunoglobulins - were secreted to this space [Fig.4]. Immunoglobulins encrusted the basal membrane of thyrocytes.The thyroid cells staying in contact with plasma cells were active: with a big amount of euchromatin in the nucleus, numerous secretory vesicles, and abundant microvilli [Fig.4].

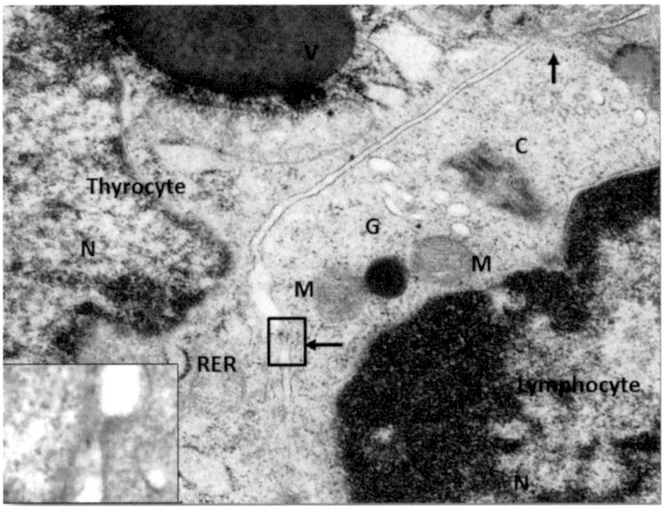

Figure 3. The lymphocyte between thyroid follicles in Hashimoto's thyroiditis. The lymphocyte is connected with the thyrocyte by an immune synapse limited by zonula adherens without cell membrane fusion (pSMAC). The space (cSMAC) is visible in the center of the immune synapse. The lymphocyte organelles are polarized under the synapse: centriole, mitochondria, granules, and Golgi complex. Signs of damage are present in the thyrocyte: enlarged cisterns of rough endoplasmic reticulum. C-centriole, M-mitochondria, G-Golgi system, L-lysosome, RER- rough endoplasmic reticulum, N-nucleus. TEM magm.25 000x

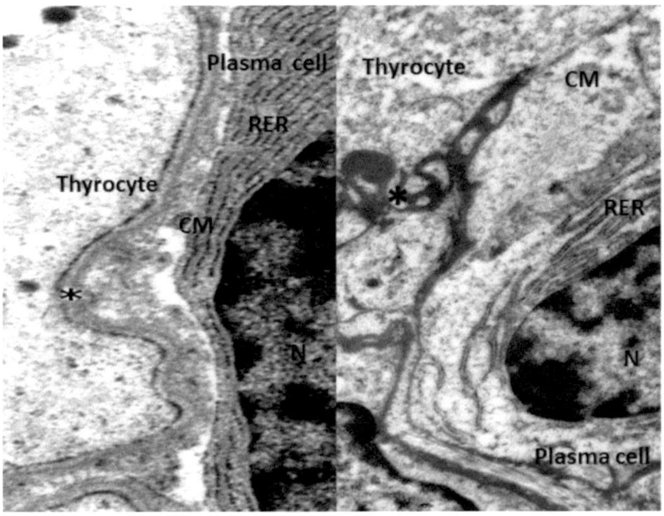

Figure 4. The plasma cells in contact with thyrocytes in Graves' disease. a) The space of the immune synapse in which electron dense substances, probably antibodies, are secreted. Enlarged cisterns of endoplasmic reticulum were observed in the thyrocyte. RER-rough endoplasmic reticulum, CM cell membrane, * immunoglobulins. TEM magn. 25 000x. b)The advanced phase of the immune reaction: the deposits of immunoglobulins in the space between the thyrocyte and plasmocyte. The space of the immune synapse is limited by zonula adherens. CM – cell membrane, RER – rough endoplasmic reticulum, * immunoglobulins deposit. TEM magn. 25 000x

In Hashimoto's thyroiditis, polarization of plasma cells was observed; the centrioles and Golgi system, mitochondria and well-developed rough endoplasmic reticulum were observed in the part connected with thyrocytes. In some areas of the contact places, secretion of substances with medium electron density from plasma cells to thyrocytes was observed [Fig.5]. The plasma cells adhered in a large area to thyrocytes, and the thyrocytes exhibited features of damage and destruction: fragmentation of the endoplasmic reticulum, edema of mitochondria, and condensation of the chromatin in the nucleus. In advanced stages, destruction and fragmentation of thyrocytes were observed.

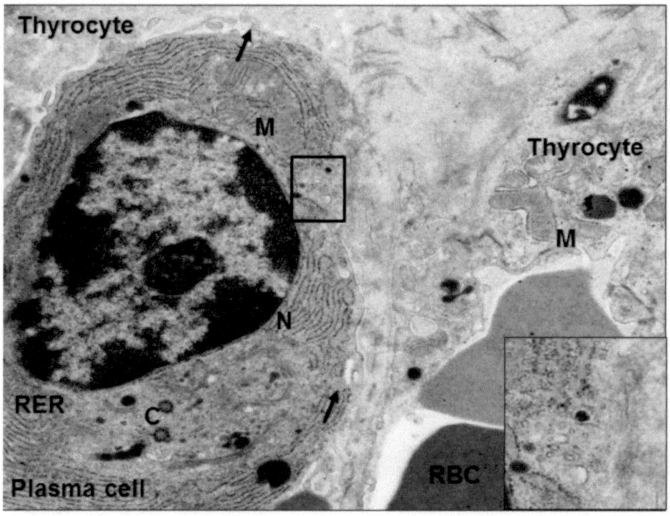

Figure 5. The plasma cell in contact with thyrocyte in Hashimoto's thyroiditis. The immune synapse is composed of a surrounding adhesion zone (pSMAC) in the central part of the site of exocytosis of electron dense substances and vesicles from plasma cell. Polarization of the organelle is visible in the plasma cell: centrioles, lysosomes, and mitochondria in the region of immune synapse. The thyrocyte is damaged with edema of mitochondria and destruction of endoplasmic reticulum. C-centriole, M-mitochondrium, RER- rough endoplasmic reticulum, N-nucleus. TEM magm.25 000x

5. Discussion

The immune synapses occurring in the thyroids of patients with Graves' disease were similar to the synapse described by Dustin [23]. Dynamic studies with planar bilayers further showed that the immune synapse was formed through a nascent intermediate in which activating TCR clusters are formed first in the pSMAC and then move to the cSMAC region in an F-actin-dependent process in a few minutes to form the pattern [7].

In the connection between thyrocytes and T-cells, the zonula occludens in Graves' disease and zonula adherens in Hashimoto's thyroiditis seem to be the peripheral pSMAC and the space in the center can correspond to the central supramolecular activation complex cSMAC.

An interesting observation is the difference in polarization of lymphocytes in immune synapses. The lymphocyte stimulating thyrocytes in Graves' disease were not polarized, but the cytotoxic lymphocytes in Hashimoto's thyroiditis had polarized organelles in the cytoplasm.

The polarization of the T-cell, i.e. formation of a center with a centriole, mitochondria, and Golgi complex suggested special organization of the cellular tubules and filaments. Actin filaments (F-actin) play a critical role throughout the various stages of T cell activation. In the steady state, actin polymerization at the leading edge and cytoskeletal contraction at the lamelliopodium mediate rapid migration [24].The microtubule organizing center (MTOC) and microtubule network of the cell provide a molecular way for vesicle movement and structural support for polarized cell functions. Within seconds after TCR stimulation, the MTOC mobilizes and polarizes to the immune synapse in T cells. Polarization is important for efficient trafficking and directed secretion of cytolytic granules and cytokines for secretion at the synapse [25-27]

Previous studies [28-30] report that mitochondria accumulate at the immunological synapse following T-cell stimulation. The fusion factor DRP1 (dynamin-related protein 1) regulates mitochondria positioning close to the peripheral supramolecular activation cluster (pSMAC), which together with the central SMAC forms the immune synapse in T cells [19]. The immune synapse controls calcium signals and calcium-dependent T-cell functions [31]. Our observations *in vivo* are similar to pictures from the electron microscope from investigations in cell culture published by Tsun [32].

Probably, the polarization of organelles in the cytotoxic lymphocytes observed is connected with transport of cytotoxic substances from these cells to thyrocytes.

Stinchcombe [33] observed NK cells conjugated with B-cells with glycolipid-pulsed CD1-bearing targets. High-resolution electron micrographs of the immunological synapse formed between NK and iNKT cytolytic cells with their targets revealed that, in both NK and iNKT cells, the centrioles could be found associated (or 'docked') with the plasma membrane within the immunological synapse. Secretory clefts were visible within the synapses formed by both NK and iNKT cells, and secretory lysosomes were polarized along microtubules leading towards the docked centrosome. The Golgi apparatus and recycling endosomes were also polarized towards the centrosome at the plasma membrane within the synapse [33]. It seems that the polarization process is connected with the cytotoxic interactions between T-cells and thyrocytes in Hashimoto's thyroiditis.

The immune synapse between plasma cells and APCs has been seldom described. Batista described the immunological synapse between plasma cells and antigen presenting cells [34]. We observed two types of immune synapses between plasma cells and thyrocytes in AITD. In Graves' disease, they are the stimulating synapses: immunoglobulins encrusting the basal membrane of the thyrocyte were secreted in the central space of the synapse and were probably connected with TSH- receptors. In the last phase of this process, deposits of immunoglobulins were visible. The similar change were observed in kidney [35,36]. In glomerulonephritis, subendothelial complement deposits [36,37] and sun epithelial (similar to situation in thyroid)

http://dx.doi.org/10.5772/53009

immunoglobulins deposits [35, 36] were observed. In Hashimoto's thyroiditis, the plasma cells were polarized and formed the microtubule organizing center (MTOC) consisting of centrioles, mitochondria and Golgi apparatus and probably microtubules and microfilaments. The peripheral zonula adherens surrounded the place of immunoglobulin secretion, but the immunoglobulins penetrated to thyrocytes and probably led to damage to these cells [38].

6. Conclusions

- Immune synapses between T-cells and plasma cells with thyroid's epithelial cells were found in AITD.
- In the ultrastructure of the synapse, peripheral zonula occludens or zonula adherens and a central space were observed in all types of the immune synapses.
- The lymphocytes forming the cytotoxic synapse were characterized by presence of a microtubule-organizing center.

Acknowledgements

This work was supported by Grant 2P05E04327 from the Polish Ministry of Science and Higher Education.

Author details

Iwona Ben-Skowronek[1] and Roman Ciechanek[2]

*Address all correspondence to: skowroneki@interia.pl

*Address all correspondence to: ciechanek.r@wp.pl

1 Department of Paediatric Endocrinology and Diabetology, Medical University in Lublin,, Poland

2 Division of Surgery, Provincial Specialist Hospital in Lublin,, Poland

Competing interests. The authors declare that they have no competing interests.

Ethics. The investigation was accepted by the local Ethical Committee at the Medical University in Lublin. All children's parents signed an informed consent before autopsy or surgical operation.

References

[1] Poo WJ, Conrad L, Janeway Jr. CA. Receptor-directed focusing of lymphokine release by helper T cells. Nature.1988. 332:378–380.

[2] Kupfer A, Swain SL, Singer SJ. The specific direct interaction of helper T cells and antigen-presenting B cells. II. Reorientation of the microtubule organizing center and reorganization of the membrane-associated cytoskeleton inside the bound helper T cells. J. Exp. Med.1987. 165:1565–1580.

[3] Kupfer A, Singer SJ. The specific interaction of helper T cells and antigen-presenting B cells. IV. Membrane and cytoskeletal reorganizations in the bound T cell as a function of antigen dose. J. Exp. Med.1989. 170:1697–1713. doi:10.1084/jem.170.5.1697.

[4] Grakoui A, Bromley SK, Sumen C, Davis MM., Shaw AS, Allen PM, Dustin ML. The immunological synapse: a molecular machine controlling T cell activation. Science 1999, 285 (5425): 221–227.

[5] Davis DM, Chiu I, Fassett M, Cohen GB, Mandelboim O, Strominger,JL. The human natural killer cell immune synapse. Proc Natl Acad Sci U S A 1999, 96 (26): 15062–7.

[6] Griffiths GM, Tsun,A, Stinchcombe JC. The immunological synapse: a focal point for endocytosis and exocytosis. J Cell Biol. 2010 (189) 3:390-408.

[7] Monks CR, Freiberg BA, Kupfer H., Sciaky N, Kupfer A. Three-dimensional segregation of supramolecular activation clusters in T cells. Nature 1998, 395:82–86.

[8] Dustin ML. The cellular context of T cell signaling. Immunity 2009, 30:482–492.

[9] Campi G, Varma R, Dustin ML. Actin and agonist MHC–peptide complex–dependent T cell receptor microclusters as scaffolds for signaling. J. Exp. Med. 2005,202:1031–1036.

[10] Yokosuka T, Sakata-Sogawa K, Kobayashi W, Hiroshima M, Hashimoto-Tane A, Tokunaga M, Dustin ML, Saito T. Newly generated T cell receptor microclusters initiate and sustain T cell activation by recruitment of Zap70 and SLP-76. Nat. Immunol.2005, 6:1253–1262.

[11] Varma R, Campi G, Yokosuka T, Saito T, Dustin ML. T cell receptor-proximal signals are sustained in peripheral microclusters and terminated in the central supramolecular activation cluster. Immunity 2006, 25:117–127.

[12] Depoil D, Fleire S, Treanor BL, Weber M, Harwood NE, Marchbank KL, Tybulewicz VL, Batista FD. CD19 is essential for B cell activation by promoting B cell receptor-antigen microcluster formation in response to membrane-bound ligand. Nat. Immunol 2008, 9:63–72.

[13] Beal AM, Anikeeva N, Varma R, Cameron TO, Vasiliver-Shamis G, Norris PJ, Dustin ML, Sykulev Y. Kinetics of early T cell receptor signaling regulate the pathway of lytic granule delivery to the secretory domain. Immunity 2009. 31:632–642.

[14] Jenkins MR, Tsun A , Stinchcombe JC, Griffiths GM. The strength of T cell receptor signal controls the polarization of cytotoxic machinery to the immunological synapse. Immunity. 2009.31:621–631.

[15] Das V, Nal B, Dujeancourt A, Thoulouze MI, Galli T, Roux P, Dautry-Varsat A, Alcover A. Activation-induced polarized recycling targets T cell antigen receptors to the immunological synapse; involvement of SNARE complexes. Immunity. 2004. 20:577–588.

[16] Stinchcombe JC, Barral DC, Mules EH, Booth S, Hume AN, Machesky LM, Seabra MC, Griffiths GM. Rab27a is required for regulated secretion in cytotoxic T lymphocytes. J. Cell Biol.2001. 152:825–834.

[17] Stinchcombe JC, Griffiths GM. Secretory mechanisms in cell-mediated cytotoxicity. Annu. Rev. Cell Dev. Biol.2007. 23:495–517.

[18] Stinchcombe JC, Majorovits E, Bossi G, Fuller S, Griffiths GM. Centrosome polarization delivers secretory granules to the immunological synapse. Nature. 2006.443:462–465.

[19] Junker C, Hoth M. Immune synapses: mitochondrial morphology matters. EMBO Journal 2011, 30:1187-1189.

[20] Mempel TR, Henrickson SE, Von Andrian UH. T-cell priming by dendritic cells in lymph nodes occurs in three distinct phases. Nature. 2004;427:154–59.

[21] Hosseini BH, Louban I, Djandji D, Wabnitz GH, Deeg J, Bulbuc N, et al. Immune synapse formation determines interaction forces between T cells and antigen-presenting cells measured by atomic force microscopy. Proc Natl Acad Sci USA. 2009;106:17852–17857.

[22] Scholer A, Hugues S, Boissonnas A, Fetler L, Amigorena S. Intercellular adhesion molecule-1-dependent stable interactions between T cells and dendritic cells determine CD8+ T cell memory. Immunity. 2008;28:258–70.

[23] Dustin ML. The immunological synapse. Arthritis Res Therapy. 2002. 4 (Suppl 3): 119-125.

[24] Giannone G, Dubin-Thaler BJ, Rossier O, Cai Y, Chaga O, et al. Lamellipodial actin mechanically links myosin activity with adhesion-site formation. Cell. 2007;128:561–75.

[25] Geiger B, Rosen D, Berke G. Spatial relationships of microtubule-organizing centers and the contact area of cytotoxic T lymphocytes and target cells. J Cell Biol. 1982;95:137–43.

[26] Kupfer A, Dennert G, Singer SJ. Polarization of the Golgi apparatus and the microtubule-organizing center within cloned natural killer cells bound to their targets. Proc Natl Acad Sci USA. 1983;80:7224–28.

[27] Kupfer A, Mosmann TR, Kupfer H. Polarized expression of cytokines in cell conjugates of helper T cells and splenic B cells. Proc Natl Acad Sci USA. 1991;88:775–79.

[28] Quintana A, Schwindling C, Wenning AS, Becherer U, Rettig J, Schwarz EC, Hoth M. T cell activation requires mitochondrial translocation to the immunological synapse. Proc Natl Acad Sci USA. 2007. 104: 14418–14423.

[29] Contento RL, Campello S, Trovato AE, Magrini E, Anselmi F, Viola A. Adhesion shapes T cells for prompt and sustained T-cell receptor signaling. EMBO J 2010.29: 4035–4047.

[30] Baixauli F, Martín-Cófreces NB, Morlino G, Carrasco YR, Calabia-Linares C, Veiga E, Serrador JM, Sánchez-Madrid F. The mitochondrial fission factor dynamin-related protein 1 modulates T-cell receptor signaling at the immune synapse. EMBO J 2011.30: 1238–1250.

[31] Kummerow C, Junker C, Kruse K, Rieger H, Quintana A, Hoth M The immunological synapse controls local and global calcium signals in T lymphocytes. Immunol Rev . 2009.231: 132–147.

[32] Tsun A, Qureshi I, Stinchcombe JC, Jenkins JR, de la Roche M, Kleczkowska J, Zamoyska R, Griffiths GM. Centrosome docking at the immunological synapse is controlled by Lck signaling. J. Cell Biol.2011;192:663-674, (10.1083/jcb.201008140).

[33] Stinchcombe JC, Salio M, Cerundala V, Pende D, Arico M, Griffiths GM. Centriole polarization to the immunological synapse direct secretion from cytolytic cells of both the innate and adaptive immune systems. BMC Biology 2011, 9-45.

[34] Batista, F.D., D. Iber, M.S. Neuberger. B cells acquire antigen from target cells after synapse formation. Nature.2001. 411:489–494.

[35] Qiu Y, Korteweg C, Chen Z, Li J, Luo J, Huang G and Gu J. Immunoglobulin G expression and its colocalization with complement proteins in papillary thyroid cancer. Modern Pathology 2012; 25, 36–45

[36] Howie AJ. Handbook of Renal Biopsy Pathology. Springer 2nd edition 2008:175-182.

[37] Licht C, Hoppe B. Complement defects in children which result in kidney diseases: diagnosis and therapy. In Complement and kidney disease. Edited by Zipfel PF. Basel-Boston-Berlin 2006 Bikhauser Verlag: 184-197.

[38] Rebuffat SA, Nguyen B,Robert B, Castex F, Peraldi Roux S. Antiperoxidase Antibody-Dependent Cytotoxicity in Autoimmune Thyroid Disease. J Clin Endocrinol Metab, 2008;93;3: 929-934

Section 2

Infectious Agents and Host Inflammatory Response

Chapter 7

Microbiome and Autoimmunity

Natalie Cherepahina, Zaur Shogenov,
Mariya Bocharova, Murat Agirov,
Jamilyia Tabaksoeva, Mikhail Paltsev and
Sergey Suchkov

Additional information is available at the end of the chapter

http://dx.doi.org/10.5772/54128

1. Introduction

Most of the currently known infections represent a persistent and stepwise development of the canonical chronic diseases of infectious origin (CDIO) associated with conditionally pathogenic microorganisms, i.e., viruses, intracellular parasites and other representatives of the endogenous microbiome, particularly, those manifesting with atypical properties. Pathogens are able to interact between themselves and to cause a disease, and the pathogens' genomes break the subtle regulation of microbial ecosystems (*microbiomes*) (Suchkov et al., 2007).

The aforementioned studies have led to a reappraisal of Koch's postulates to announce that he had shown theoretically more then a hundred years before: one microbe causes one disease. Interactions of microbial pathogens with specific tools of the patient's immune machinery in due the course of the infectious process give rise to different types of *micro-biocenosis* to manifest a broad range of activities of the microbiome-related pathogens including their ability to suppress the immune response.

The key role of immune-related and microbial factor in CDIO pathogenesis is evidently proved today. However, a comparison of types of the patient's individual immune responses and the features of *microbial landscapes* with the clinical manifestations of the disease (*clinical pattern*) by singling out postinfectious clinical-and-immunological syndrome (PICIS) as a pathogenically oriented category and a fundamental term is appearing to be a more complicated objective to be cleared.

As many authors established, for CDIO-related specific form of PICIS has clinical and prognostic significance and informative and thus predictive value, because, for sure, PICIS determines to a considerable degree the extant of progressing and chronization of the underlying disease whilst determining risks of complications.

Postinfectious secondary immunodeficiency syndrome (PIFSI) is a *monosyndromal* and predominant form of PICIS in patients with CDIO.

More than in a third of cases another form of PICIS could be formed and thus observed, accompanying by postinfectious autoimmune syndrome (PIFA) reflecting the involvement of immune-mediated autoaggression, or PIFASID as an associated form of immune imbalance.

The susceptibility to one or another form of CDIO-associated PICIS depends on a number of genetically determined factors, which play a crucial role in formation of the patient's immune resources *via* cooperation between mechanisms of innate and adaptive immunity (Fig. 1).

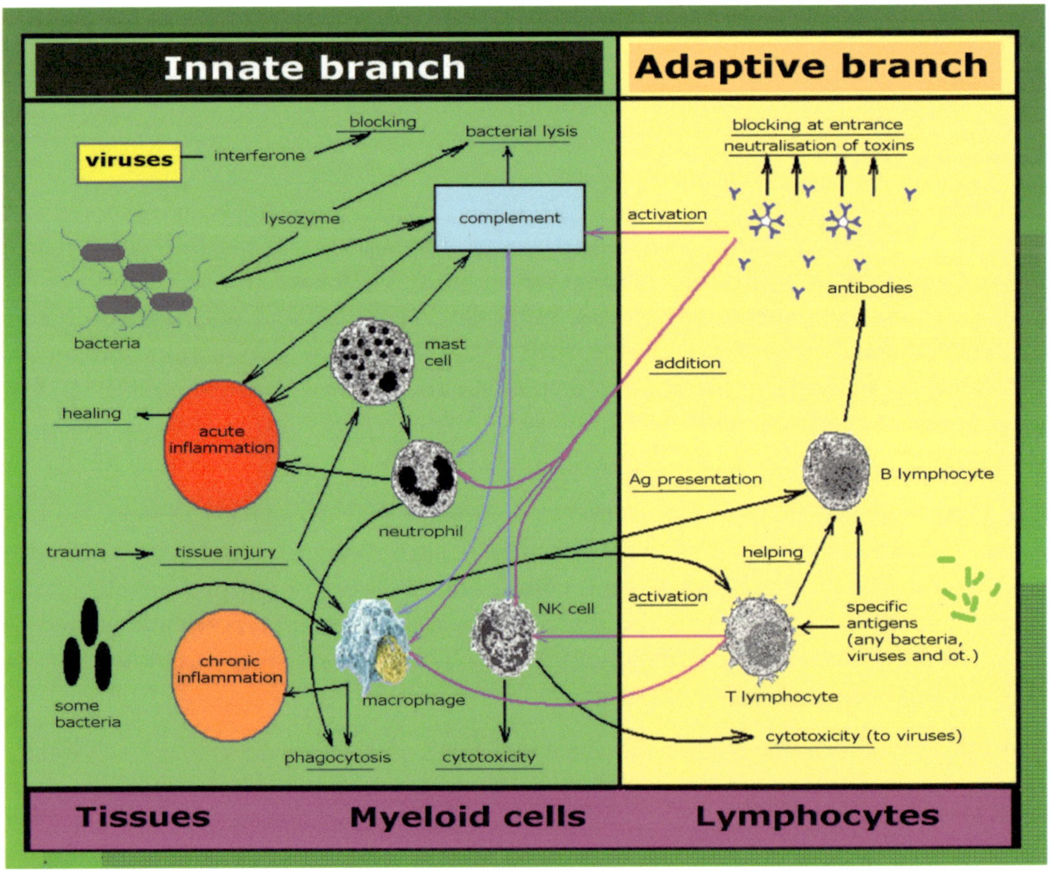

Note: NK, natural killer

Figure 1. Main features of innate and adaptive immunity

Unfortunately, the role of these mechanisms in the development and chronization of infectious diseases is still obscure, which deprives a doctor of the possibility to improve the currently available models of CDIO chronization with the ultimate goal to develop the most advanced treatment-and-rehabilitation in a package of the preventive treatment protocols, and their implementation into routine and daily clinical practice (Paltsev et al., 2009a).

The key role in the chronization and thus complications of such diseases, and thus the development of the associated immune disorders is played by:

i. properties of the infectious agent;

ii. type of a patient's immune response.

The microbial factor may promote development of a vast array of the associated immune disorders and thus forms of immune-mediated pathologies (PICIS), particularly, owing the microorganisms to gain, in the running course of the disease evolution, a large arsenal of intrinsic tools enabling microbes to escape from attacks of immune-mediated weapon, to attenuate and the latter whilst getting them weakened or to influence the dynamics of the clinical manifestations of PICIS itself. Actually, the severity and duration of CDIO depends on the interaction between the microbiome and the antimicrobial immunity machinery (Paltsev et al., 2009b).

2. PICIS and its role in the state-of-the-art model of immunopathogenesis of chronic infectious diseases

The PICIS variants include:

1. postinfectious secondary immunodeficiency syndrome (PIFSIS);
2. postinfectious autoimmune syndrome (PIFAS);
3. PIFAS coupled with PIFSIS (PIFASID) (Suchkov et al., 2004).

The occurrence and thus incidence of these syndromes in CDIO patients differs statistically depending on the form of a type of the primary infection and the stage of the destructive inflammatory process in the targeted organs or tissues. For example, the initial (including *subclinical*) stages of any clinical courses of CDIO are usually concomitant with a predominant (>50%) formation of PIFSIS, while the quotes of PIFAS and PIFASID do not exceed 20%.

This situation changes with further development and chronization of the infectious process and its transformation from a subclinical into the clinical stage, viz., the incidence of autoimmune syndromes increases substantially. In intermediate stages of chronization, the quotes of PIFAS reach 50%, whilst in the final stages of chronization similar indices of PIFASID reach 60%.

It may thus be concluded that PIFSIS is not only the outcome of the infectious process, but, rather, the major factor responsible for provoking complications and raising thus a chronic relapsing course. The role of *progression* and *chronization* of the disease is determined, in a large measure, by the form of PICIS or, rather, of PIFAS and PIFASID, which reflect the manifestations and thus a pattern of postinfectious autoaggression (Suchkov et al., 2004).

3. *Microbiome* and its role in the state-of-the-art model of CDIO pathogenesis

A crucial role in CDIO pathogenesis is played by primary and superinfectious factors endowed with the ability to generate large microbial associates. Therefore, the features of the patient's microbiome are key etiopathogenic links for realization of the infection-associated chronization phenomenon.

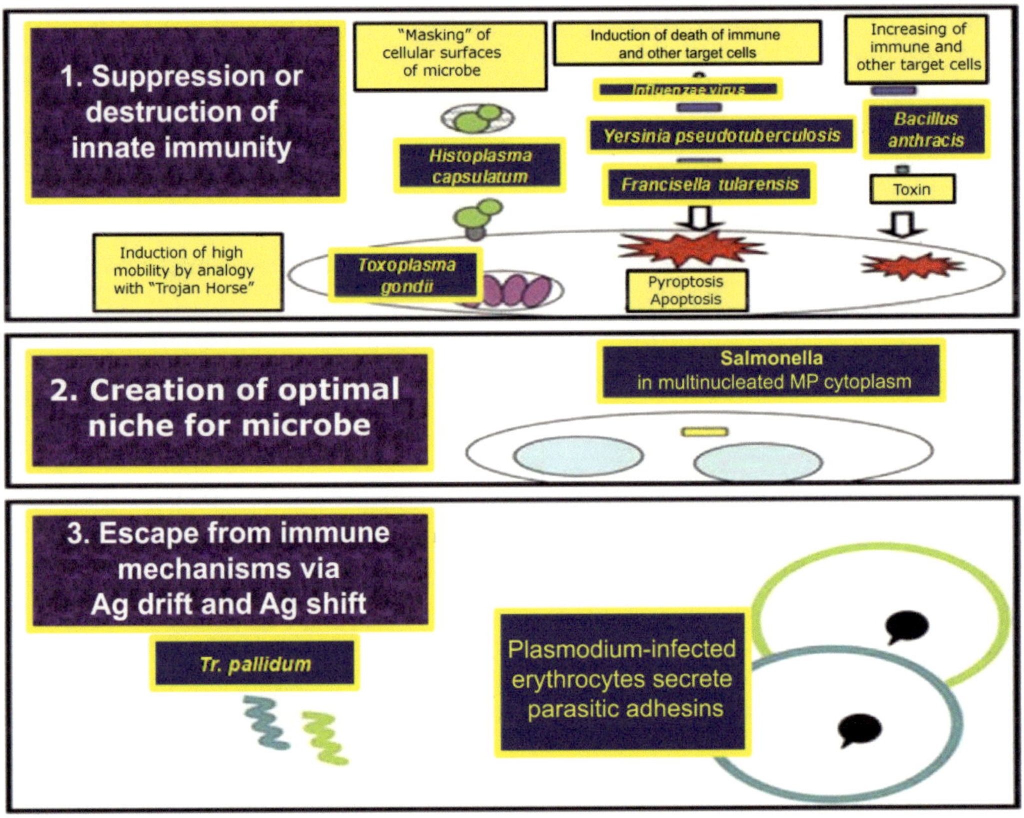

Notes: *Ag*, antigen

Figure 2. Scenarios of interactions between a microbial pathogen and the patient's antimicrobial immune response illustrating an escape from the immune supervision to survive

Moreover, in a course of their evolution microorganisms acquire a vast array of molecular and cellular tools enabling them to escape from the intrinsic control of the immune system

http://dx.doi.org/10.5772/54128

over the microbiome itself, to switch off mechanisms of the control over the microbiome, or to initiate changes underlying the *resistance* phenomenon (Fig. 2). As a result of the antagonistic interactions between a microbe and the antimicrobial immunity machinery, the immune response is either not elicited at all or is only partly activated giving rise to manifestations of PIFSIS, or progressing in a form provoking either PIFAS or PIFASID. This is concomitant with the formation of membrane films by clinical isolates of pathogenic microorganisms escaping from the control of antimicrobial agents.

In 30% of cases, the causative agent is not cultivated, but, rather, is converted into the *L*-form, which does not exclude the presence of an "invisible" pathogen in the course of the instrumental and laboratory diagnostics procedures, and implies the latent progress of the infectious process. The latter presents particular interest because the conversion of some microorganisms into the latent (*cryptic* or *sleeping*) form is one of the ways to chronization by escaping from the proper immune response.

4. Features of microbial spectra in CDIO patients

Conventional (predominantly, *gram*-negative) bacterial flora is detected in the majority of CDIO patients, though the results of the recent studies testify not only to the growth of *gram*-negative microorganisms, but also to a dramatic increase in the number of superinfectious pathogens of viral and parasitic origin.

The results of our recent studies suggest that the most frequently occurring human infections may conventionally be divided into two main categories:

1. susceptibility to relapsing infections provoked by pyogenic bacteria (*S. pneumoniae, S. aureus*, etc.) with a minimum *mimicking* resource increases dramatically in patients whose disorders are linked with antibody (Ab), complement and phagocytosis deficiency, PIFSI being the predominant form of PICIS;

2. a particular susceptibility to viral and intracellular pathogens endowing with a high *mimicking* potential increases in patients with disturbances in primary cell-mediated immunity (Fig. 3)

Fluorescence has been used to show that the process of intraintestinal hatching of *Trichuris muris* is critically dependent on the attachment of an enterobacterium to the polar operculum of the egg (*Panel A*). Hatched worms attach to the bowel wall and induce activation of type 2 helper T (Th2) cells, which in turn inhibit the proliferation and differentiation of type 17 helper T (Th17) and regulatory T (Treg) cells. In contrast, worm development was halted and specific immune responses were altered in mice that were depleted of gram-negative enterobacteria by antibiotics (*Panel B*), underscoring the influence of the intraintestinal environment on intestinal immune responses.

At the same time intracellular pathogens interfere in cell nucleus during DNA transcription. One of the key mechanisms by which microbes achieve the immunosuppressive effects is by subverting one of the body's most prolific nuclear receptors, the vitamin D receptor (VDR). Defects in VDR signaling transduction have previously been linked to bacterial infection and chronic inflammation. Each pathogen that decreases VDR expression makes it easier for other pathogens themselves to slow immune activity even further, creating a snowball effect.

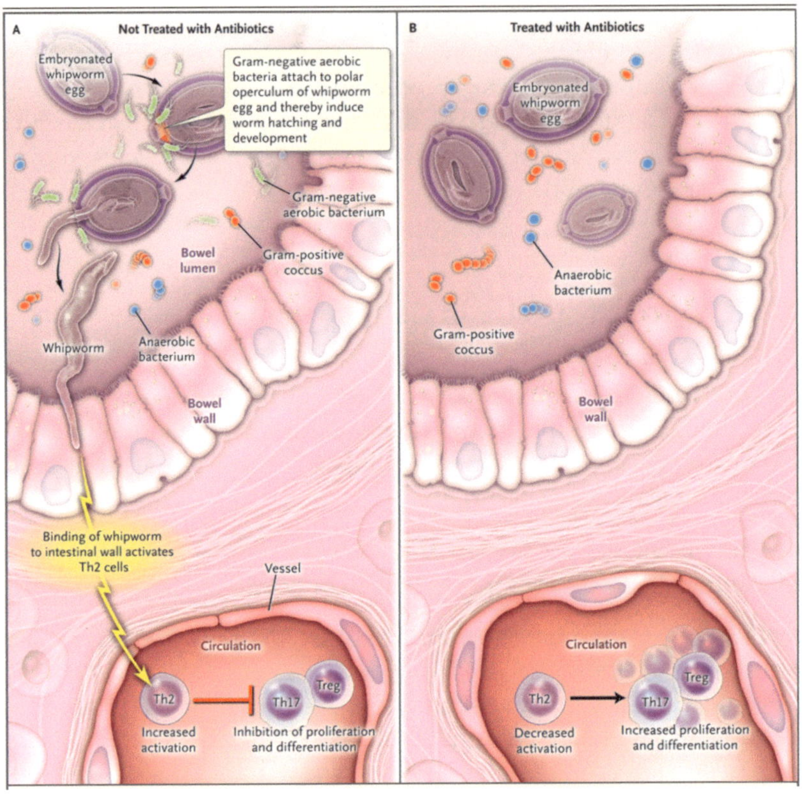

Figure 3. Hatching Parasites

However, a complete set of mechanisms by which persistent intracellular microbes slow innate immune activity has yet to be definitively determined (Proal A. D. et al. 2011). In such patients, these microorganisms provoke fast progressing infections associated with PIFA or moderate PIFSI with an impending transformation of PIFSI into PIFASID.

Microbiomes detected and properly assessed in the course of chronization and progression of CDIO are characterized by a high degree of multiplicity and variability, which have every right to be regarded as clinically important chronization criteria regardless of the nosological form of the disease. At the same time, the intrinsic architectonics of microbiomes varies widely depending on the microbial category:

1. in some cases (ICIIP and COPD/CP), the dominant is common to all microbial categories (including the total virulent resource/TVR);

2. for other categories (e.g., CPN), the bacterial dominant (which is TVR-limited) displays, contrary to ICIIP and COPD/CP, a "gap" in both specific ratio and virus variety;

3. in certain disorders (e.g., chronic myocarditis/CM), the specific ratio of bacteria and their TVR tend to minimum against the background of an absolute viral dominant.

5. Features of interactions between patient's antimicrobial immunity and etiopathogens during PICIS formation in the course of disease progression

The main feature of the defense immune response to the infective pathogen is formation of two subpopulations of regulatory T helper cells (Th cells). Effector CD4+ Th cells divide into Th-1, Th-2, Th-3 and Th-17 subpopulations depending on cytokines secreted, transcription factors and signal pathways. Th1 cells trigger effector mechanisms of cell-mediated immunity, and Th2 cells are responsible for antibody (Ab) formation (Mc Guirk et al., 2002) (Fig. 4).

Th3 cells (or regulatory Treg-cells) are the other clone of cells expressing CD4+ and CD25+. They are able to regulate functions of Th1/Th2 subpopulations and to maintain immune homeostasis (Sakaguchi, 2004; Shevach, 2002).

Th3 cells come from thymic CD4+ progenitor cells in the presence of IL-2 and TNF-β. Naive At the periphery CD4+ T cells can be converted by the signals transmitted through STATS in the presence of TNF-β into inducible Treg expressing transcription factor FoxP3 (Koenen, 2008). These cells are characterized also by low level of IL-2 and IFN-γ production and high level of IL-10, IL-35, TGF- β production. Two regulatory or proinflammatory cytokines, IL-10 and TNF-β, mediate suppression of the immune responses against autoAgs and thus prevention of autoimmune diseases.

Note: Ag, Lc, IL, NK, GM-CSF, TNF, IFN, LT, MP, antigen, leukocyte, interleukin, natural killer cell, granulocyte-monocyte colony-stimulating factor, tumor necrosis factor, interferon, leukotriene, macrophage, respectively; Th, T helper cell.

The development of autoimmune diseases was previously associated only with Th1 cells, but absence of IFN-γ not only prevents development of autoimmunity in mice, but accelerates process. This fact has lead to discovery of a separate subclone of T cells, differing from Th1 cells and capable of inducing local inflammation and autoimmunity.

This clone (Th17) is derived from naive CD4+ T cells in response to stimulation with IL-6, IL-23, IL-1β, TGF-β (Stochinger et al., 2007). IL-6 and IL-23 activate STAT3, which enhances the expression of transcription factors RORyt RORy, which in turn increase the expression of major cytokines of the clones - IL17A; IL17F; IL21; IL22 (Dyachenko & Dyachenko, 2010).

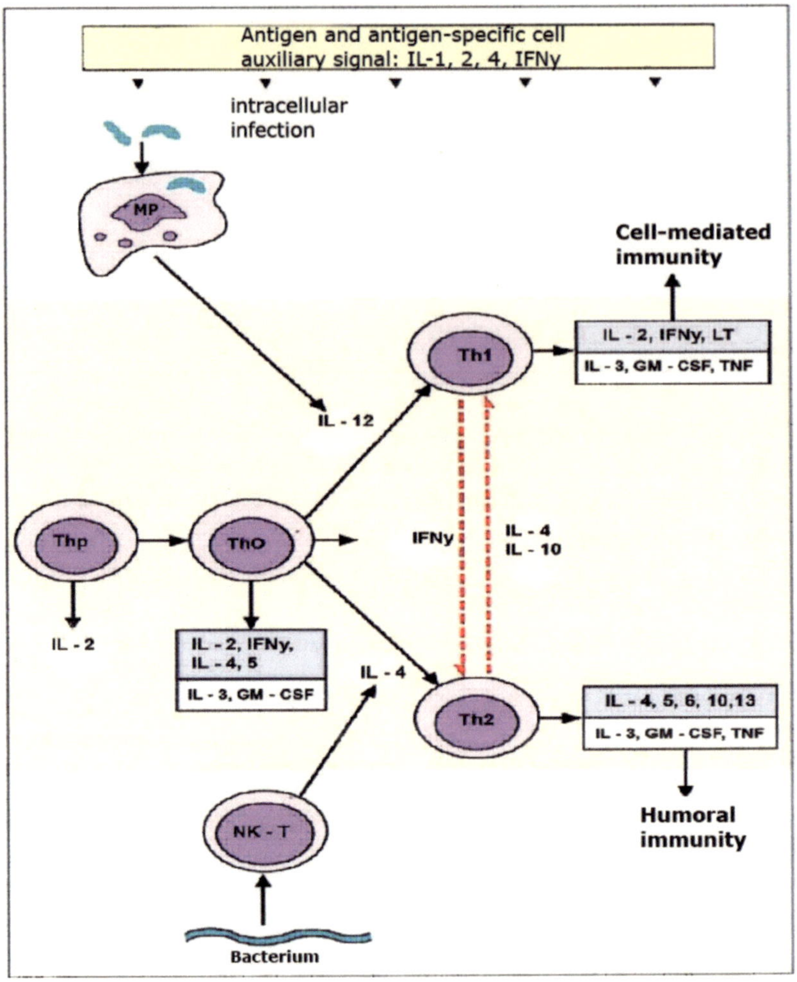

Figure 4. Ag-specific differentiation of T cells in two main-line directions and formation of regulatory Th1, Th2 cells

Thus, the differentiation of T cells is a result of the coordinated activity of cytokines and transcription factors. At the same time TGF-β produced by dendritic cells and macrophages may send differentiation of naive T cells both in the direction of Treg cells (CD4 + CD25 + FoxP3+), and in the direction of Th17 cells producing IL-17 (Aarvak, 2009; Chabaud et al.. 2001).. It occurs as a result of the expression of transcription factor FoxP3 and RORyt, which are important for the differentiation of Treg or Th17cells, respectively.

High concentrations of TGF-β stimulate production of FoxP3, which block the expression of genes associated with RORyt, resulting in the differentiation of naive CD4 + T-cells in ROR-yt, and it leads to the differentiation of Th17 cells and expression of IL-17 (Volpe et al., 2008; Zhou et al., 2008).. It is believed that FoxP3 rivals with RORyt through physical interaction, while the inflammatory mediators IL-6 and IL-21 implement their inhibitory effect on post-translational level (Zhou et al., 2008).

Th17 cell line plays an important role in protection against a variety of microorganisms, have a strong proinflammatory effect by expressing IL-17. IL-17 promotes an expansion and recruitment of innate-related immune cells such as neutrophils enhances the inflammatory nuclear reactions together with TLR-ligands, IL-1β, TNF-α and stimulates the production of beta defensives and other antimicrobial peptides (Vojdani et al., 2006a, Vojdani et al., 2006b, Vojdani et al., 2006c, Chung et al., 2009; McGeachy et al., 2009). IL-17RA (its receptor) has common characteristics with classical receptors of innate immunity, and its intracellular tail domain transmits a signal over a general inflammatory transduction pathway, thus linking the innate and adaptive immunity.

The role of Th17 is not clear in case of viral and parasitic infections. Thus, for instance, Th17-induced response inhibits apoptosis of virus-infected cells and contributes to the persistence of the virus. Tissue infiltrated with activated Th17 lymphocytes producing significant amounts IL-17, IL-26, IL-21, IL-22, TNF-α and lymphotoxin-B in chronic inflammation (Yu et al;., 2009; Cho et al., 2004). Production of these cytokines is inversely related with the production of Th-1 and Th-2 cytokines.

Localization of etiopathogen, i.e., out-or intracellular, is a factor determining the development of a particular immune response and, therefore, one or other form of PICIS as a result of specific immune response (Mazo et al., 2007; Litvinov et al., 2008; Zhmurov et al., 2000; Rumyantsev & Goncharova, 2000).

The latter circumstance is important not only to the pathogenesis, but also from a clinical point of view, since much of the pathogens that have the ability to escape from immune response, also create unpredictable risks of complications and difficulties with the choice of treatment scheme. Herewith therapy should be personalized, taking into account the spectra of producing cytokines: IFN-y (Th1); IL-4, IL-5, IL-13 (Th2); IL-17 (Th17). The aim of such therapy may be the modulation effects caused in separate factors, cytokines, and transcription factors.

In so doing, the crucial factor responsible for the development of one or another type of the immune response and, accordingly, one or another form of PICIS is extra- and intracellular localization of the etiopathogen. The latter is important not only from the pathogenic, but also from the clinical point of view, because a considerable amount of pathogens escaping from the immune response involve unpredictable complications and difficulty in the choice of treatment strategies (Antonov & Tsinzerling, 2001; Borisov, 2000; Kukhtevich et al., 1997; Morozov, 2001 Paukov, 1996).

According to our original data, at least three forms of PICIS, viz., PIFSI, PIFA and PIFA-SID, are identified in the paradigm of immune pathologies associated with the underlying disease.

PIFSIS is a dominant monosyndromal form of associated immune pathologies. In other cases, we deal with the formation of a different clinical immunologic syndrome reflecting autoimmune PIFA aggression. In some patients, a combination of PIFSIS and PIFAS gives rise to the appearance of the bisyndromal form of immunopathology (PIFASID).

6. Forms of PICIS

6.1. PIFSI

Abatement of antimicrobial protective mechanisms due to deficiency of innate immunity concomitant with imbalances in the adaptive branch is a crucial feature of PIFSIS, which manifests itself as a chronic disease (presumably, of bacterial and mixed origin). Suppression of the activity of its effector links markedly weakens the patient's response to the infecting pathogen resulting in the persistence of the pathogenic microorganism, or superinfection with conditionally pathogenic microorganisms maintaining low-intensity processes.

6.2. PIFAS

Many proteins from pathogens share structural similarities with human proteins, and those can also contribute to autoantibody (autoAb) production (Fig. 5). Lekakh et al. found that polyspesific autoAbs harvested from sera of healthy donors were able to cross-react with DNA and lipopolysaccharides of bacterial strains including *Escherichia coli, Pseudomonas aeruginosa, Shigella boydii, and Salmonella.* Furthermore, since human Abs are polyspecific, it is likely that some of them produced to target pathogens may mistakenly target human proteins, causing 'collateral damage' (Khitrov et al., 2007).

In the course of CDIO progression, a portion of autoreactive cytotoxic T lymphocytes (CTL) able to interact with cross-reacting microbial Ags associated with pathogen-conditioned infection undergo activation under the influence of various factors including molecular *mimicry* (Khitrov et al., 2007a; Fujinami et al., 2006; Rose & Mackay, 2000; Benoist & Mathis, 2001).

The consequences of this phenomenon manifest themselves during recognition of autoepitopes by autoreactive CTL as a result of which PIFAS acquires an ability to attack any organ or tissue in the infected host. The risk of development of this syndrome increases dramatically with increasing morbidity from infectious diseases and at high rates of pathogen flows, as, e.g. in mixed infections (Sanaev et al., 2007; Cherepakhina et al., 2010a).

At present, there exist three explanations for the associative interplay between the infection and the risks of PIFAS occurrence based on activation of autoreactive clones of T and B cells:

a. activation of microbial superAgs;

b. leakage of cryptic (intramolecular) autoepitopes;

c. molecular mimicry (Bauer et al., 2001; Bingen-Bidois et al., 2002; Blackwell et al., 1987; Carballido et al., 2003; Dantzer & Wollman, 2003).

http://dx.doi.org/10.5772/54128

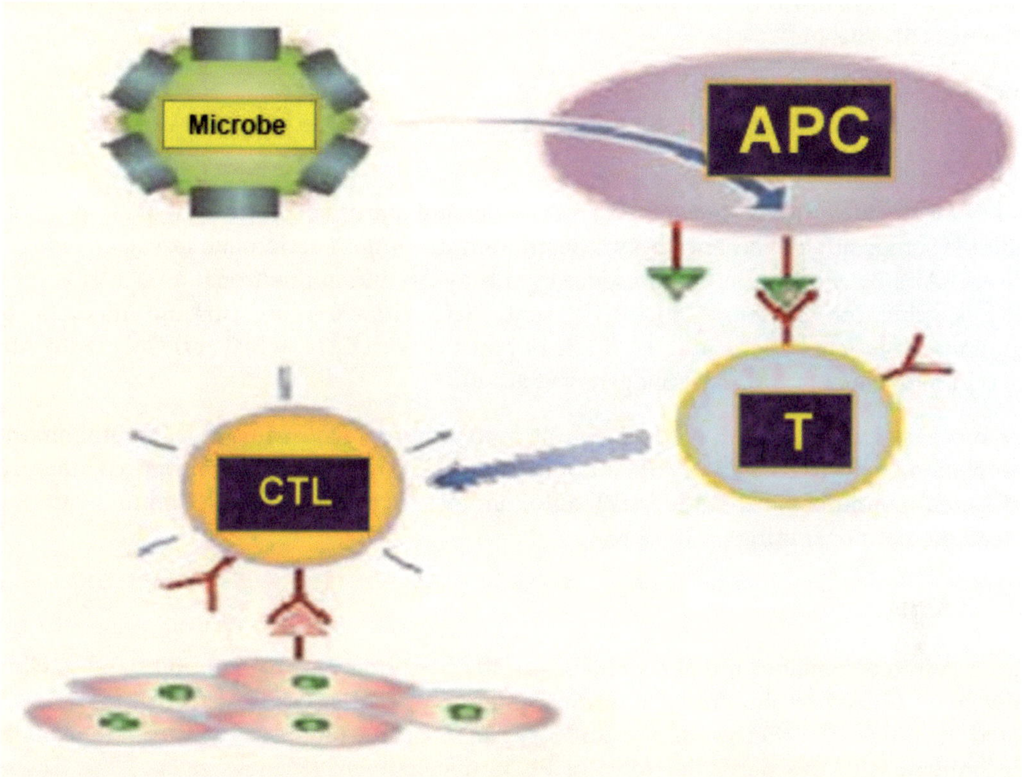

Note: The presence, in microbial pathogens, of Ags cross-reacting with or mimicking patient's Ags attenuates the patient's protective response by changing the direction of the infectious process. Activation of self-reactive CTL and production of Abs able to cross-react with both microbial epitopes and epitopes of the infected patient Abs in the paradigm of molecular/Ag mimicry underlies PIFA. Ag, antigen; Ab, antibody; APC, antigen-presenting cell; T, T lymphocyte; CTL, cytotoxic T lymphocyte; PIFAS, postinfectious autoimmunity syndrome

Figure 5. Molecular (Ag) mimicry and its role in PIFA induction

The aforementioned pathogenic mechanisms are not mutually exclusive and play an essential role in certain (early, as a rule) stages of the CDIO development as well as in PIFAS associated with the underlying disease. In other words, the induction stimuli for PIFA at the initiation point are as follows:

a. Ag features of the microbial pathogen;

b. tropism of the infectious pathogen to cells, organs and tissues against which the cytopathic effect is specifically directed (Sanaev et al., 2008; Cherepakhina et al., 2009).

Contrary to PIFSIS, in patients with PIFAS all the three categories of antimicrobial Abs (antibacterial, antiviral, antiparasitic) have high incidence. If the incidence and high titers of antibacterial and antiviral Abs are approximately equal in the majority of patients, antiparasitic Abs are present in maximum titers in some forms of the disease (e.g. CPN and CM), but are absent in others (ICIIP), most probably due to specific peculiarities of the underlying disease rather than mechanisms of PIFA formation (Vinnitskij, 2002; Kolesnikov et al., 2001; Cherepakhina et al., 2010b).

Autoaggression provoked by an improper cooperation between both branches of immunity as a result of adaptive branch hyperfunction is a dominant feature of PIFAS (Shogenov et al.,2006).

Its key factors include a wide variety of anti-organ and anti-tissue auto-Abs able to promote multiple seropositivity and appearance of autoimmune inflammation markers (e.g., anti-B7-HI-auto-Ab). By illustration, the presence of antimyelin and antineuronal auto-Abs is typically specific for patients with ICIIP; anti-THG auto-Abs are specific markers of autoimmune inflammations in renal tissue of patients with CPN, while anti-CMC auto-Abs are typical of patients with CM (Shogenov et al., 2010).

The most informative PIFAS models include autoimmune myocarditis (AIM), autoimmune encephalomyelitis (AEM) and ICIIP, autoimmune hepatitis (AIH), autoimmune colienteritis (ACE), autoimmune pancreatitis (AIP), autoimmune gastritis (AIG), autoimmune (streptococcal) glomerulonephritis (AGN), etc.

6.3. PIFASID

This syndrome combines the abnormalities of the both branches of immunity and is clinically characterized by the presence of mixed immunopathology (PIFAS+PIFSIS). The associated disorders in effector and regulatory links of the adaptive branch are usually concomitant with this particular form of PICIS development (Manges et al., 2004; Cherepakhina et al., 2010c).

7. Clinical and immunological criteria of PICIS and state-of-the-art algorithms of immunogenetic diagnostics of CDIO

The recommended diagnostic ideology relies on the combination of two categories of screening procedures, viz.:

1. pathogenesis-oriented diagnosis of PICIS forms;
2. etiotropic diagnosis of microbial factors as the major PICIS provoker during chronization and progression of the infectious disease.

We have elaborated several criteria for substantiated clinical diagnosis of PICIS.

The following criteria should be taken into consideration during screening of abnormalities (immune complex test)

1. *innate branch:* selective phagocytosis and natural cytotoxicity (NCT) indexes, base functions of dendritic (DC) and Ag-presenting (APC) cells, in some cases, complement components;

2. *adaptive branch: selective* typing of effector and (in cases only) regulatory links of immunity combined with blood serotyping on antitarget auto-Abs and identification of Abs against mimicking Ag determinants (Khaitov & Pinegin, 2000; Bach, 2005).

The criteria for etiotropic diagnostics (construction/design of the microbial landscape map) taking account of newest advances in developing molecular and biological technologies, including achievements of metabolomics and metagenomics include the following:

1. spectrum and localization of microbial gene pools;

2. serological profile of antimicrobial Abs.

It may be inferred from the aforementioned that the therapeutic management of such patients should include not only eradication of the infectious agent, but also immunocorrection (in fact, the elimination of PICIS), which is especially important in patients with relapses and frequent alternation of exacerbation and remission periods.

8. Conclusion

Many currently known infectious pathologies are characterized by persistent growth of the CDIO link associated with conditionally pathogenic microorganisms, viruses, intracellular parasites and other endogenous pathogenic microorganisms, particularly those manifesting atypical properties (such as multiple resistance to antimicrobial drugs). At the same time, patients with such pathologies manifest not only low-level immune reactivity, but also inadequate immune responsiveness to the infectious process.

Numerous studies have shown that concrete forms of PICIS have clinical and prognostic significance for CDIO, because it is PICIS that determines, in a large measure, the progression and chronization of the underlying disease and predicts the risk of complications.

PIFSI is a *monosyndromal* and dominant form of PICIS in patients with chronic infectious pathologies.

At the same time, a different form of PICIS characteristic of immune autoaggression of PIFASID or an associated form of immunopathology was recorded in more than 30% of cases. Under these conditions, the form of PICIS and, correspondingly, the degree of immune disorders in patients with CDIO correlate, in an associative manner, with the severity of the clinical course of the disease and the specific peculiarities of *microbiocoenosis* and their interaction with the immune system of the patient. Therefore, any neglect of the results of the interaction between the microbial factor and the host organism implies the risk of appearance of novel specific resistant forms of microorganisms that weaken the immune responsiveness of the host organism and complicate the clinical course of the disease by promoting its chronization and by worsening prognosis. A certain contribution to aggravation and progression of the pathology is made by uncontrolled intake of antibiotics with a vast array of immunosuppressive properties and other pharmacological activities.

Recent progress in the study of the pathogenesis of autoimmune diseases may open up fresh opportunities for the recovery of lost or defective immune system functions, development and implementation of autoimmune diseases in the clinic qualitatively new treatment-and-rehabilitation technologies based on the use of the most advanced applied molecular biology and immunology strategies.

Author details

Natalie Cherepahina*, Zaur Shogenov, Mariya Bocharova, Murat Agirov, Jamilyia Tabaksoeva, Mikhail Paltsev and Sergey Suchkov

Federal Medical-Biological Agency, Moscow State Medical University, I.V. Kurchatov National Center for Science and Technologies, I.M. Sechenov First Moscow State Medical University, Moscow State Medical & Dentistry University, Russia

References

[1] Aarvak T. (1999). IL-17 is produced by some proinflammatory Th1/Th0 cells but not by Th2 cells. *J.Immunol.* Vol.162, No.3, (February 1999). pp. 1246-1251, ISSN 0022-1767

[2] Antonov V.P. & Tsinzerling V.A. Contemporary status of the problem of chronic and slow neuroinfections. (2001). *Archieves of Pathology (in Russian).* Vol.63(1), (January 2001), pp. 47-51, ISSN 0004-1955

[3] Bach J. F. Infections and autoimmunity. *Rev. Med. Interne.* Vol.1, (October 2005), pp. 32-34, ISSN 0248-8663

[4] Bauer J.; Rauschka H. & Lassmann H. Inflammation in the nervous system: the human perspective. *Glia,* Vol.36, No.2, (November 2001), pp. 235-243, ISSN 1098-1136

[5] Benoist C. & Mathis D. Autoimmunity provoked by infection: how good is the case for T cell epitope mimicry? *Nat. Immunol.* Vol.2, No.9, (September 2001), pp. 797-801, ISSN 1529-2908

[6] Bingen-Bidois M.; Clermont O. & Bonacorsi S. Phylogenetic analysis and prevalence of urosepsis strains of Escherichia coli bearing pathogenicity island-like domains. *Infect Immun.* Vol. 70, No.6, (June 2002), pp. 3216-3226, ISSN 1098-5522

[7] Blackwell C.C.; May S.J. & Brettle R.P. Secretor state and immunoglobulin levels among women with recurrent urinary tract infections. *J Clin Lab Immunol.* Vol.22, No. 3, (1987), pp. 133-137, ISSN 0141-2760

[8] Borisov I.A. Pyelonephritis. (2000). In: *Nephrology,* Tareeva I.E. (Ed.), pp. 383-399, Medicine, ISBN 5-225-04195-7, Moscow, Russia

[9] Carballido J.A.; Alvarez-Mon M. & Olivier C. Inflammatory pathology in urology. Standardization. *Actas Urol Esp.* Vol.27, No.3, (March 2003), pp. 173-179, ISSN 0210-4806

[10] Chabaud M.; Lubberts E. & Joosten L. (2001). IL-17 derived from juxta-articular bone and synovium contributes to joint degradation in rheumatoid arthritis. *Arthritis Res.* Vol.3, No.3, (January 2001), pp. 168-177, ISSN 1478-6354

[11] Cherepakhina N. E.; Maksimenko D. M. & Suchkov S.V. (2010). Microbial landscape and its value for the modern model of immunopathogenesis of chronic relapsing infectious diseases. *Proceedings of the III World asthma & COPD forum and World forum of pediatrics (in Russian).* pp. 99-102, ISBN 978-88-7587-558-9, Dubai, UAE, April 24-27, 2010

[12] Cherepakhina N.E.; Maksimenko D.M. & Suchkov S.V. (2010). Strategy of immunotherapy and immunorehabilitation of chronic relapsing infectious. *International Journal on Immunorehabilitation (in Russian).* Vol.12, No.2, (May 2010), p. 139, ISSN 1562-3629

[13] Cherepakhina N.E.; Shogenov Z.S. & Elbeik T. (2009). Postinfectious clinical-and-immunologic syndrome and its place in clinical practice. *Therapeutic Archives (in Russian).* Vol.81(1), No.12, (December 2009), pp. 71-78, ISSN 0040-3660

[14] Cherepakhina N.E.; Tabaksoeva D.A. & Suchkov S.V. (2010). Associative relation of microbial factor and postinfectious clinical-and-immunologic syndrome in case of chronic relapsing diseases. *Clinical Microbiology and Antimicrobial Chemotherapy (in Russian).* Vol.12, No.2, suppl.1, (2010), p. 54, ISSN 1684-4386

[15] Cho M.L.; Yoon C.H. & Hwang S.Y. (2004). Effector function of type II collagen-stimulated T cells from rheumatoid arthritis patients: cross-talk between T cell and synovial fibrodlasts. *Arthritis Reum.* Vol.50, No.3, (March 2004), pp. 776-784, ISSN 0004 -3591

[16] Chung Y. & C. Dong. (2009). Don't leave home without it: the IL-23 visa to Th-17 cells. *Nature Immunol.*-Vol.10, No.3, (March 2009), pp.236-238, ISSN 1529-2908

[17] Dantzer R. & Wollman E.E. Relationships between the brain and the immune system. *J Soc Biol.* Vol.197, No.2, (2003), pp. 81-88, ISSN 0037-766X

[18] Dyachenko P., Dyachenko A. (2010). The role of Th17-cells in the pathogenesis of autoimmune diseases. *Bulletin of the Sumy State University, Medicine,* Vol.2, No.2 (October 2010), p.14-22, ISSN 1817-9215

[19] Fujinami R. S.; von Herrath M. G. & Christen U. Molecular mimicry, bystander activation, or viral persistence: infections and autoimmune disease. *Clin. Microbiol. Rev.* Vol.19, No.1, (January 2006), pp. 80-94, ISSN 0893-8512

[20] Khaitov R. M. & Pinegin B.V. Contemporary conceptions of safeguard of host organism against infection. *Immunol(in Russian). og* Vol.1, (January 2000), pp. 61-64, ISSN 0206-4952

[21] Khitrov A.N.; Shogenov Z.S. & Suchkov S.V. (2007). Molecular mimicry phenomenon and its place in postinfectious autoimmune syndrome (PIFA) pathogenesis. *Molecular Medicine (in Russian)*. Vol.4, (2007), pp. 24-32, ISSN 1728-2918

[22] Khitrov A.N.; Shogenov Z.S. & Tretyak E.B. (2007). Postinfectious immunodeficiency and autoimmunity: pathogenic and clinical values and implications. *Expert Review of Clinical Immunology (in Russian)*. Vol.3, No.3, (May 2007), pp. 323-331, ISSN 1744-666X

[23] Koenen H.J.; Smeets R.L. & Vink P.M. (2008). Human CD25highFoxp3pos regulatory T cells differentiate into IL-17-producing cells. *Blood.* Vol.112, No.6, (September 2008), pp. 2340-2352, ISSN 0006-4971

[24] Kolesnikov A.P.; Khabarov A.S. & Kozlov V.A. (2001). Diagnostics and differentiated treatment of secondary immunodeficiencies. *Therapeutic Archives (in Russian)*. Vol. 73(4), (April 2001), pp. 55-59, ISSN 0040-3660

[25] Kukhtevich A.V.; Gordovskaya N.B. & Kozlovskaya N.L. Pyelonephritis. *Russian Medical Journal*. Vol.5, No.23, (December 1997), pp. 54-62, ISSN 0869-7760

[26] Litvinov V.A.; Cherepakhina N.E. & Suchkov S.V. (2008). Chronic pyelonephritis: features of immunopathogenesis and principles of clinical immunogenetic diagnostics. *Physician (in Russian)*. Vol.1, (January 2008), pp. 12-17, ISSN 0236-3054

[27] Manges A. R.; Dietrich P. S. & Riley L.W. Multidrug-resistant Escherichia coli clonal groups causing community-acquired pyelonephritis. *Clin Infect Dis*. Vol.38, No.3, (February 2004), pp. 329-334, ISSN 0934-9723

[28] Mazo E.B.; Vinnitskij L.I. & Litvinov V.A. (2007). Chronic pyelonephritis: features of immunopathogenesis and its' clinical and diagnostical values. *Therapeutic Archives (in Russian)*. Vol.79(1), (January 2007), pp. 85-89, ISSN 0040-3660

[29] McGeachy M.J.; Chen Y. & Tato C.M. (2009). The interleukin 23 receptors essential for the terminal differentiation of interleukin 17-producing effector T helper cells in vitro. *Nature Immunol* Vol.10, No.3 (March 2009) pp. 314-324, ISSN 1529-2908

[30] McGuirk P. & Mills K.H. Pathogen-specific regulatory T cells provoke a shift in the Th1/Th2 paradigm in immunity to infectious diseases. (2002). *Trends in Immunology*. Vol.23, No.9, (September 2002), pp. 450-455, ISSN 1471-4906

[31] Morozov A.V. Chronic infection of urinary tract (pathogenesis, diagnostic and treatment principles). *Russian Medical Journal (in Russian)*. Vol.9, No.23, (December 2001), pp. 1074-1077, ISSN 0869-7760

[32] Paltsev M.A. Clinical and immune-mediated syndrome (CAIMS) in clinical practice: features and strategies in immune and molecular diagnostics. (2009). *New Horizons in Allergy, Asthma & Immunology* pp. 177-181, ISBN 978-88-7587-505-3, Dubai, UAE, April 24-27, 2009

[33] Paltsev M.A.; Cherepakhina N.E. & Suchkov S.V. (2009). Postinfectious clinical immunologic syndrome: foundations of etiopathogenesis and strategy of immunogeno-

diagnostics. *Bulletin of the Russian Academy of Medical Sciences (in Russian)*. Vol.10, (October, 2009), pp. 25-31, ISSN 0869-6047

[34] Paukov V.S. Immunology and morphology of chronic inflammation. *Achieves of Patholog (in Russian)*. Vol.58(1), (January 1996), pp. 28-33, ISSN 0869-7760

[35] Proal A.D.; Albert P.J. & Blaney G.P. (2011). Immunostimulation in the era of the metagenome. Cellular & Molecular Immunology. Vol.3, No.3, (May 2011), p. 1–13, ISSN 1672-7681

[36] Rose N.R. & Mackay I.R. Molecular mimicry: a critical look at exemplary instances in human diseases . *Cell Mol. Life Sci.* Vol.57, No.4 (April 2000), pp. 542-551, ISSN 1420-682X

[37] Rumyantsev A.S. & Goncharova I.S. Etiology and pathogenesis of pyelonephritis. *Nephrology(in Russian)*. Vol.4, No.3, (2000), pp. 40-52, ISSN 1561-6274

[38] Sakaguchi S. (2004). Naturally arising CD4+ regulatory T cells for immunologic self-tolerance and negative control of immune responses. *Annu.Rev.Immunol.* Vol.22, (April 2004), pp.531-562, ISSN 0732-0582

[39] Sanaev A.O.; Kachkov I.A. & Vinnitskij L.I. (2007). Modern aspects of immunotherapy at intracranial infectious inflammatory diseases therapy by example of brain abscesses. *Allergology and Immunology (in Russian)*. Vol.8, No.4, (2007), pp. 384-387, ISSN 1562-3637

[40] Sanaev A.O.; Kachkov I.A. & Vinnitskij L.I. (2008). Immunomonitoring and immunorehabilitation in case of intracranial infectious inflammatory diseases. *Russian Journal of Immunology (in Russian)*. Vol.2(11), No.1, (2008), pp. 78-82, ISSN 1028-7221

[41] Shevach E.M. (2002). CD4+CD25+ suppressor T cells: more questions than answers. *Nat.Rev.Immunol.* Vol.2, No.6 (June 2002), pp. 389-400, ISSN 1474-1733

[42] Shogenov Z.S.; Akhmedilova K.A. & Tabaksoeva D.A. Features of immunopathogenesis and chronization of myocarditis as the basis of immunogenetic diagnostic and immunogenetic monitoring protocols development. *Russian cardiology journal (in Russian)*. Vol.6(86), (November 2010), pp. 76-87, ISSN 1560-4071

[43] Shogenov Z.S.; Cherepakhina N. E. & Suchkov S.V. (2006). Immunogenetic diagnostics and postinfectious immunodeficiency syndrome in physicians' practice. *Clinical Laboratory Diagnostics (in Russian)*. Vol.11, (November 2006), pp. 36-43, ISSN 0869-2084

[44] Stochinger B. & Veldhoen M. (2007). Differentiation and function of Th17 T cells. *Curv.Opin.Immunol.* Vol.19, No.3, (June 2007), pp. 281-286, ISSN 0952-7915

[45] Suchkov S.V.; Blagoveschenskij S.V. & Vinnitskij L.I. (2004). Modern aspects of immunopathogenesis and immunocorrection in patients with intracranial infectious inflammatory diseases. *Allergology and Immunology (in Russian)*. Vol.5, No.2, (2004), pp. 323-330, ISSN 1562-3637

[46] Suchkov S.V.; Shogenov Z.S. & Khitrov A.N. (2007). Postinfectious autoimmune syndrome: features of pathogenesis and modern protocols of clinical immunogenodiagnostics. *Therapeutic Archives (in Russian)*. Vol.79, No.4, (April 2007), pp. 71-76, ISSN 0040-3660

[47] Vinnitskij L.I. Diagnostic facilities of contemporary immune technologies in surgical clinic. (2002) *Allergology and Immunology (in Russian)*. Vol.3, No.1, (2002), pp. 198-203, ISSN 1562-3637

[48] Vojdani A. & Erde J. (2006a). Regulatory T cells, a potent for CAM researchers: the ultimate antagonist (I). *eCAM*, Vol.3, No.1, (March 2006). pp. 25-30, ISSN 1741-427X

[49] Vojdani A. & Erde J. (2006b). Regulatory T cells, a potent for CAM researchers: modulating allergic and infections disease pathology (II). *eCAM*, Vol.3, No.2, (June 2006). pp. 209-215, ISSN 1741-427X

[50] Vojdani A. & Erde J. (2006c). Regulatory T cells, a potent for CAM researchers: modulating tumor immunity (III). *eCAM*, Vol.3, No.3, (September 2006). pp. 309-316, ISSN 1741-427X

[51] Volpe E.; Servant N. & Zollinger R. (2008). A critical function for transforming growth factor-beta, interleukin 23 and proinflammatory cytokines in driving modulating human Th-17 responses. *Nat. Immunol.* Vol.9, No.6, (June 2008), pp.650-657, ISSN 1529-2908

[52] Yu. J.J. (2008). Interleukin-17: a novel inflammatory cytokine that bridges innate and adaptive immunity. *Front.Biosci.* Vol.13 (January 2008), pp. 170-177, ISSN 1093-9946

[53] Zhmurov V.A.; Oskolkov V.A. & Malishevskij M.V. (2000). Correlation between immunogenetic markers and metabolic processes at chronic pyelonephritis. *Urology (in Russian)*. Vol.3, (2000), pp. 9-13, ISSN 0042-1154

[54] Zhou L.; Lopes J.E. & Chong M.M.W. (2008). TGF-β-induced Foxp3 inhibits Th17 cell differentiation by antagonizing RORt function. *Nature*. Vol.453, (May 2008), pp. 236-240, ISSN

Chapter 8

Environmental Factors and Type 1 Diabetes Mellitus in Pediatric Age Group

Giuseppe d'Annunzio, Andrea Accogli,
Ramona Tallone, Sara Bolloli and Renata Lorini

Additional information is available at the end of the chapter

http://dx.doi.org/10.5772/53267

1. Introduction

Type 1 diabetes mellitus (T1DM) is the most common endocrinopathy in pediatric age group, due to an autoimmune process characterized by a selective destruction of insulin producing pancreatic β-cells progressing over different stages [1]. T1DM develops in genetically susceptible subjects by activation of so far uncharacterized environmental factors that trigger an inflammatory process with infiltration of pancreatic islets and subsequent loss of β-cells. Despite the growing incidence of T1DM, the causative mechanisms are not completely defined up to now, and the identification of factors triggering the immune process represents a challenge for clinical immunologists, with practical, diagnostic and therapeutic implications [2,3]. The clinical onset of T1DM is preceded by an asymptomatic period characterized on pathology grounds by insulitis, i.e. an infiltration of the pancreatic islet of Langerhans by CD4+, CD8+ T lymphocytes (both Th1 and Th2 subsets), B lymphocytes, macrophages and dendritic cells. T lymphocytes can differentiate into 2 major subsets: Th1, producing IL-2 and IFN-γ, and Th2, secreting mainly IL-4. All these cells produce cytokines which can be directly cytotoxic to β-cells or play an indirect role on β-cell destruction influencing some cells of the immune system, then resulting in either acceleration or arrest of the immune attack [4]. Worldwide T1DM incidence has grown more than two to three fold during the last decades, particularly in Finland, where T1DM incidence has increased from 12 to 63 cases per 100,00 [5]. A raising incidence has also been reported in Italy, where Sardinia Region shows an incidence rate similar to Finland, therefore is called "Hot Spot" [6,7]. Interestingly, this rise of incidence was not followed by a parallel increased frequency of the major risk genes [8]. T1DM can be defined as a polygenic disease, and the genes mainly involved include

Major Histocompatibility Complex (MHC) class II (DR and DQ) on chromosome 6, responsible for 40% of genetic risk, and insulin gene located on chromosome 11. Moreover thanks to whole genome screening techniques more than 15 loci have been identified. In particular, an allele of the gene for a negative regulator of T-cell activation, i.e. Cytotoxic T Lymphocyte Antigen 4 (CTLA-4), on chromosome 2q33, and a variant of PTNP22 gene encoding LYP (a suppressor of T cell activation) and ILrRA gene are considered as other important susceptibility loci [8]. Recently, the prevalence of MHC class II genes seems to be decreasing [9]. Moreover, studies in identical twins showed a concordance rate ranging from 27 to 61%, otherwise lower in non-identical twins (3.8-12%) [10]. Despite the growing incidence of T1DM, the causative mechanisms are not completely defined up to now. The paradigm of autoimmune dysregulation has not offered a clear explanation for its raising incidence.

The reported discrepancy between higher incidence of T1DM without concomitant shift in the frequency of susceptibility genes, suggests that environmental factors play a key role in the development of the autoimmune process leading to clinical onset of the disease [11]. Moreover the shift to younger age at T1DM clinical onset is caused by environmental risk factors accelerating the on-going β-cell destructive process up to clinical disease even in children with lower levels of genetic risk otherwise exposed to such factor [12-14].

The high T1DM incidence is a phenomenon of the 20th century, even if the disease has been described already in antiquity. This increasing incidence and its difference among neighboring regions strengthens the role of multiple environmental factors in the pathogenesis of T1DM. In the present chapter the main environmental factors involved in T1DM pathogenesis according to the most relevant scientific evidence will be considered. The main topics are: perinatal and socioeconomic factors, hygiene hypothesis, dietary components both in mother and in children, gut permeability, infectious agents, vaccinations, obesity and Accelerator Hypothesis, epigenetic.

2. Perinatal factors

Environmental risk factors combined with genetic susceptibility are thought to contribute to the development of autoimmune destruction of pancreatic β-cells. The rapid increasing incidence of T1DM, especially in the youngest age group [15], cannot be explained by genetic factors. It has been postulated that gestational or perinatal events could trigger T1DM.

2.1. Infections

It has been reported that certain infections during pregnancy contribute to an increased risk of T1DM in the offspring. The first report of a link between infection and diabetes was the exposure to rubella in intrauterine life. Studies showed that about 20% of children born with congenital rubella develop T1DM during infancy [16,17]. Other reports describe an increased risk of T1DM if the mother has had an enterovirus infection during pregnancy [18,19]. Anyway these studies are not confirmed by all investigators [20,21] and whether enterovirus infection during the first trimester of pregnancy is associated with increased risk for T1DM in the offspring remains controversial up to now [21]. Not only congenital infections are associated with the risk of T1DM, but also perinatal infections are discussed as protective factors or triggers of the disease [22]. Certain studies reported that two infections in the first year of life seem to be protective against T1DM, while neonatal respiratory diseases are associated with a increased risk of disease [22].

2.2. In utero and postnatal dietary exposure

To explain the growing incidence in T1DM within the first year of life, it has been hypothesized that certain dietary nutrients could be protective for islet autoimmunity. Maternal intake of vitamin D is significantly associated with a decreased risk of islet autoimmunity in offspring, independent from HLA genotype, family history of T1DM, presence of gestational diabetes mellitus and ethnicity (adjusted HR=0.37; 95% CI 0.17-0.78). Instead, vitamin D intake via supplements, ω-3 fatty acid and ω-6 fatty acids intake during pregnancy are not associated with appearance of islet autoimmunity in offspring [23]. There is also an increased interest in nutritional factors in the first months of life as risk factors for T1DM. Some authors reported that children exposed to cereals between 0 and 3 months of life were more likely to develop islet cell auto-antibodies compared to those who were exposed during the fourth through sixth month [24]. Another study showed that ingestion of gluten-containing foods before 3 months of age was associated with increased islet cell autoimmunity compared to children who received only breast milk until 3 months of life. Then other studies showed that a high intake of cow's milk could have a protective effect [25]. On the other hand, some authors claim that milk protein carries an increased risk of T1DM [26,27]. It is also been reported a correlation between a high intake of nitrosamines, nitrites and nitrates and T1DM [25,28][Table 1].

		HR*	CI**
Protective effect	Vitamin D intake	0.49;95%	(0.17-0.78)
Increased risk	Inadequate prenatal care	0.53;95%	(0.40-0.71)
	Medicaid insurance	0.67;95%	(0.58-0.77)
	Unmarried mother	0.79;95%	(0.69-0.91)
	Mother's age ≥ 25 yrs	1.28;95%	(1.13-1.45)
	Mother's BMI ≥ 30 kg/m^2	1.29;95%	(1.01-1.64)
	Mother's age ≥ 35 yrs	1,32;95%	(1.01-1.64)

HR*: Hazard Ratio; CI**: Confidence Interval

Table 1. Maternal factors and T1DM risk.

2.3. Birth-weight

An association between birth weight and risk for T1DM has been postulated. A meta-analysis study of 12.807 cases of T1DM found an increased risk in children heavier at birth: children with birth weight from 3,5 to 4 Kg showed an increased risk of 6% (OR 1.06; 95% CI 1.01-1.11) (p=0.02) and children with birth weight over 4 Kg have an increased risk of 10% (OR 1.10; 95% CI 1.04-1.19) (p=0.003), compared to children weighing 3 to 3,5 Kg at birth [29]. Several studies support this link [30], while others did not find any association with T1DM [31].

2.4. Caesarean section

Another controversial question is the role of caesarean section. A meta-analysis study of 9.938 cases reported a 20% increase in the risk of childhood-onset T1DM (adjusted OR 1.19, 95% CI 1.04-1.36, p=0.01) [32], while other authors did not find any association between caesarean delivery and risk for T1DM [33].

2.5. Other perinatal factors

It is also been investigated the association between blood incompatibility and risk for T1DM: ABO incompatibility was related to an increased risk for the disease in some studies [34], while others found an association just only with Rhesus immunization [33].

A report have shown that also neonatal jaundice of unknown cause confers an increased risk for T1DM [34].

Another topic discussed is about the stress events. Some authors found an increased risk of T1DM in children diagnosed between 5 to 9 years of age who experienced stress events [25], while others showed that stressful events during the first two years of life increased the risk of the disease, probably by affecting the autoimmune pathogenetic process [35]. Finally, some investigators have reported a decreased risk for T1DM in children of prenatal smokers [36,37].

3. Social factors

Other factors such as maternal age may contribute to increase the risk for T1DM. It is been observed an increased incidence of disease in children born to older mother [25,34,38,39]. These data are confirmed by a population-based case-control study in Washington State on children younger than 19 years from 1987 to 2005, an increased OR in children of mothers older than 25 years (age 25-34 HR=1.28; 95% CI 1.13-1.45; age≥35 HR=1.32; 95% CI 1.10-1.58) has been reported [31]. Risk for T1DM is also been related with maternal weight: mother with a BMI of 30 Kg/m^2 or higher had an increased ORs for the disease (BMI≥30: OR 1.29; CI 1.01-1.64). Pregnancy-related factors also include birth order: the first-born child has the highest risk for T1DM and the risk decreases with number of children born [38,40]. Several studies have found an inverse association between increasing number of siblings and risk of T1DM [31,37,41,42]. An inverse correlation has also been observed with lower economic status or care access, such as unmarried mother (OR 0.79; 95% CI 0.69-0.91), inadequate prenatal care (OR 0.53; 95% CI 0.40-0.71), or Medicaid Insurance (OR 0.67; 95% CI 0.58-0.77) [31]. Another widely discussed topic is tobacco exposure, as influencing immune system, and represents a risk factors for T1DM. It's been questioned if the decrease of passive smoking in children may be a predisposing factor for the increasing incidence of T1DM, in according with the hygiene hypothesis. To clarify this aspect, ABIS, a population-based prospective long term cohort study, revealed no difference in prevalence of immunological markers (GAD and IA-2 antibodies) between tobacco smoke-exposed and non-exposed children [43].

3.1. Hygiene hypothesis

Recently, attention has been focused on lifestyle changes as a major factor in the rise of T1DM frequency, as well as other immune or allergic diseases [44]. Improved hygiene and living conditions decreased the frequency of childhood infections, leading to a modulation of the developing immune system and increasing risk for autoimmune and allergic diseases such as T1DM and asthma [45]. This theory, called "Hygiene Hypothesis", finds its roots in the 1870 when Charles Harris Blackley noticed that aristocrats and city dwellers were more likely to get hay fever than farmers [46]. One century later, in 1966, Leibowitz and colleagues noted that in Israel the incidence of multiple sclerosis (MS) was positively related to levels of sanitation [47]. More recently, Correale et al. showed that patients with multiple sclerosis who become infected with helminths have a strikingly reduced rate of disease progression [48]. However, the term "Hygiene Hypothesis" was proposed in 1989 by Strachan, who noted that hay fever was less frequent in families with many siblings [49].

In accordance to hygiene hypothesis, several studies report the lowest incidence of T1DM in areas with poorest hygiene condition [50,31]. These data are supported by the experiments in non-obese diabetic (NOD) mice (mice that spontaneously develop a condition resembling T1DM) and in BB rats, in which caesarean delivery and isolated living conditions increased the incidence of diabetes from 40% to 80%. In humans, several studies reported a significant inverse correlation between the incidence of T1DM and certain socioeconomic index (unemployment, lack of a car, crowded housing conditions, and living in rental housing rather than purchased property) [50,51]. In the people living in Washington state from 1987 to 2005, D'Angeli and colleagues found a negative association between T1DM and some indicators of lower economic status or care access, such as an unmarried mother (OR 0.79%; 95% CI 0.69-0.91), inadequate prenatal care (OR 0.53%; 95% CI 0.40-0.71), or Medical insurance (OR, 0.67; 95% CI 0.58-0.77) [31]. Young children with older brothers and sisters and sharing the bedroom, as well as those who attended a day-care centre during the first six months of life showed a lower incidence of T1DM later in life than children who did not attend a day-care centre and who had no older siblings [52].

3.1.1. *Hygiene hypothesis and autoimmunity*

A topic discussion of our day is whether the reduced exposure to certain infections, as result of improving socioeconomic conditions, may be responsible for the increased incidence in diabetes and other autoimmune conditions such as systemic lupus erythematosous and multiple sclerosis [45,53-55]. As regards the rise in the disease in Western Europe and the USA during the twentieth century strikingly correlates with the decline of helminths infections, particularly E. vermicularis [56]. Experimental studies showed in Non-Obese Diabetic (NOD) mice, infected with mycobacterium or helminthes, a reduced frequency of T1DM [54,57-58]. Moreover, infection of 4-5 week-old NOD mice with Schistosoma mansoni or injection of soluble eggs (SEA) seems to prevent diabetes clinical onset. One possible explanation is that helminths antigens are able to induce either IL-10 production by dendritic cells and activation of Natural Killer T cells (NKTs) and Regulatory T cells (TRegs). Considering the role of IL-10 in delaying or inhibiting the host immune response and limiting tissue pathology [59-61], exogenous administration of IL-10 inhibits the development of diabetes in NOD mice [62]. Moreover, some bacterial infections can inhibit diabetes development in NOD mice. In mice infected with S. typhimurium the protective mechanism could be the key role of dendritic cells in modulating the trafficking of diabetogenic T cells to the pancreas [63]. Another way by which bacteria and viruses could protect against autoimmune disorders is related to Toll-Like Receptor (TLRs). In fact, when TLRs bind bacterial ligands, stimulate mononuclear cells to produce several cytokines, which down-regulate the autoimmune response. Wen and colleagues showed that Specific-Pathogen Free (SPF) NOD mice are protected from the disease when knocked-out from the MyD88 gene, encoding an adaptor for multiple TLRs [64]. Modification of the immune system in knocked out MyD88 seriously impairs the interactions between the immune system and microbiota. Due to these positive results after treatments with a mycobacterium extract [65], helminthiases treatment and probiotics [66,67] in patients with atopic dermatitis and multiple sclerosis, have recently been reported [68,69]. Instead, vaccination with bacille Calmette-Guèrin produced negative results in patient with T1DM [70,71].

Nowadays a topic discussion is about the role of gut bacteria in the control of autoimmune diseases. In fact changes in the composition of the gut flora influence the development of autoimmune and allergic diseases. It has been observed that the use of lactobacilli, derived from the gut, decreases the incidence of diabetes in NOD mice [72]. More recently, Takiishi et al. showed that treatment of NOD mice with Lactococcus lactis, a common and food-grade commensally bacterium genetically modified, which is able to secrete IL-10 and human pro-insulin auto-antigen, can revert autoimmune diabetes in newly diagnosed NOD mice, by increasing frequency of TRegs [73]. Dan Litman's group showed that a single commensally bacteria, i.e. segmented filamentous bacteria (SFB), is able to drive the appearance of CD4+ T helper cells producing interleukin 17 (IL-17) and IL-22 (Th17 cells) in the lamina propria, thereby influencing the microbiota equilibrium [74]. On the other hand, colonization of germ-free mice with a defined intestinal flora resulted in Treg generation, expansion and activation in the lamina propria [75]. Based on these encouraging results in animal models, the use of probiotics to delay or prevent T1DM in humans has become an area of inter-

http://dx.doi.org/10.5772/53267

est. The PRODIA study, currently ongoing in Finland, is investigating whether, the use of probiotics during the first 6 months of life decreases the clinical onset of T1DM in children with genetic susceptibility [76].

4. Dietary components

4.1. Feeding and risk of T1DM

The T1DM is a chronic disease characterized by a preclinical phase in which environmental exposure, such as food, can contribute to the development of the autoimmune process of pancreatic β-cells destruction. Recent studies have focused upon the role of breastfeeding, introduction of cow's milk, wheat/cereals/gluten, vitamin D and E, ω-3 fatty acids [77]. Some studies suggest that already during pregnancy, low maternal consumption of vegetables may influence the future of the unborn [78,79].

4.2. The influence of breastfeeding

The influence of breastfeeding on the development of diabetes remains a controversial issue; for some it seems to have a protective role, for others, a predisposing role, for others no effect [80]. Gerstein conducted in 1993 a meta-analysis of retrospective case-control studies showing that breast-feeding for short periods (<3 months) is associated with the development of T1DM, with an odds ratio (OR) of 1.43 [81]. A Finnish study has shown that early introduction of cow milk-based formula was associated with an increased risk of β-cell autoimmunity in genetically predisposed children, but the duration of breastfeeding was not associated with an increased risk of autoimmunity in children with first-degree relatives with T1DM in Germany, Australia and USA. The risk of diabetes seems to be higher in patients with first-degree relatives with T1DM, and this risk is increased in carriers of HLA genotype [82-84]. The positive correlation between short duration of breastfeeding and the development of diabetes has been studied in non-diabetic children at the age of 5 years, evaluating the presence of circulating antibodies predictive of the disease [Auto-Antibodies to Insulin (IAA), Glutamic Acid Decarboxylase Antibodies (GADA) and Protein Tyrosine Phosphatase-like (IA-2A)]. This study demonstrates the long-term increased risk of developing T1DM with the early introduction of formula milk. A protective role of breast milk which, for the presence of cytokines and growth factors, promote the maturation of the intestinal mucosa and the development of the immune system has been suggested [85]. Conflicting results can be explained by observing the many differences in feeding practices between the different countries. There is variation between countries and cultures in the proportion of babies first introduced to milk-based formula and there are differences in the kind of complementary food that infants who are not first exposed to milk-based formula [85].

4.3. Introduction of gluten

It has been known as T1DM is connected with other autoimmune diseases, such as thyroiditis or celiac disease. Two prospective studies in USA and Germany showed a high risk for the development of β-cells auto-immunity when gluten's introduction happens before the fourth month rather than after the seventh; moreover this risk is similar when gluten ingestion starts before the third month [24,86]. Several studies were aimed to explain the etiology of this phenomenon. Simpson et al. compared the levels of antibodies to a wheat storage globulin homologue of Glo-3A, which is a non-gluten component of the wheat protein matrix. They have shown that in children with islet auto-immunity, the antibody titer was directly linked to the early introduction of gluten, and inversely to breastfeeding duration [87]. Not all authors agree with this association; a prospective analysis from the DIPP study did not show a correlation between early or late introduction of gluten and subsequent development of pancreatic β-cells autoimmunity [88]. Mojibian et al. hypothesized that the passage of gliadin (a polypeptide of the wheat) through the intestinal epithelial barrier may trigger an inflammatory response, and then an autoimmune disease, in genetically predisposed individuals. The passage of protein molecules is facilitated by inflammation produced by intestinal infections. The location of an uncovering receptor for Coxsackie and Adenovirus at the level of tight junctions may explain the development of T1DM. The bowel inflammation and T-cells activation by gluten could activate and potentiate β-cell auto-immunity, like viral infections [89]. Recently a study in NOD mice demonstrated that there is a statistically significant protection from diabetes in mice that received gluten-free diet [90].

4.4. Vitamin D and E

Some studies have shown an increased risk of developing diabetes in children with low intake of vitamin D. An European case-control study has quantified the reduction in risk with an OR of 0.67 (95% CI 0.53-0.86) in children supplemented with vitamin D [Table 2]. Also a Finnish study showed a protective role of vitamin D, with an OR equal to 0.12 (95% CI 0.03-0.51), comparing children who received regular doses of 2000 IU/day rather than 400 IU/day, and an OR of 3 (95% CI 1.0-9.0) comparing children with an irregular supplementation rather no supplementation with vitamin D [91,92]. Simpson et al. followed from 1993 to 2011 2,664 children at increased risk of T1DM, monitoring the intake of vitamin D and blood levels of 25(OH)D. They have shown that vitamin supplementation is not associated with an increased protection from autoimmune phenomena [93]. Vitamin D deficiency predisposes individuals to type 1 and type 2 diabetes, and receptors for its activated form 1α25-dihydroxyvitamin D3 have been identified in β-cells and immune cells. In some populations, T1DM is associated with certain polymorphisms within the vitamin D receptor gene. In studies in non-obese diabetic mice, pharmacological doses of 1α25-dihydroxyvitamin D3, or its structural analogues, have been shown to delay the onset of diabetes, mainly through immune modulation [94]. Human studies reported that vitamin D is able to modulate the immune response by suppressing pro-inflammatory cytokines and promoting the secretion of anti-inflammatory ones [23]. Therefore it seems appropriate the supplementation with vitamin D in countries with an increased risk of deficiency, especially if T1DM incidence is high. Other authors emphasized the important role of vitamin E for its antioxidant function; Vitamin E ameliorates oxidative stress in T1DM patients and improves antioxidant defense system [95].

		HR	CI
European study	Vitamin D intake	0.67;95%	(0.53-0.86)
Finnish study	Vitamin D intake (2000UI/d)	0.12;95%	(0.03-0.90)
	Vitamin D intake (400UI/d)	3.00;95%	(1.0-9.0)

Table 2. Child's diet and T1DM risk: protective effect with Vitamin D supplementation

4.5. ω-3 fatty acids and other factors

An observational study in children at high risk of T1DM reported that ω-3 fatty acid intake is not associated with progression to overt disease; however the protective influence of ω-3 fatty acids remains controversial. On the other hand, ω-6 fatty acids seem to exert an opposite role. It has been argued that use of cod liver oil in the first year of life reduces the risk of the disease. The case-control study DAISY [Diabetes AutoImmunity Study in the Young] demonstrates that use of ω-3 fatty acids, between 1 and 6 years, exerts a risk reduction with an hazard ratio of 0.45 [96,97]. The immunomodulatory role of ω-3 fatty acids is quite similar to the role exerted by Vitamin D. Conversely, ω-6 fatty acids like arachidonic acid promote the pro-inflammatory cytokine prostaglandin E_2 with subsequent development of β-cell autoimmunity in genetically predisposed subjects [23]. Recently, an interesting case-control study of 298 Italian children aged 0-15 years (145 affected by T1DM) showed a significant association, dose-response, between frequency of T1DM and meat consumption. The association proposed by Benson et al. between T1DM and daily consumption of water containing nitrates, nitrites and nitrosamines is intriguing [98,99].

5. Gut permeability

In the recent years a topic discussion is about the link between T1DM and gut. The role of gut as a regulator of T1DM was first suggested in animal studies. Changes affecting the gut immune system modulated the incidence of diabetes. In particular structural changes, such as a decreased expression of tight junctions (TJ) proteins claudin-1 and occludin, together with increased gut permeability were noted in the intestinal morphology of Bio-Breeding (BB) rats, compared with Wistar rats [100,101]. These data are supported by the observations that early onset of autoimmune diabetes in BB-rats was associated with high gut permeability [102] and in NOD-mouse increased intestinal permeability precedes the clinical onset of T1DM [103]. In humans, studies showed that gut permeability, measured by the lactulose-mannitol test, is increased in T1DM patients [104,105] and can precede clinical onset [106]. These results are supported by the discovery of high serum zonulin concentrations, a novel member of tight-junction protein that correlates with increased ratios in sugar permeability testing, in patients with T1DM [105] and in subjects at risk of T1DM i.e. β-cell autoantibody-positive individuals [106]. Based on these findings, Wats et al. showed that the administration of zonulin antagonist reduced the cumulative incidence of T1DM in diabetic-prone rats [107]. It has also been hypothesized that changes in the normal flora may contribute to the development of T1DM by affecting intestinal permeability. Duodenal administration of Lactobacillus plantarum increased the expression of epithelial TJ proteins occluding and Zo-1 in the biopsies obtained by human volunteers [108]. Moreover, antibiotic treatment that impairs intestinal bacteria, protects from autoimmune diabetes in BB-rat model [109]. In DP-rats (Diabetes-prone rats), the onset of T1DM could be delayed by the administration after weaning of Lactobacillus johnsonii, isolated from DR-rats (Diabetes Resistant Bio-Breed rats) [110]. The composition of intestinal microbiota may not only affect permeability but may also have immune-modulating effects. Recent studies suggest for intestinal microbiota an important regulator role of Th17 immunity in the gut [74]. It has been reported that Lactobacillus johnsonii enhances Th17 differentiation of T cells upon TCR stimulation [112]. The up-regulation of IL-17 immunity in the mucosal surface has been shown to activate an antimicrobial response together with mucosal repair mechanisms and support of the gut barrier [111]. Also virus, such as rotavirus and enterovirus act as promoters of the diabetogenic gut environment with high intestinal permeability, enhanced immune activation, and via the gut-pancreas link, causing activation of β-cell autoimmunity in pancreatic lymph nodes [112]. It is also discussed the role of antiviral cytokines that damage barrier function [113] or the direct effect of virus, as suggested for Rotavirus and Coxsackie viruses [114,115]. The increased gut permeability in T1DM patients may be due to the uptake of dietary antigens causing improper immune activation and intestinal inflammation. Studies suggested that early exposure to dietary wheat may trigger β-cell auto-immunity in children at genetic risk [24,86]. In vitro, gliadin-stimulation of small intestinal biopsies taken from patients with T1DM, caused increase in T-cells and their activation markers, i.e. CD-25 and ICAM-1, promoting intestinal inflammation [116]. Gliadin may also induce an increase in intestinal permeability and zonulin released by binding to the chemokine receptor CXCR3 expressed by epithelial cells and T cells [117]. It has been noted that dietary prevention of diabetes in NOD-mice with a gluten-free diet was associated with a decrease in the number of ceacal bacteria [118]. In humans, epidemiological studies suggest that the short breastfeeding time and early feeding of cow milk (CM) proteins in the infancy increase the risk of diabetes [119]. This may be due to the lack of breastfeeding role of support epithelial and immunological maturation of gut, such as the gut closure [120] and the IgA system [121]. It has been hypothesized that CM may contain diabetogenic factors, such as immunogenic bovine insulin, that could trigger insulin-specific immunity in the gut and, in the context of impaired oral tolerance, contribute to expansion of this immune response against β cells [122]. Weaning to a hydrolyzed casein formula decreased the gut permeability [102] and led to lower expression of IFN-γ [123] in islet infiltrating lymphocytes of BB-rats, resulting in a 50% reduction in the development of autoimmune diabetes [102]. In humans, recent results of the TRIGR pilot study, have showed that weaning to hydrolyzed casein decreased the risk of β-cell autoimmunity by 40% in the infants at genetic risk [124]. In the FINDIA pilot study, the use of bovine-insulin-free whey-based formula, during the first 6 months of life, decreased the appearance of β-cell auto-antibodies by 3 age [125].

6. Infections

6.1. Background

Several studies in humans and animal models have supported the hypothesis that infectious agents, in particular some viruses, can be considered as one among the environmental agents able to elicit or enhance the autoimmune response characterizing T1DM [44]. On the other hand viral infections could exert a protective role against auto-immunity [126]. This opposite scenario might be explained by the type of infecting virus, the immune status of the host and the timing of infection [127]. A possible explanation could be the significant changes in human living standards (i.e. sewage treatment, availability of microbiologically pure water) during the last century, followed by reduced repeated exposure to fecal-oral transmitted agents particularly early in life.

The major obstacle in clinical research is represented by the limited availability human samples. In fact the pancreas is very difficult to access, and routine biopsy aimed to study the role of viruses in the target organ cannot be proposed, since the majority of newly-diagnosed patients are children.

However five lines of evidence link virus to T1DM [128]:

1. Some viruses are able to destroy β-cells and cause mononuclear infiltration
2. Experimental animal models report development of T1DM in mice infected with different strains of Picornaviruses
3. Some viral infections in humans have been followed by T1DM (i.e. congenital rubella)
4. Direct isolation of viruses from humans or animals with T1DM has been documented
5. Virus DNA or RNA are able to initiate antiviral immune response which cross-reacts with insulin or other components within or on the surface of β-cells.

6.2. Viruses and β-cells

Viruses can directly damage β-cells or induce a strong cellular immune response leading to progressive lack of insulin and development of clinical signs and symptoms of the disease. Besides direct cytotoxic effect, other mechanisms involved in β-cell destruction are molecular mimicry and bystander activation [129].

The hypothesis that viral infections are capable of triggering islet auto-reactivity has been proven by several evidences both in humans and in animal models. The host immune response to viruses consists of the secretion of interferon-γ, acting as initiator of inflammation. In the pancreas interferon-γ up-regulates MHC class I molecules on β-cells, making them vulnerable to autoimmune attack [130]. Up-regulation of MHC class I molecules is followed by lymphocytic infiltration in β-cells, as reported also in humans [131]. Moreover viral particles or even isolate live virus have been detected in pancreas from patients deceased at clinical onset of T1DM.

Another evidence strengthening the association between viruses and T1DM is the identification of 4 protective genetic variations of IFIH1 gene, responsible for interferon production after viral infection [132]. Individuals with IFIH1 predisposing alleles have higher IFIH1 levels, while individuals with protective alleles have lower IFIH1 levels. After a HEV infections, the predisposed group showed increased stimulating capacity of dendritic cell, with production of pro-inflammatory cytokines and development of T1DM. The opposite scenario has been reported in the protected group.

The key role of viruses as trigger of autoimmune response may result from molecular similarities between viral antigens and host cell auto-antigens, otherwise defined as "Molecular Mimicry". These similarities are responsible for a break of the immune tolerance to endogenous auto-antigens. In particular, analogies between an epitope of Coxsackie B virus (P2-C 35-43) and an epitope of GAD 65 auto-antigen (GAD 65 258-266) has been reported also in humans [133]. Molecular mimicry is able to enhance or accelerate autoimmune process, however it does not start auto-immunity.

Another link between viruses and auto-immunity is the so called "Bystander Activation". Pre-existing auto-reactive T-cell precursors, activated by viral infections, become auto-aggressive and induce the autoimmune response. Bystander activation has been reported in animal model infected by Coxsackie B4 virus who later develop T1DM [134]. Molecular mimicry and bystander activation are not mutually exclusive.

The direct viral infection and lysis of β-cells has been reported in the so-called "Fulminant Diabetes" (FD). FD accounts for about 20% of diabetes mellitus in Japan and is characterized by extremely rapid and severe destruction of pancreatic β-cells in absence of insulitis, but with high titers of anti-enterovirus IgA, compatible with recurrent HEV infections [135].

Several viruses have been linked to T1DM, i.e Coxsackie, Mumps, Rubella, Cytomegalovirus, Retroviruses and Rotaviruses [136-139], otherwise several evidences link enteroviruses, in particular Coxsackie B4 virus to T1DM [140].

6.3. Coxsackie viruses and T1DM

Human EnteroViruses (HEV) [141] are small, non-enveloped viruses (30 nm), characterized by an icosahedric capsid consisting of 60 capsomers; one capsomer comprises 4 structural proteins (VP1, VP2, VP3, VP4). HEV belong to the Picornaviridiae family and 5 different species are recognized: Poliovirus and HEV A, B, C, D. Enteroviruses are ubiquitous and transmitted by faecal-oral route, and characterized by a great genetic variability and consequent broad spectrum of tissue tropism and pathological effects. HEV infections are usually asymptomatic or characterized by fever, malaise, sometimes respiratory involvement or cutaneous Rash. More severe diseases such as meningitis, encephalitis and pericarditis have been reported.

Six different serotypes characterize Coxsackie virus B (CVB 1-6); the B4 serotype is defined "diabetogenic" [142]. Affected patients harbor enterovirus RNA homologous to that of Coxsackie B4 in peripheral blood mononuclear cells [143], and in small intestine samples, suggesting a persistent enterovirus infection [144].

Recently direct evidence of Coxsackie B4 enterovirus infection in human β-cells with reduced insulin secretion and islet inflammation mediated by natural killer cells has been provided [145-147].

6.4. Viruses: foes or friends?

It has been reported a protective role of viral infection in the development of T1DM. Studies in animal models report a protective effect of enterovirus infections when contracted precociously, before weaning, which disappears if the infection occurs thereafter [148]. A virus with protective effect exerts a inflammatory profile very different if compared to diabetogenic one, with opposite consequences on autoimmune reaction. The kind of virus, its β-cell affinity, and the timing of infection play a crucial role in T1DM occurrence. In fact proliferation virus-induced auto-reactive T cells after recurrent infections with protective viruses determine protection from β-cell autoimmune destruction with deviation of the auto-inflammatory response, a trafficking of auto-reactive T cells and a stimulation of Treg cells [127].

7. Vaccines and risk of T1DM

The role of vaccine in the development of T1DM has been matter of debate. In fact there is a temporal association between increased incidence of the disease after improvement of living conditions and reduction of infectious diseases in childhood, thanks to the widespread use of vaccines. Moreover, some vaccines prevent or induce T1DM in animal models. Furthermore, it has been postulated that only early vaccinations (i.e. within the first month of life) could prevent T1DM [149]. The same author reported a clusters of cases of T1DM 2-4 years post-immunization with pertussis, MMR, and BCG vaccine, but it remains to define the link between the haemophilus-vaccine and T1DM [150]. On the other hand, a large epidemiological study on all children born in Denmark from 1990 and 2000, for whom correct information about vaccine schedule and clinical diagnosis of T1DM 2 to 4 years after vaccination, revealed no significant association between vaccines and development of T1DM. Moreover, no evidence of any clustering of cases after vaccination with any kind of vaccine [151]. This nationwide cohort, together to the prospective and independent ascertainment of vaccination history and the time of T1DM diagnosis overcame the risk of selection bias and recall bias [151]. De Stefano et al., in a case-control study, didn't support an association between any of the recommended childhood vaccines and increased risk of T1DM [152]. Similar results have been reported in a retrospective cohort study in active components of US Military between 2002-2008 [153]. Another retrospective cohort study in Sweden examining the risk of autoimmune and neurological disorders in people vaccinated against pandemic influenza A demonstrated no changes in the frequency of several autoimmune diseases, including T1DM [154].

The possibility that vaccination may increase the risk of T1DM has been evaluated in a few epidemiologic studies. Classen has provided the only evidence of a possible increased risk, but the nature of the evidence is strictly ecological, involving comparisons between countries or between different time periods in the same country. Such comparisons, however, may be influenced by many factors unrelated to vaccination, i.e. genetic predisposition. Moreover, similar ecological analyses did not found significant correlations between diabetes and BCG, pertussis, and mumps vaccine.

Recently, in Japan a case of fulminant T1DM has been reported after influenza vaccination [155]. On the other hand the absence of autoimmunity in this form of diabetes is recognized. The role of vaccinations in T1DM deserves attention. Even if vaccinations are not triggers of autoimmune process leading to overt diabetes, it is otherwise possible that in genetically predisposed subjects vaccine exposure could anticipate the clinical symptoms and therefore being associated to T1DM.

8. Obesity as environmental factor

In the past decades a worldwide rising incidence of the disease has been reported [157], with a significant trend toward earlier age at diagnosis than previously observed [158]. This shift to a younger age at T1DM diagnosis could be explained by exposure to higher doses of several environmental factors, like viral infections, polluted air, and more recently, sedentary lifestyle [159-160]. In particular, physical inactivity results in obesity, whose incidence within pediatric age is dramatically rising [156,160,161]. In younger children obesity-induced insulin resistance exerts in metabolic β-cells up-regulation, accelerating their loss through glucotoxicity, and can potentially bring forward the earlier age of diabetes clinical onset, according to the so-called Accelerator Hypothesis [162].

8.1. Accelerator hypothesis

The Accelerator Hypothesis, firstly postulated by Wilkins, argues that diabetes mellitus is a unique disorder of insulin resistance set against different genetic backgrounds, rather than two distinct diseases (type 1 and type 2), and focuses on the tempo of β-cell loss [162]. Therefore the concept of tempo might explain the commonality between type 1 and type 2 diabetes, which are distinguished only by the rate of β-cell loss and by the specific accelerator involved [163]. Three main accelerators play a pathogenetic role: the first is the intrinsic potential for β-cell apoptosis, a necessary but insufficient step in the development of diabetes. The second accelerator is insulin resistance secondary to obesity, and represents the link between type 1 and type 2 diabetes. Insulin resistance increases insulin secretory demands on β-cells and may trigger damage in these metabolically up-regulated cells by increasing antigen presentation. Insulin resistance is characterized by a decreased ability of insulin to stimulate the use of glucose by the muscle and adipose tissue, where the suppression of lipase controlled by insulin is impaired [164]. The consequent excessive supply of free fatty acids further affects glucose transportation in the skeletal muscles, and inhibits insulin activity [165]. In the liver, insulin resistance leads to increased hepatic glucose production, initially compensated by increased insulin secretion. If the process persists, glucotoxicity can occur, leading to chronic hyperglycemia and clinical diabetes [166]. The third accelerator is genetic susceptibility, predisposing to β-cell autoimmunity [167]. Several studies support the role of the Accelerator Hypothesis, showing that BMI increasing and precocious weight gain are inversely related to age at diagnosis of T1DM [168-173]. Noteworthy, other reports don't agree with the primary pathogenic role of obesity [174,175]. Recently another study in a large cohort of patients from the Mediterranean area makes this theory controversial and unproven up to now [176].

In our previous report in a limited cohort of 174 Italian patients from Genoa (northern Italy) we demonstrated that obesity is not a common finding in younger children at T1DM diagnosis [177].

In particular, the obesogenic environment, i.e. sedentary lifestyle, which promotes insulin resistance and other metabolic consequences deserves attention.

On the other hand, some studies don't support the role of Accelerator Hypothesis. In fact, data from UK compared BMI at T1DM diagnosis with age at diagnosis in South Asian and white children and did not find significant differences. The authors concluded that BMI could be too crude as indicator of insulin resistance, and that other specific indicators should be considered [178].

In a large cohort of Mediterranean patients diagnosed with T1DM between 1990 and 1994 BMI-SDS has not significantly increased. In addition a positive association between BMI-SDS and age at diagnosis has been also reported [176].

It is plausible that Accelerator Hypothesis does or not does become manifest because of the genetic background and environmental factors, including the prevalence of overweight and obesity.

All studies include children BMI to define obesity; however, this measurement seems to be a too crude measure of insulin resistance, as well as of percentage fat mass and its distribution and for the critical variable of cardiovascular fitness, which is the major determinant of insulin sensitivity.

9. Epigenetic

The study of epigenetic in the pathogenesis of autoimmune diseases represents a new challenge and a fascinating field for clinicians and researchers, particularly as regards T1DM. It is recognized that genetic background is only one aspect in T1DM pathogenesis, and the role of environment, gender and aging deserves equally attention. In fact genetic background is responsible for susceptibility or protection from clinical onset of the disease. Moreover, genome wide association studies discovered significant associations underlying immune tolerance breakdown only in a relatively small group of patients, leading to the concept of "Missing Heritability" [179]. Furthermore the low concordance rate of T1DM in monozygotic twins reinforces the concept that external additional factors play a crucial role, and the link between genetic susceptibility and environment as trigger of auto-immunity can be represented by epigenetic [180].

In contrast to genetic alterations, epigenetic changes determine and/or perpetuate an heritable change in gene expression without a change in DNA sequence. Epigenetic mechanisms are involved in eukaryotic gene regulation through modification in chromatin structure in part packaging DNA, in part as modulating gene expression. Epigenome can be defined as a cell specific and stable pattern of gene expression determined by epigenetic mechanisms. Epigenetic mechanisms are involved in cell type development and function, since they are able to determine stable gene expression or repression. Another important feature of epigenetic mechanisms consists of determining metabolic plasticity to cells, with subsequent adaptation to environmental modifications [181].

The main epigenetic abnormalities include DNA methylation and histone modifications, leading to spatial and temporal changes in gene regulation. Studies in identical twins showed that the appearance of epigenetic differences increase with age and the most significant epigenetic differences have been occurred in those twins who spent less time together [182].

As regards T1DM pathogenesis, epigenetic role is by modulating lymphocyte maturation and cytokine expression, both involved in the development of autoimmune attack to β-cells [183]. In particular T-helper lymphocyte differentiation is under epigenetic control [184]. Another mechanism by which epigenetic modifications play a role in T1DM pathogenesis is by influencing β-cell development and repair. In fact glucose and insulin regulate methylation process which takes place in the cell via elevated homocysteine and homocysteine remethylation, with a concomitant reduced capacity to remove homocysteine by means of transulfuration processes [185]. Homocysteine can be re-methylated to form methionine. The maintenance of methylation patterns in DNA and histone are linked to cellular methyl group metabolism, which is influenced by nutritional intake of folate [185]. Maternal nutrition state can influence newborn metabolic phenotype through epigenetic modifications. In fact the relationship between nutritional status and epigenetic is crucial during embryogenesis, intrauterine life and perinatal period, influencing offspring's pancreas vascularisation and development [186]. Furthermore Dutch people exposed to famine during intrauterine life in the years of the Second World War experienced higher frequency of type 2 diabetes and cardiovascular risk in adulthood [187]. As regards a direct epigenetic involvement in T1DM pathogenesis few data are available. On the other hand a possible contribution is represented by food intake, for methyl donors (i.e. methionine and choline) and cofactors (i.e. folic acid and vitamin B12) which are important for DNA and histone methylation.

10. Conclusions

Even if diabetes mellitus is a condition described in the ancient Egypt, no specific etiologic factor has been defined up to now. Fascinating case reports and large multicenter studies demonstrated the complexity of pathogenetic events characterizing autoimmune diseases.

Several environmental factors, old and new, play a crucial role in the development of T1DM, being as protective as dangerous, and their interplay with genetic susceptibility can explain the difficulty to find a single causative agent [188].

On the other hand the study of environmental factors increases the knowledge of natural history of the disease, and allows the recognition and knowledge of those protective agents which can delay the clinical onset of the disease and represent the basis for primary prevention programs.

Author details

Giuseppe d'Annunzio, Andrea Accogli, Ramona Tallone, Sara Bolloli and Renata Lorini

Pediatric Clinic, University of Genoa, IRCCS G. Gaslini Institute, Genoa, Italy

References

[1] Eizirik DL, Colli ML, Ortis F. The role of inflammation in insulitis and beta-cell loss in type 1 diabetes. Nature Reviews Endocrinology 2009; 5(4):219-226.

[2] Devendra D, Liu E, Eisenbarth GS. Type 1 diabetes: recent developments. British Medical Journal 2004; 328(7442):750-754.

[3] Eisenbarth GS. Type 1 diabetes: molecular, cellular and clinical immunology. Advances in Experimental Medicine and Biology 2004; 552:306-310.

[4] Atkinson MA, Gianani R. The pancreas in human type 1 diabetes: providing new answers to age-old questions. Current Opinion in Endocrinology, Diabetes and Obesity 2009; 16(4):279-285.

[5] Patterson CC, Dahlquist GG, Gyürüs E, Green A, Soltész G; EURODIAB Study Group. Incidence trends for childhood type 1 diabetes in Europe during 1989-2003 and predicted new cases 2005-20: a multicentre prospective registration study. Lancet 2009; 373(9680):2027-2033.

[6] Bruno G, Maule M, Merletti F, Novelli G, Falorni A, Iannilli A, Iughetti L, Altobelli E, d'Annunzio G, Piffer S, Pozzilli P, Iafusco D, Songini M, Roncarolo F, Toni S, Carle F, Cherubini V. RIDI Study Group. Age-period-cohort analysis of 1990-2003 incidence time trends of childhood diabetes in Italy: the RIDI study. Diabetes 2010; 59(9): 2281-2287.

[7] Songini M, Lombardo C. The Sardinian way to type 1 diabetes. Journal of Diabetes Science and Technology 2010; 4(5):1248-1255.

[8] Barrett JC, Clayton DG, Concannon P, Akolkar B, Cooper JD, Erlich HA, Julier C, Morahan G, Nerup J, Nierras C, Plagnol V, Pociot F, Schuilenburg H, Smyth DJ, Ste-

vens H, Todd JA, Walker NM, Rich SS. Type 1 Diabetes Genetics Consortium. Genome-wide association study and meta-analysis find that over 40 loci affect risk of type 1 diabetes. Nature Genetics 2009; 41(6):703-707.

[9] Fourlanos S, Varney MD, Tait BD, Morahan G, Honeyman MC, Colman PG, Harrison LC. The rising incidence of type 1 diabetes is accounted for by cases with lower-risk human leukocyte antigen genotypes. Diabetes Care 2008; 31(8):1546-1549.

[10] Redondo MJ, Jeffrey J, Fain PR, Eisenbarth GS, Orban T. Concordance for islet autoimmunity among monozygotic twins. The New England Journal of Medicine 2008; 359(26):2849-2850.

[11] Gillespie KM. Type 1 diabetes: pathogenesis and prevention. Canadian Medical Association Journal 2006; 175(2):165-170.

[12] Dahlquist G. Environmental risk factors in human type 1 diabetes: an epidemiological perspective. Diabetes Metabolism Review 1995; 11:37-46.

[13] Gale EA. Spring harvest? Reflections on the rise of type 1 diabetes. Diabetologia 2005; 48:2245–2250.

[14] Dahlquist G. Can we slow the rising incidence of childhood-onset autoimmune diabetes? The overload hypothesis. Diabetologia 2006; 49:20-24.

[15] Dahlquist G, Mustonen L. Analysis of 20 years of prospective registration of childhood onset diabetes time trends and birth cohort effects. Swedish Childhood Diabetes Study Group. Acta Paediatrica 2000; 89(10):1231-1237.

[16] Ginsberg-Fellner F, Witt ME, Fedun B, Taub F, Dobersen MJ. Diabetes mellitus and autoimmunity in patients with congenital rubella syndrome. Reviews of Infectious Diseases 1985; 7:170-176.

[17] Menser MA., Forrest JM., Bransby RD. Rubella infection and diabetes mellitus. Lancet 1978; 1:57-60.

[18] Dahlquist G, Ivarsson S, Lindberg B, Forsgren M. Maternal enteroviral infection during pregnancy as a risk factor for childhood IDDM. Diabetes 1995; 44:408-413.

[19] Hyöty H, Hiltunen M, Knip M, Laakkonen M, Vähäsalo P, et al. A prospective study of the role of coxsackie B and other enterovirus infections in the pathogenesis of IDDM. Childhood Diabetes in Finland (DiMe) Study Group. Diabetes 1995; 44:652-657.

[20] Fuchtenbusch M, Irnstetter A, Jager G, Ziegler AG. No evidence for an association of coxsackie virus infections during pregnancy and early childhood with development of islet autoantibodies in offspring of mothers or fathers with type 1 diabetes. Journal of Autoimmunity 2001; 17:333-340.

[21] Viskari HR, Roivainen M, Reunanen A, et al. Maternal first-trimester enterovirus infection and future risk of type 1 diabetes in the exposed fetus. Diabetes 2002; 51:2568-2571.

[22] Blom L, Nyström L, Dahlquist G. The Swedish childhood diabetes study: Vaccinations and infections as risk determinants for diabetes in childhood. Diabetologia 1991; 34:176-181.

[23] Fronczak CM, Barón AE, Chase HP, Ross C, Brady HL, Hoffman M, Eisenbarth GS, Rewers M, Norris JM. In utero dietary exposures and risk of islet autoimmunity in children. Diabetes Care 2003 Dec; 26(12):3237-3242.

[24] Norris JM, Barriga K, Klingensmith G, Hoffman M, Eisenbarth GS, Erlich HA, Rewers M. Timing of initial cereal exposure in infancy and risk of islet autoimmunity. Journal of American Medical Association 2003; 290:1713-1720.

[25] Dahlquist G, Blom L, Lönnberg G. The Swedish Childhood Diabetes Study – a multivariate analysis of risk determinants for diabetes in different age groups. Diabetologia 1991; 34:757-762.

[26] Akerblom HK, Savilahti E, Saukkonen TT, Paganus A, Virtanen SM, Teramo K. The case for elimination of cow's milk in early infancy in the prevention of Type 1 diabetes: the Finnish experience. Diabetes Metabolism Reviews 1994; 9(4):269-278.

[27] Vaarala O, Knip M, Paronen J, Hämäläinen AM, Muona P, Väätäinen M, Ilonen J, Simell O, Akerblom HK. Cow's milk formula feeding induces primary immunization to insulin in infants at genetic risk for type 1 diabetes. Diabetes 1999; 48(7):1389-1394.

[28] Dahlquist GG, Blom LG, Persson LA, Sandström AI, Wall SG. Dietary factors and the risk of developing insulin dependent diabetes in childhood. British Medical Journal 1990; 300:1302-1306.

[29] Cardwell CR, Stene LC, Joner G, Davis EA, Cinek O, Rosenbauer J, Ludvigsson J, Castell C, Svensson J, et al. Birthweight and the risk of childhood-onset type 1 diabetes: a meta-analysis of observational studies using individual patient data. Diabetologia 2010; 53(4):641-651.

[30] EURODIAB Substudy 2 Study Group. Rapid early growth is associated with increased risk of childhood type 1 diabetes in various European populations. Diabetes Care 2002; 25:1755-1760.

[31] D'Angeli MA, Merzon E, Valbuena LF, Tirschwell D, Paris CA, Mueller BA. Environmental factors associated with childhood-onset type 1 diabetes: an exploration of the hygiene and overload hypotheses. Archives of Pediatrics & Adolescent Medicine 2010; 164(8):732-738.

[32] Cardwell CR, Stene LC, Joner G, Cinek O, Svensson J, Goldacre MJ, Parslow RC, Pozzilli P, Brigis G, Stoyanov D, Urbonaite B, Sipetić S, Schober E, Ionescu-Tirgoviste C, Devoti G, de Beaufort CE, Buschard K, Patterson CC. Caesarean section is associated with an increased risk of childhood-onset type 1 diabetes mellitus: a meta-analysis of observational studies. Diabetologia 2008; 51(5):726-735.

[33] Stene LC, Magnus P, Lie RT, Sovik O, Joner G, Norwegian Childhood Diabetes Study Group. No association between preeclampsia or cesarean section and incidence of

type 1 diabetes among children: a large, population-based cohort study. Pediatric Research 2003; 54:487-490.

[34] Dahlquist G, Källén B. Maternal-child blood group incompatibility and other perinatal events increased the risk for early-onset type 1 (insulin-dependent) diabetes mellitus. Diabetologia 1992; 35:671-675.

[35] Thernlund GM, Dahlquist G, Hansson K, Ivarsson SA, Ludvigsson J, Sjöblad S, Hägglöf B. Psychological stress and the onset of IDDM in children. Diabetes Care 1995; 18(10):1323-1329.

[36] Marshall AL, Chetwynd A, Morris JA, Placzek M, Smith C, Olabi A, Thistlethwaite D. Type 1 diabetes mellitus in childhood: a matched case control study in Lancashire and Cumbria, UK. Diabetic Medicine 2004; 21(9):1035-1040.

[37] Svensson J, Carstensen B, Mortensen HB, Borch-Johnsen K. Danish Study Group of Childhood Diabetes. Early childhood risk factors associated with type 1 diabetes- is gender important? European Journal of Epidemiology 2005; 20:429-434.

[38] Stene LC, Magnus P, Lie RT, Søvik O, Joner G. Norwegian childhood Diabetes Study Group. Birth weight and childhood onset type 1 diabetes: population based cohort study. British Medical Journal 2001; 322:889-892.

[39] Dahlquist GG, Patterson C, Soltesz G. Perinatal risk factors for childhood type 1 diabetes in Europe. The EURODIAB Substudy 2 Study Group. Diabetes Care 1999; 22:1698-1702.

[40] Bingley PJ, Douek IF, Rogers CA, Gale EA. Influence of maternal age at delivery and birth order on risk of type 1 diabetes in childhood: prospective population based family study. Bart's-Oxford Family Study Group. British Medical Journal 2000; 321:420-424.

[41] Cardwell CR, Carson DJ, Patterson CC. Parental age at delivery, birth order, birth weight and gestational age are associated with the risk of childhood Type 1 diabetes: a UK regional retrospective cohort study. Diabetic Medicine 2005; 22(2):200-206.

[42] Haynes A, Bower C, Bulsara MK, Finn J, Jones TW, Davis EA. Perinatal risk factors for childhood type 1 diabetes in western Australia—a population-based study (1980–2002). Diabetic Medicine 2007; 24:564-570.

[43] Johansson A, Hermansson G, Ludvigsson J. ABIS Study Group. Tobacco exposure and diabetes-related autoantibodies in children: results from the ABIS Study. Annals of the New York Academy of Sciences 2008; 1150:197-199.

[44] Bach JF. The effect of infections on susceptibility to autoimmune and allergic diseases. The New England Journal of Medicine 2002; 347(12):911-920.

[45] Bach JF. Six questions about the hygiene hypothesis. Cellular Immunology 2005; 233(2):158-161.

[46] Blackley CH (1873) Experimental Researches on the Causes and Nature of Catarrhus Aestivus (Hay-fever and Hay-asthma), Baillière Tindall and Cox

[47] Leibowitz U, Antonovsky A, Medalie JM, Smith HA, Halpern L, Alter M. Epidemiological study of multiple sclerosis in Israel. II. Multiple sclerosis and level of sanitation. Journal of Neurology, Neurosurgery and Psychiatry 1966; 29(1):60-68.

[48] Correale J, Farez M. Association between parasite infection and immune responses in multiple sclerosis. Annals of Neurology 2007; 61(2):97-108.

[49] Strachan DP. Hay fever, hygiene, and household size. British Medical Journal 1989; 299:1259-1260.

[50] Patterson CC, Carson DJ, Hadden DR. Epidemiology of childhood IDDM in Northern Ireland 1989-1994: low incidence in areas with highest population density and most household crowding. Northern Ireland Diabetes Study Group. Diabetologia 1996; 39(9):1063-1069.

[51] Staines A, Bodansky HJ, McKinney PA, Alexander FE, McNally RJ, Law GR, Lilley HE, Stephenson C, Cartwright RA. Small area variation in the incidence of childhood insulin-dependent diabetes mellitus in Yorkshire, UK: links with overcrowding and population density. International Journal of Epidemiology 1997;26(6):1307-1313.

[52] McKinney PA, Okasha M, Parslow RC, Law GR, Gurney KA, Williams R, Bodansky HJ. Early social mixing and childhood Type 1 diabetes mellitus: a case-control study in Yorkshire, UK. Diabetic Medicine 2000; 17(3):236-242.

[53] Dunne DW, Cooke A. A worm's eye view of the immune system: consequences for evolution of human autoimmune disease. Nature Reviews Immunology 2005; 5:420–6.

[54] Cooke A, Tonks P, Jones FM, O'Shea H, Hutchings P, Fulford AJ, Dunne DW. Infection with Schistosoma mansoni prevents insulin dependent diabetes mellitus in non-obese diabetic mice. Parasite Immunology 1999; 21:169-176.

[55] Cooke A, Zaccone P, Raine T, Phillips JM, Dunne DW. Infection and autoimmunity: are we winning the war, only to lose the peace? Trends in Parasitology 2004; 20:316-321.

[56] Gale EAM. A missing link in the hygiene hypothesis? Diabetologia 2002; 45:588-594.

[57] Bras A, Aguas AP. Diabetes-prone NOD mice are resistant to Mycobacterium avium and the infection prevents autoimmune disease. Immunology 1996; 89:20-25.

[58] Saunders KA, Raine T, Cooke A, Lawrence CE. Inhibition of autoimmune type 1 diabetes by gastrointestinal helminth infection. Infection and Immunity 2007; 75:397-407.

[59] Mangan NE, Fallon RE, Smith P, Van Rooijen N, McKenzie AN, Fallon PG. Helminth infection protects mice from anaphylaxis via IL-10-producing B cells. The Journal of Immunology 2004; 173:6346-6356.

[60] Gaubert S, Viana da Costa A, Maurage CA, Lima EC, Fontaine J, Lafitte S, Minoprio P, Capron A, Grzych JM. X-linked immunodeficiency affects the outcome of Schistosoma mansoni infection in the murine model. Parasite Immunology 1999; 21:89-101.

[61] Wohlleben G, Trujillo C, Muller J, Ritze Y, Grunewald S, Tatsch U, Erb KJ. Helminth infection modulates the development of allergen-induced airway inflammation. International Immunology 2004; 16:585-596.

[62] Phillips JM, Parish NM, Drage M, Cooke A. Cutting edge: interactions through the IL-10 receptor regulate autoimmune diabetes. The Journal of Immunology 2001; 167:6087-6091.

[63] Raine T, Zaccone P, Mastroeni P, Cooke A. Salmonella typhimurium infection in nonobese diabetic mice generates immunomodulatory dendritic cells able to prevent type 1 diabetes. The Journal of Immunology 2006; 177:2224-2233.

[64] Wen L, Ley RE, Volchkov PY, Stranges PB, Avanesyan L, Stonebraker AC, Hu C, Wong FS, Szot GL, Bluestone JA, Gordon JI, Chervonsky AV. Innate immunity and intestinal microbiota in the development of Type 1 diabetes. Nature 2008 23; 455(7216):1109-1113.

[65] Arkwright PD, David TJ. Intradermal administration of a killed Mycobacterium vaccae suspension (SRL 172) is associated with improvement in atopic dermatitis in children with moderate-to-severe disease. Journal of Allergy and Clinical Immunology 2001; 107(3):531-534.

[66] Kalliomäki M, Salminen S, Arvilommi H, Kero P, Koskinen P, Isolauri E. Probiotics in primary prevention of atopic disease: a randomised placebo-controlled trial. Lancet 2001; 357(9262):1076-1079.

[67] Isolauri E, Arvola T, Sütas Y, Moilanen E, Salminen S. Probiotics in the management of atopic eczema. Clinical and Experimental Allergy 2000; 30(11):1604-1610.

[68] Fleming JO, Isaak A, Lee JE, Luzzio CC, Carrithers MD, Cook TD, Field AS, Boland J, Fabry Z. Probiotic helminth administration in relapsing-remitting multiple sclerosis: a phase 1 study. Multiple Sclerosis Journal 2011; 17:743-754.

[69] Lynch NR, Hagel I, Perez M, Di Prisco MC, Lopez R, Alvarez N. Effect of anthelmintic treatment on the allergic reactivity of children in a tropical slum. Journal of Allergy and Clinical Immunology 1993; 92:404-411.

[70] Allen HF, Klingensmith GJ, Jensen P, Simoes E, Hayward A, Chase HP. Effect of Bacillus Calmette-Guerin vaccination on new-onset type 1 diabetes. A randomized clinical study. Diabetes Care 1999; 22(10):1703-1707.

[71] Elliott JF, Marlin KL, Couch RM. Effect of bacille Calmette-Guérin vaccination on C-peptide secretion in children newly diagnosed with IDDM. Diabetes Care 1998; 21(10):1691-1693.

[72] Calcinaro F, Dionisi S, Marinaro M, Candeloro P, Bonato V, Marzotti S, Corneli RB, Ferretti E, Gulino A, Grasso F, et al. Oral probiotic administration induces interleu-

kin- 10 production and prevents spontaneous autoimmune diabetes in the non-obese diabetic mouse. Diabetologia 2005; 48 1565-1575.

[73] Takiishi T, Korf H, Van Belle TL, Robert S, Grieco FA, Caluwaerts S, Galleri L, Spagnuolo I, Steidler L, Van Huynegem K, Demetter P, Wasserfall C, Atkinson MA, Dotta F, Rottiers P, Gysemans C, Mathieu C. Reversal of autoimmune diabetes by restoration of antigen-specific tolerance using genetically modified Lactococcus lactis in mice. The Journal of Clinical Investigation 2012; 122(5):1717-1725.

[74] Ivanov II, Atarashi K, Manel N, Brodie EL, Shima T, Karaoz U,Wei D, Goldfarb KC, Santee CA, Lynch SV. Induction of intestinal Th17 cells by segmented filamentous bacteria. Cell 2009; 139:485-498.

[75] Geuking MB, Cahenzli J, Lawson MA, Ng DC, Slack E, Hapfelmeier S, McCoy KD, Macpherson AJ. Intestinal bacterial colonization induces mutualistic regulatory T cell responses. Immunity 2011; 34(5):794-806.

[76] Ljungberg M, Korpela R, Ilonen J, Ludvigsson J, Vaarala O. Probiotics for the prevention of beta cell autoimmunity in children at genetic risk of type 1 diabetes—the PRODIA study. Annals of the New York Academy of Sciences 2006; 1079:360-364.

[77] Norris JM. Infant and childhood diet and type 1 diabetes risk: recent advances and prospects. Current Diabetes Report 2010; 10(5):345-349.

[78] Brekke HK, Ludvigsson J. Daily vegetable intake during pregnancy negatively associated to islet autoimmunity in the offspring--the ABIS study. Pediatric Diabetes 2010; 11(4):244-250.

[79] Virtanen SM, Uusitalo L, Kenward MG, Nevalainen J Uusitalo U,Kronberg-Kippilä C, Ovaskainen ML, Arkkola T, Niinistö S, Hakulinen T, Ahonen S, Simell O, Ilonen J,Veijola R, Knip M. Maternal food consumption during pregnancy and risk of advanced β-cell autoimmunity in the offspring. Pediatric Diabetes 2011; 12(2):95-99.

[80] Knip M, Virtanen SM, Akerblom HK. Infant feeding and the risk of type 1 diabetes. The American Journal Of Clinical Nutrition 2010; 91(5):1506S-1513S.

[81] Gerstein HC. Cow's milk exposure and type I diabetes mellitus. A critical overview of the clinical literature. Diabetes Care 1994; 17(1):13-19.

[82] Brekke HK, Ludvigsson JF, van Odijk J, Ludvigsson J. Breastfeeding and introduction of solid foods in Swedish infants: the All Babies in Southeast Sweden study. British Journal of Nutrition 2005; 94(3):377-382.

[83] Castaño L, Eisenbarth GS. Type 1 diabetes: a chronic disease of human, mouse and rat. Annual Review of Immunology 1990; 8:647-679.

[84] Couper JJ, Steele C, Beresford S, Powell T, McCaul K, Pollard A, Gellert S, Tait B, Harrison LC, Colman PG. Lack of association between duration of breast-feeding or introduction of cow's milk and development of islet autoimmunity. Diabetes 1999; 48(11):2145-2149.

[85] Holmberg H, Wahlberg J, Vaarala O, Ludvigsson J, ABIS Study Group. Short duration of breast-feeding as a risk-factor for beta-cell autoantibodies in 5-year-old children from the general population. British Journal of Nutrition 2007; 97(1):111-116.

[86] Ziegler AG, Schmid S, Huber D, Hummel M, Bonifacio E. Early infant feeding and risk of developing type 1 diabetes-associated autoantibodies. Journal of American Medical Association 2003; 290(13)1721-1728.

[87] Simpson M, Mojibian M, Barriga K, Scott FW, Fasano A, Rewers M, Norris JM. An exploration of Glo-3A antibody levels in children at increased risk for type 1 diabetes mellitus. Pediatric Diabetes 2009; 10(8):563-572.

[88] Virtanen SM, Kenward MG, Erkkola M, Kautiainen S, Kronberg-Kippilä C, Hakulinen T, Ahonen S, Uusitalo L, Niinistö S, Veijola R, Simell O, Ilonen J,Knip M. Age at introduction of new foods and advanced beta cell autoimmunity in young children with HLA-conferred susceptibility to type 1 diabetes. Diabetologia 2006; 49(7): 1512-1521.

[89] Mojibian M, Chakir H, Lefebvre DE, Crookshank JA, Sonier B, Keely E, Scott FW. Diabetes-specific HLA-DR-restricted proinflammatory T-cell response to wheat polypeptides in tissue transglutaminase antibody-negative patients with type 1 diabetes. Diabetes 2009; 58(8):1789-1796.

[90] Funda DP, Kaas A, Tlaskalová-Hogenová H, Buschard K. Gluten-free but also gluten-enriched (gluten+) diet prevent diabetes in NOD mice; the gluten enigma in type 1 diabetes. Diabetes/Metabolism Research and Reviews 2008; 24(1):59-63.

[91] The EURODIAB Substudy 2 Study Group. Vitamin D supplement in early childhood and risk for Type I (insulin-dependent) diabetes mellitus. Diabetologia 1999; 42(1): 51-54.

[92] Hyppönen E, Läärä E, Reunanen A, Järvelin MR, Virtanen SM. Intake of vitamin D and risk of type 1 diabetes: a birth-cohort study. Lancet 2001; 358(9292):1500-1503.

[93] Simpson M, Brady H, Yin X, Seifert J, Barriga K, Hoffman M, Bugawan T, Barón AE, Sokol RJ, Eisenbarth G, Erlich H, Rewers M, Norris JM. No association of vitamin D intake or 25-hydroxyvitamin D levels in childhood with risk of islet autoimmunity and type 1 diabetes: the Diabetes Autoimmunity Study in the Young (DAISY). Diabetologia 2011; 54(11):2779-2788.

[94] Mathieu C, Gysemans C, Giulietti A, Bouillon R. Vitamin D and diabetes. Diabetologia 2005; 48(7):1247-1257.

[95] Gupta S, Sharma TK, Kaushik GG, Shekhawat VP. Vitamin E supplementation may ameliorate oxidative stress in type 1 diabetes mellitus patients. Clinical Laboratory Science 2011; 57(5-6):379-386.

[96] Stene LC, Thorsby PM, Berg JP, Rønningen KS, Joner G; Norwegian Childhood Diabetes Study Group. Peroxisome proliferator-activated receptor-gamma2 Pro12Ala

polymorphism, cod liver oil and risk of type 1 diabetes. Pediatric Diabetes 2008; 9(1): 40-45.

[97] Norris JM, Yin X, Lamb MM, Barriga K, Seifert J, Hoffman M, Orton HD, Barón AE, Clare-Salzler M, Chase HP, Szabo NJ, Erlich H, Eisenbarth GS, Rewers M. Omega-3 polyunsaturated fatty acid intake and islet autoimmunity in children at increased risk for type 1 diabetes. Journal of American Medical Association 2006; 29(12): 1420-1428.

[98] Muntoni S, Mereu R, Atzori L, Mereu A, Galassi S, Corda S, Frongia P, Angius E, Pusceddu P, Contu P, Cucca F, Congia M, Muntoni S. High meat consumption is associated with type 1 diabetes mellitus in a Sardinian case-control study. Acta Diabetologica 2012 [Epub ahead of print].

[99] Benson VS, Vanleeuwen JA, Taylor J, Somers GS, McKinney PA, Van Til L. Type 1 diabetes mellitus and components in drinking water and diet: a population-based, case-control study in Prince Edward Island, Canada. Journal of the American College of Nutrition 2010; 29(6):612-624.

[100] Graham S, Courtois P, Malaisse WJ, Rozing J, Scott FW, Mowat AM. Enteropathy precedes type 1 diabetes in the BB rat. Gut 2004; 53:1437-1444.

[101] Neu J, Reverte CM, Mackey AD, Liboni K, Tuhacek-Tenace LM, Hatch M, Li N, Caicedo RA, Schatz DA, Atkinson M. Changes in intestinal morphology and permeability in the biobreeding rat before the onset of type 1 diabetes. Journal of Pediatric Gastroenterology and Nutrition 2005; 40(5):589-595.

[102] Visser JT, Lammers K, Hoogendijk A, Boer MW, Brugman S, Beijer-Liefers S, Zandvoort A, Harmsen H, Welling G, Stellaard F, Bos NA, Fasano A, Rozing J. Restoration of impaired intestinal barrier function by the hydrolysed casein diet contributes to the prevention of type 1 diabetes in the diabetes-prone BioBreeding rat. Diabetologia 2010; 53(12):2621-2628.

[103] Lee AS, Gibson DL, Zhang Y, Sham HP, Vallance BA, Dutz JP. Gut barrier disruption by an enteric bacterial pathogen accelerates insulitis in NOD mice. Diabetologia 2010; 53:741-748.

[104] Kuitunen M, Saukkonen T, Ilonen J, Akerblom HK, Savilahti E. Intestinal permeability to mannitol and lactulose in children with type 1 diabetes with the HLA-DQB1*02 allele. Autoimmunity 2002; 35:365-368.

[105] Sapone A, de Magistris L, Pietzak M, Clemente MG, Tripathi A, Cucca F, Lampis R, Kryszak D, Cartenì M, Generoso M, Iafusco D, Prisco F, Laghi F, Riegler G, Carratu R, Counts D, Fasano A. Zonulin upregulation is associated with increased gut permeability in subjects with type 1 diabetes and their relatives. Diabetes 2006; 55(5): 1443-1449.

[106] Bosi E, Molteni L, Radaelli MG, Folini L, Fermo I, Bazzigaluppi E, Piemonti L, Pastore MR, Paroni R. Increased intestinal permeability precedes clinical onset of type 1 diabetes. Diabetologia 2006; 49(12):2824-2827.

[107] Watts T, Berti I, Sapone A, Gerarduzzi T, Not T, Zielke R, Fasano A. Role of the intestinal tight junction modulator zonulin in the pathogenesis of type I diabetes in BB diabetic-prone rats. Proceedings of National Academy of Sciences of the U.S.A 2005; 102:2916-2921.

[108] Jalonen T, Isolauri E, Heyman M, Crain-Denoyelle AM, Sillanaukee P, Koivula T. Increased beta-lactoglobulin absorption during rotavirus enteritis in infants: relationship to sugar permeability. Pediatric Research 1991; 30:290-293.

[109] Brugman S, Klatter FA, Visser JT, Wildeboer-Veloo AC, Harmsen HJ, Rozing J, Bos NA. Antibiotic treatment partially protects against type 1 diabetes in the Bio-Breeding diabetes-prone rat. Is the gut flora involved in the development of type 1 diabetes? Diabetologia 2006; 49(9):2105-2108.

[110] Valladares R, Sankar D, Li N, Williams E, Lai KK, Abdelgeliel AS, Gonzalez CF, Wasserfall CH, Larkin J, Schatz D, Atkinson MA, Triplett EW, Neu J, Lorca GL. Lactobacillus johnsonii N6.2 mitigates the development of type 1 diabetes in BB-DP rats. PLoS One 2010; 5(5):e10507.

[111] Blaschitz C, Raffatellu M. Th17 cytokines and the gut mucosal barrier. Journal of Clinical Immunology 2010; 30:196-203.

[112] Vaarala O. Is the origin of type 1 diabetes in the gut? Immunology and Cell Biology 2012; 90(3):271-276.

[113] Hirata Y, Broquet AH, Menche´n L, Kagnoff MF. Activation of innate immune defense mechanisms by signaling through RIG-I/IPS-1 in intestinal epithelial cells. Journal of Immunology 2007; 179:5425-5432.

[114] Coyne CB, Shen L, Turner JR, Bergelson JM. Coxsackievirus entry across epithelial tight junctions requires occludin and the small GTPases Rab34 and Rab5. Cell Host & Microbe 2007; 2:181-192.

[115] Nava P, López S, Arias CF, Islas S, González-Mariscal L. The rotavirus surface protein VP8 modulates the gate and fence function of tight junctions in epithelial cells. Journal of Cell Science 2004; 117:5509-5519.

[116] Auricchio R, Paparo F, Maglio M, Franzese A, Lombardi F, Valerio G, Nardone G, Percopo S, Greco L, Troncone R. In vitro-deranged intestinal immune response to gliadin in type 1 diabetes. Diabetes 2004; 53(7):1680-1683.

[117] Lammers KM, Lu R, Brownley J, Lu B, Gerard C, Thomas K, Rallabhandi P, Shea-Donohue T, Tamiz A, Alkan S, Netzel-Arnett S, Antalis T, Vogel SN, Fasano A. Gliadin induces an increase in intestinal permeability and zonulin release by binding to the chemokine receptor CXCR3. Gastroenterology 2008; 135(1):194-204.

[118] Hansen AK, Ling F, Kaas A, Funda DP, Farlov H, Buschard K. Diabetes preventive gluten-free diet decreases the number of caecal bacteria in non-obese diabetic mice. Diabetes Metabolism Research and Reviews 2006; 22:220-225.

[119] Vaarala O, Atkinson MA, Neu J. The "perfect storm" for type 1 diabetes: the complex interplay between intestinal microbiota, gut permeability, and mucosal immunity. Diabetes 2008; 57:2555-2562.

[120] Catassi C, Bonucci A, Coppa GV, Carlucci A, Giorgi PL. Intestinal permeability changes during the first month: effect of natural versus artificial feeding. Journal of Pediatric Gastroenterology and Nutrition 1995; 21:383-386.

[121] Piirainen L, Pesola J, Pesola I, Komulainen J, Vaarala O. Breastfeeding stimulates total and cow's milk-specific salivary IgA in infants. Pediatric Allergy and Immunology 2009; 20:295-298.

[122] Vaarala O. Is it dietary insulin? Annals if the New York Academy of Science 2006; 1079:350-359.

[123] Scott FW, Cloutier HE, Kleemann R, Wöerz-Pagenstert U, Rowsell P, Modler HW, Kolb H. Potential mechanisms by which certain foods promote or inhibit the development of spontaneous diabetes in BB rats: dose, timing, early effect on islet area, and switch in infiltrate from Th1 to Th2 cells. Diabetes 1997; 46(4):589-598.

[124] Knip M, Virtanen SM, Seppä K, Ilonen J, Savilahti E, Vaarala O, Reunanen A, Teramo K, Hämäläinen AM, Paronen J, Dosch HM, Hakulinen T, Akerblom HK; Finnish TRIGR Study Group. Dietary intervention in infancy and later signs of beta-cell autoimmunity. The New England Journal of Medicine 2010; 363(20):1900-1908.

[125] Vaarala O, Ilonen J, Ruohtula T, Pesola J, Virtanen SM, Härkönen T, Koski M, Kallioinen H, Tossavainen O, Poussa T, Järvenpää AL, Komulainen J, Lounamaa R, Akerblom HK, Knip M. Removal of Bovine Insulin From Cow's Milk Formula and Early Initiation of Beta-Cell Autoimmunity in the FINDIA Pilot Study. Archives of Pediatrics & Adolescent Medicine 2012 Mar 5 [epub ahead of print].

[126] Filippi CM, Estes EA, Oldham JE, von Herrath MG. Immunoregulatory mechanisms triggered by viral infections protect from type 1 diabetes in mice. Journal Clinical Investigation 2009; 119(6):1515-1523.

[127] Filippi CM, von Herrath MG. Viral trigger for type 1 diabetes: pros and cons. Diabetes. 2008; 57(11):2863-2871.

[128] Pietropaolo M, Trucco M. Viral elements in autoimmunity of type 1 diabetes. Trends Endocrinology and Metabolism 1996; 7:139-144.

[129] Barbeau WE. What is the key environmental trigger in type 1 diabetes - Is it viruses, or wheat gluten, or both? Autoimmunity Review. 2012 May 22 [Epub ahead of print].

[130] Thomas HE, Parker JL, Schreiber RD, Kay TW. IFN-gamma action on pancreatic beta cells causes class I MHC upregulation but not diabetes. Journal of Clinical Investigation 1998; 102(6):1249-1257.

[131] Bottazzo GF, Dean BM, McNally JM, MacKay EH, Swift PG, Gamble DR. In situ characterization of autoimmune phenomena and expression of HLA molecules in the pancreas in diabetic Insulitis. The New England Journal of Medicine 1998; 313(6): 353-360.

[132] Nejentsev S, Walker N, Riches D, Egholm M, Todd JA. Rare variants of IFIH1, a gene implicated in antiviral responses, protect against type 1 diabetes. Science. 2009; 324(5925):387-389.

[133] Atkinson MA, Bowman MA, Campbell L, Darrow BL, Kaufman DL, Maclaren NK. Cellular immunity to a determinant common to glutamate decarboxylase and coxsackie virus in insulin-dependent diabetes. Journal of Clinical Investigation 1994; 94(5):2125-2129.

[134] Horwitz MS, Ilic A, Fine C, Rodriguez E, Sarvetnick N. Presented antigen from damaged pancreatic beta cells activates autoreactive T cells in virus-mediated autoimmune diabetes. Journal of Clinical Investigation 2002; 109(1):79-87.

[135] Imagawa A, Hanafusa T. Fulminant type 1 diabetes--an important subtype in East Asia. Diabetes Metabolism Research Review 2011; 27(8):959-964.

[136] Smelt MJ, Faas MM, de Haan BJ, Draijer C, Hugenholtz GC, de Haan A, Engelse MA, de Koning EJ, de Vos P. Susceptibility of human pancreatic β cells for cytomegalovirus infection and the effects on cellular immunogenicity. Pancreas 2012; 41(1):39-49.

[137] Honeyman MC, Coulson BS, Stone NL, Gellert SA, Goldwater PN, Steele CE, Couper JJ, Tait BD, Colman PG, Harrison LC. Association between rotavirus infection and pancreatic islet autoimmunity in children at risk of developing type 1 diabetes. Diabetes. 2000;49(8):1319-1324.

[138] Ginsberg-Fellner F, Witt ME, Fedun B, Taub F, Dobersen MJ, McEvoy RC, Cooper LZ, Notkins AL, Rubinstein P. Diabetes mellitus and autoimmunity in patients with the congenital rubella syndrome. Reviews of Infectious Diseases 1985; 1:S170-176.

[139] Banatvala JE, Bryant J, Schernthaner G, Borkenstein M, Schober E, Brown D, De Silva LM, Menser MA, Silink M. Coxsackie B, mumps, rubella, and cytomegalovirus specific IgM responses in patients with juvenile-onset insulin-dependent diabetes mellitus in Britain, Austria, and Australia. Lancet 1985; 1(8443):1409-1412.

[140] Green J, Casabonne D, Newton R. Coxsackie B virus serology and Type 1 diabetes mellitus: a systematic review of published case-control studies. Diabetic Medicine 2004; 21(6):507-514.

[141] Tauriainen S, Oikarinen S, Oikarinen M, Hyöty H. Enteroviruses in the pathogenesis of type 1 diabetes. Seminars in Immunopathology 2011; 33(1):45-55.

[142] Tracy S, Drescher KM, Jackson JD, Kim K, Kono K. Enteroviruses, type 1 diabetes and hygiene: a complex relationship. Reviews in Medical Virology 2010; 20(2): 106-116.

[143] Oikarinen S, Martiskainen M, Tauriainen S, Huhtala H, Ilonen J, Veijola R, Simell O, Knip M, Hyöty H. Enterovirus RNA in blood is linked to the development of type 1 diabetes. Diabetes 2011; 60(1):276-279.

[144] Hober D, Sauter P. Pathogenesis of type 1 diabetes mellitus: interplay between enterovirus and host. Nature Reviews in Endocrinology 2010; 6(5):279-289.

[145] Dotta F, Censini S, van Halteren AG, Marselli L, Masini M, Dionisi S, Mosca F, Boggi U, Muda AO, Prato SD, Elliott JF, Covacci A, Rappuoli R, Roep BO, Marchetti P. Coxsackie B4 virus infection of beta cells and natural killer cell insulitis in recent-onset type 1 diabetic patients. Proceedings of the National Academic of Sciences of the U.S.A 2007; 104(12):5115-5120.

[146] Grieco FA, Sebastiani G, Spagnuolo I, Patti A, Dotta F. Immunology in the clinic review series; focus on type 1 diabetes and viruses: how viral infections modulate beta cell function. Clinical Experimental Immunology 2012; 168(1):24-29.

[147] Schulte BM, Lanke KH, Piganelli JD, Kers-Rebel ED, Bottino R, Trucco M, Huijbens RJ, Radstake TR, Engelse MA, de Koning EJ, Galama JM, Adema GJ, van Kuppeveld FJ. Cytokine and chemokine production by human pancreatic islets upon enterovirus infection. Diabetes. 2012; 61(8):2030-2036.

[148] Tracy S, Drescher KM. Coxsackievirus infections and NOD mice: relevant models of protection from, and induction of, type 1 diabetes. Annals of the New York Academy of Sciences 2007; 1103:143-151.

[149] Classen JB, Classen DC. The timing of pediatric immunization and the risk of insulin-dependent diabetes mellitus. Infectious Disease Clinical Practice 1997; 6:449-454.

[150] Classen JB, Classen DC. Clustering of cases of type 1 diabetes mellitus occurring 2-4 years after vaccination is consistent with clustering after infections and progression to type 1 diabetes mellitus in autoantibody positive individuals. Journal of Pediatric Endocrinology and Metabolism 2003; 16 (4):495-508.

[151] Hviid A, Stellfeld M, Wohlfahrt J, Melbye M. Childhood vaccination and type 1 diabetes. The New England Journal of Medicine 2004;350:1398-1404.

[152] DeStefano F, Mullooly JP, Okoro CA, Chen RT, Marcy SM, Ward JI, Vadheim CM, Black SB, Shinefield HR, Davis RL, Bohlke K; Vaccine Safety Datalink Team. Childhood vaccinations, vaccination timing, and risk of type 1 diabetes mellitus. Pediatrics 2001; 108(6):E112.

[153] Duderstadt SK, Rose CE Jr, Real TM, Sabatier JF, Stewart B, Ma G, Yerubandi UD, Eick AA, Tokars JI, McNeil MM. Vaccination and risk of type 1 diabetes mellitus in active component U.S. Military, 2002-2008. Vaccine 2012; 30(4):813-819.

[154] Bardage C, Persson I, Ortqvist A, Bergman U, Ludvigsson JF, Granath F. Neurological and autoimmune disorders after vaccination against pandemic influenza A (H1N1) with a monovalent adjuvanted vaccine: population based cohort study in Stockholm, Sweden. British Medical Journal 2011; 343:d5956.

[155] Yasuda H, Nagata M, Moriyama H, Kobayashi H, Akisaki T, Ueda H, Hara K, Yokono K. Development of fulminant Type 1 diabetes with thrombocytopenia after influenza vaccination: a case report. Diabetic Medicine 2012; 29(1):88-9.

[156] Daneman D. Type 1 diabetes. Lancet 2006;367:847-58.

[157] The DIAMOND Project Group. Incidence and trends of childhood type 1 diabetes worldwide 1990-1999. Diabetic Medicine 2006; 23:857-866.

[158] Evertsen J, Alemzadeh R, Wang X. Increasing incidence of pediatric type 1 diabetes mellitus in Southeastern Wisconsin: relationship with body weight at diagnosis. PLoS One 2009; 4(9):e6873.

[159] Libran IM, Pietropaolo M, Arslanian SA, La Porte RE, Becker DJ: Changing prevalence of overweight children and adolescents at onset of insulin-treated diabetes. Diabetes Care. 2003;26:2871-2875.

[160] TEDDY Study Group. The Environmental Determinants of Diabetes in the Young (TEDDY) Study. Annals of the New York Academy of Sciences 2008; 1150:1-13.

[161] Centro Nazionale per la Prevenzione e il Controllo delle Malattie (CCM). Okkio alla Salute, sistema di indagini sui rischi e comportamenti in età 6-17 anni. Ministero della Salute, Ministero della Pubblica Istruzione. 2008. www.epicentro.iss.it

[162] Wilkin TJ. The accelerator hypothesis: weight gain as the missing link between type I and type II diabetes. Diabetologia. 2001; 44:914-922.

[163] Wilkin TJ: The accelerator hypothesis: a review of the evidence for insulin resistance as the basis for Type 1 as well Type II diabetes. International Journal of Obesity 2009; 33:716-726.

[164] Accili D. The struggle for mastery in insulin action: From triumvirate to republic. Diabetes 2004; 53:1633-1642.

[165] Boden, G. Role of fatty acids in the pathogenesis of IR in NIDDM. Diabetes 1997; 46:3-10.

[166] Kaiser N, Leibowitz G, Nesher R. Glucotoxicity and β-cell failure in T2DM. Journal of Pediatric Endocrinology and Metabolism 2003; 16:5-22.

[167] Daneman D. Is the 'Accelerator Hypothesis' worthy of our attention? Diabetic Medicine 2005; 22:115-117.

[168] Kibirige M, Metcalf B, Renuka R, Wilkin TJ. Testing the Accelerator Hypothesis (1): the relationship between body mass and age at onset of type 1 diabetes. Diabetes Care 2003; 26:2865-2870.

[169] Betts P, Mulligan J, Ward P, Smith B, Wilkin TJ. Increasing body weight predicts the earlier onset of insulin-dependent diabetes in chidhood: testing the 'accelerator hypothesis'(2). Diabetic Medicine 2005; 22:144-151.

[170] Knerr I, Wolf J, Reinehr T, Stachow R, Grabert M, Schober E, Rascher W, Holl RW; DPV Scientific Initiative of Germany and Austria. The 'accelerator hypothesis': relationship between weight, height, body mass index and age at diagnosis in a large cohort of 9,248 German and Austrian children with type 1 diabetes mellitus. Diabetologia 2005; 48:2501-2504.

[171] Kordonouri O, Hartmann R. Higher body weight is associated with earlier onset of type 1 diabetes in children: confirming the 'Accelerator Hypothesis'. Diabetic Medicine 2005; 22:1778-1784.

[172] Clarke SL, Craig ME, Garnett SP, Chan AK, Cowell CT, Cusumano JM, Kordonouri O, Sambasivan A, Donaghue KC. Higher Increased adiposity at diagnosis in jounger children with type 1 diabetes does not persist. Diabetes Care 2006; 29:1651-1653.

[173] Dabelea D, D'Agostino RB Jr, Mayer-Davis EJ, Pettitt DJ, Imperatore G, Dolan LM, Pihoker C, Hillier TA, Marcovina SM, Linder B, Ruggiero AM, Hamman RF; SEARCH for Diabetes in Youth Study Group. Testing the Accelerator Hypothesis. Diabetes Care 2006; 29:290-294.

[174] Porter JR, Barrett TG. Braking the Accelerator Hypothesis? (Letter) Diabetologia 2003; 47:352-356.

[175] O'Connell MA, Donath S, Cameron FS: Major increase in type 1 diabetes-no support for the Accelerator Hypothesis. Diabetic Medicine 2007; 24:920-923.

[176] Gimenez M, Aguilera E, Castell C, De Lara N, Nicolau J, Conget I. Relationship between BMI and age at diagnosis of Type 1 Diabetes in a Mediterranean Area in the period of 1990-2004. Diabetes Care 2007; 30:1593-1595.

[177] d'Annunzio G, Emmanuele V, Pistorio A, Morsellino V, Lorini R. Increased adiposity at diagnosis in younger children with type 1 diabetes does not persist: response to Clarke et al. Diabetes Care 2007; 30:e9.

[178] Porter JR, Barrett TG. Acquired non-type 1 diabetes in childhood: subtypes, diagnosis and management. Archives of Disease in Childhood 2004; 89:1138-1144.

[179] De Santis M, Selmi C. The therapeutic potential of epigenetics in autoimmune diseases. Clinical Reviews in Allergy & Immunology 2012; 42(1):92-101.

[180] Brooks WH, Le Dantec C, Pers JO, Youinou P, Renaudineau Y. Epigenetics and autoimmunity. Journal of Autoimmunity 2010; 34(3):207-219.

[181] Meda F, Folci M, Baccarelli A, Selmi C. The epigenetics of autoimmunity. Cellular & Molecular Immunology 2011; 8(3):226-236.

[182] Fraga MF, Ballestar E, Paz MF, Ropero S, Setien F, Ballestar ML, Heine-Suñer D, Cigudosa JC, Urioste M, Benitez J, Boix-Chornet M, Sanchez-Aguilera A, Ling C, Carls-

son E, Poulsen P, Vaag A, Stephan Z, Spector TD, Wu YZ, Plass C, Esteller M. Epigenetic differences arise during the lifetime of monozygotic twins. Proceedings of the National Academy of Sciences of the USA 2005; 102(30):10604-10609.

[183] Pfleger C, Meierhoff G, Kolb H, Schloot NC; p520/521 Study Group. Association of T-cell reactivity with beta-cell function in recent onset type 1 diabetes patients. Journal of Autoimmunity 2010; 34(2):127-135.

[184] Wilson CB, Rowell E, Sekimata M. Epigenetic control of T-helper-cell differentiation. Nature reviews. Immunology 2009; 9(2):91-105.

[185] Fox JT, Stover PJ. Folate-mediated one-carbon metabolism. Vitamins and Hormones 2008; 79:1-44.

[186] Chamson-Reig A, Arany EJ, Summers K, Hill DJ. A low protein diet in early life delays the onset of diabetes in the non-obese diabetic mouse. Journal of Endocrinology 2009; 201(2):231-239.

[187] Kaati G, Bygren LO, Edvinsson S. Cardiovascular and diabetes mortality determined by nutrition during parents' and grandparents' slow growth period. European Journal of Humane Genetics 2002; 10(11):682-688.

[188] Vaarala O, Atkinson MA, Neu J. The "perfect storm" for type 1 diabetes: the complex interplay between intestinal microbiota, gut permeability, and mucosal immunity. Diabetes 2008; 57(10):2555-2562.

Chapter 9

Common Mechanisms of Pathogenesis of Tissue-Specific Autoimmune Diseases: The Edited Model to Illustrate Those for IDDM and Multiple Sclerosis

S. A. Krynskiy, A. V. Kostyakov, D. S. Kostyushev,
D. A. Gnatenko and S. V. Suchkov

Additional information is available at the end of the chapter

http://dx.doi.org/10.5772/53597

1. Introduction

Autoimmune diseases result from specific immune response to structures of the self. Such a response, resulting from activation of self-specific lymphocytes, is an inevitable side effect of the work of the immune system. However, mechanisms of central and peripheral tolerance normally prevent damage to tissues of the organism, blocking activation and proliferation of autoreactive lymphoid cells. Thus, it would be more accurate to say that autoimmune diseases result from breakdown of tolerance mechanisms that leads to chronic self-sustained response against the structures of the self. Autoimmune diseases should be discriminated from autoimmune reactions. The latter are associated with immune response against infectious pathogens and stop immediately after the pathogenic agent is eliminated. Autoimmune diseases are also quite frequently associated with cross-reactive immune response to exogenous pathogens. In fact, such a link is implicated into pathogenesis of most of those diseases. However, autoimmune diseases continue to progress even if the pathogen is cleared.

The key feature that distinguishes "normal" autoimmunity from pathological conditions is breakdown of tolerance that takes place in the latter case. This difference is illustrated by comparing characteristics of autoantibodies present in normal organism with characteristics of autoantibodies in patients with autoimmune diseases. Apart from higher titers in the patients with autoimmune diseases, antibodies in those patients also show higher avidity to target antigen and mono\oligoclonal structure, as opposed to polyclonal structure in normal samples. In normal organism, detected autoantibodies typically belong to IgM isotype, while in pathology they usually belong to IgG isotype. This has an important implication, as production of IgG antibodies can not be mediated by B-lymphocytes alone. It practically always requires involvement of antigen-specific CD4+ T-cells, which illustrates that pathogenesis of autoimmune diseases is a complex multistep process, requiring breakdown of tolerance on several levels.

	Normal samples	Samples from patients with autoimmune conditions
Isotype	IgM	IgG
Affinity	Low	High
Clonal structure	Polyclonal	Usually oligoclonal or monoclona
Titer	Low	High

Table 1. Autoantibody characteristics in normal individuals compared to those n individuals having a tissue-specific autoimmune disease.

Etiology of autoimmune diseases remains obscure, along with factors that serve as triggers for the disease. Nowadays it seems obvious that neither genetic predisposition nor environmental factors alone are sufficient for causing the disease. The common concept is that autoimmune diseases arise from complex interaction between genetic factors and environment. The conception of post-infectious autoimmune syndrome (PIFAS) defines infection as an important component of pathogenesis (Foy et al., 1996). According to this conception, autoimmune diseases develop in genetically predisposed organisms as a result of specific infection causing cross-reactive immune response affecting own cells and tissues of the organism. Later this response becomes self-sustained and can continue even in the absence of infectious agent that caused it in the first place. In accordance with this conception, evidence arises that in most cases of autoimmune conditions, the primary event of pathogenesis is infection. Arguments that support role of infection in specific autoimmune diseases can be divided into several categories: clinical (clinical findings, as in the case of acute rheumatic fever following streptococcal infections), epidemiological (obtained in epidemiological studies that fit criteria of evidence-based medicine), laboratory (based on laboratory diagnostics of infection in the past, i.e. by accessing antibody levels in biological fluids or obtaining DNA of the pathogen from tissues affected by immune response).

These criteria are applied to show correlation between presence of an infectious agent in the organism and an autoimmune condition. Once such correlation has been found, the next step is studying mechanisms that mediate induction of disease. In relation to pathogens in question, such mechanisms can be divided into specific (those that include stimulation of antigen-specific clones of lymphocytes) and non-specific (based on causing appropriate inflammatory environment for disease induction) (Goodnow et al., 2007). Deeper insight into the problem shows that several of these mechanisms have to be active to initiate an autoimmune response, and that both specific and non-specific mechanisms typically contribute to pathogenesis equally.

http://dx.doi.org/10.5772/53597

2. Mechanisms of tolerance: An overview

A number of mechanisms is at work to prevent negative effects associated with autoimmune reactions. The conception of tolerance has been introduced to explain those mechanisms. Tolerance is lack of reactivity of the immune system to antigens of the body. Tolerance is an active process that can be induced through central and peripheral mechanisms. Central tolerance refers to processes taking place during lymphocyte differentiation in central lymphoid organs, before activation (in the process of antigen-independent differentiation of lymphocytes). A classic example of central tolerance is negative selection of T-lymphocytes that takes place during their maturing in the thymus. Selection of lymphocytes in the thymus includes two stages. On the first stage cells that have low ability to react with own molecules of major histocompartibility complex (MHC) undergo apoptosis. Ability to react with own MHC is necessary for proper T-cell function, since T-cells respond only to antigen fragments presented by antigen-presenting cells (APCs) in complex with MHC molecules (B-cells, on the other hand, respond to full molecules of antigens and don't require interaction with MHC). On the second stage cells that undergo apoptosis are those that strongly react with fragments of own antigens of the body presented by MHC (the so-called negative selection). Therefore, cells that survive do have ability to react with own MHC, but not too strong an ability. Those cells also have low potential to respond to own antigen fragments. Such a complex process of selection is necessary, because T-cells have a central role in specific immune responses, and consequences of a tolerance breakdown at T-cell level would be quite grave. However, it should be noted that possibility of response to own pathogens is an inevitable side effect of the mechanisms T-cells utilize in their receptor mechanisms (requirement of interaction with own MHC molecules). In B-cells the mechanisms of selection don't differ principally from those in T-cells, however they are much less strict.

The described mechanisms aren't sufficient to fully prevent appearance of autoreactive clones in the blood. However, activation of T-cells requires several conditions to be met (apart from interaction of the antigen-specific receptor with its target). Appropriate contact between T-cell and APC is called immune synapse. A key condition for a successful activation is interaction of CD28 molecule of the T-cell with costimulatory molecules B1/B7 of the APC. Without such interaction, activation of TCR causes anergy or apoptosis of the lymphocyte. This interaction is unlikely in the absence of appropriate costimulation, which is induced by presence of non-specific molecular signals of "presence of danger" (DAMPs – Danger associated molecular patterns) or "presence of an infectious agent" (PAMPs – Pathogen associated molecular patterns). The latter include fragments of bacterial cellular wall, exogenous DNA, flagellin, etc. Those factors cause activation of APCs, increasing expression of MHC-antigen complexes and costimulatory molecules. In the event of interaction of an autoreactive T-lymphocyte with its target, the described costimulation is not expected to be active. That means that APCs would not be activated, and won't express necessary amounts of B1/B7. Expression of MHC molecules would also remain low. This mechanism of control ensures that T-cell activation seldom takes place without activation of innate immunity. As a result, autoreactive T-lymphocytes that interact with self-antigens more often than not undergo apoptosis or become anergic as a result of TCR stimulation without appropriate costimulation.

Activation of B-cells doesn't require antigen presentation in association with MHC. These cells have the ability to recognize antigens directly through BCR. However, as well as in the case of T-cells, stimulation of BCR has to be coupled with costimulatory mechanisms, or the cell would most likely undergo apoptosis. Signals inducing B-cells proliferation include interaction with PAMPs. Those are mediated by toll-like receptors (TLRs) that interact with PAMPs, and complement C3 receptor (CD21), that binds to C3 component of the complement. C3 binds to specific components of the mictobial cell wall (alternative complement activation), or to pathogens opsonised with antibodies (classic complement activation). Those mechanisms direct immune response towards reaction to microbial pathogens bearing signs of "danger".

Before the start of B-cell antigen dependent differentiation and antibody production, B-cells have to pass another checkpoint (Goodnow et al., 2007). That is interaction with T-cells specific for the same antigen, through CD40/CD40L system (Foy et al., 1996). Therefore, interaction of two antigen-specific cells, both of which have undergone multiple points of selection, is required before B-cell mediated immune response with highly-affined antibody production and memory cells formation can take place. Functional activity of the immune system is preciously regulated to minimize chances of autoimmune reaction.

Another mechanism controlling the activity of immune response is activity of regulatory T-cells (Treg). Natural Tregs have the phenotype of CD4+CD25low, and express a specific transcription factor – Foxp3. Foxp3 mediates suppressor function by inducing factors such as TGFbeta, GITR, IL-10. Upon activating, Treg cells specifically inhibit immune response. An important feature of their cells is that their TCRs show significantly higher affinity to own antigens than those in other T-cells. It is thought that cells with affinity to self-antigens higher than in most T-cells but lower than is required for negative selection may differentiate into Treg (Wan et al., 2007). There are also other types of regulatory lymphoid cells with suppressor function, such as induced Treg that form in vivo in conditions of activated CD4+-cells stimulation with IL-10, and B-regulatory cells.

An important function of mechanisms of tolerance is degenerative feedback for countering uncontrolled immune cells activation. Continuous stimulation of TCR causes negative regulation of CD 28 receptor needed for T-cell costimulation through B1 and B7 molecules of the APCs. Instead, T-cells start producing CTLA (CD 28), a molecule that is an antagonist for B1 and B7. This cuts costimulation of T-cells and causes induction of anergy.

3. Role of infection: The conception of PIFAS

Seeing that autoimmune diseases arise from lack of balance between stimulation of the immune system and activity of suppressor mechanisms, infection, especially chronic, proposes to be an important factor in the induction of autoimmune process. Even by itself,

http://dx.doi.org/10.5772/53597

chronic antigen stimulation accompanied by lymphocyte proliferation and activation of effector mechanisms significantly magnifies the chance of breakdown in tolerance mechanisms. A parallel can be drawn between autoimmune conditions and tumors of the immune system. The latter, rising from uncontrolled proliferation of lymphocytes, have been firmly associated with excessive chronic antigen stimulation (chronic infection with HIV, Hepatitis C, Epstein-Barr virus).

The conception of PIFAS distinguishes the following 5 steps in the pathogenesis of autoimmune diseases (Cherepachina et al., 2009):

1. Genetic predisposition.
2. Infectious process causing cross-reactive activation of the immune system.
3. Latent stage of the autoimmune disease characterized by production of autoantibodies and antigen-specific clones of lymphocytes. It is accompanied by morphological signs of immune inflammation (i.e., latent autoimmune insulitis preceding manifestation of autoimmune diabetes mellitus) and can be detected by accessing the proteome of the patient. Markers that can be detected in the proteome are divided into markers of immune inflammation and markers of tissue degeneration.
4. Latent stage of the disease accompanied by impairment of functional activity of the affected tissues which cab be detected by functional diagnostics or by accessing the metabolome of the patient.
5. Manifest stage of the disease.

4. Pathogenetic mechanisms of autoimmune diseases

Now we shall give a more detailed description of mechanisms that have a role in the pathogenesis of autoimmune diseases.

4.1. Molecular mimicry

The conception of molecular mimicry is one of the most common concepts in immunology. It is also the simplest hypothesis that can be applied to explain the etiology of autoimmune diseases. The conception is built on laboratory findings that show homology between amino acid sequences of infectious agents and those of proteins of the body. Activation of T-cells with TCR specific for the pathogen causes cross-reactive reaction to own antigens of the organism, and as a result, impairment of functions of target organs. For the pathogen this serves as a mechanism of evading the immune response, since self-reactive clones of lymphocytes are typically less active due to mechanisms of negative selection, and are also prone to suppression by mechanisms of peripheral tolerance. This interferes with elimination of the pathogen (Sherbet, 2009). And long-term persistence of the pathogen contributes even further to the ongoing autoimmune reaction. Such a reaction may or may not come to an end after and if the infectious agent is finally eliminated. In the latter case, the process becomes self-supporting, recruiting other mechanisms of disease progression. If secondary production of self-reactive T-lymphocyte clones takes place, as opposed to just antibody production, this usually marks the onset of autoimmune disease. An important factor here is the phenomenon of epitope spreading, which is caused by changes in conformation of antigens that are subject to immune response (see later).

4.2. Superantigens

As opposed to specific monoclonal stimulation of immune system caused by antigens, stimulation by superantigens causes polyclonal activation of cells of the immune system. Mechanisms of superantigen-mediated activation primarily affect T-cells activation. Stimulation by antigens causes activation of T-cells as a result of presentation of processed antigen by MHC molecules of the APCs. TCR binds to the peptide presented by MHC. Superantigens react directly with MHC molecules, binding to beta-unit of the molecule (Conti-Fine et al., 1997). They cause non-specific polyclonal activation of T-cells, reacting with all cells that can bind to appropriate MHC-molecule (all cells that are restricted to the haplotype of that MHC molecule). Participation of superantigens in the pathogenesis of autoimmune diseases seems to be indirect. One of the aspects is their contribution to inflammatory response and antigen presentation (mostly due to stimulation of macrophages by activated CD4+ Th1-cells). Pathogenic agents producing superantigens can also contribute to pathogenesis of autoimmune diseases by increasing the possibility of activation of autoreactive T-cells as a component of polyclonal activation.

4.3. Altered presentation of own antigens

The next component of pathogenesis is abnormal presentation of self-antigens caused by inflammatory response to infectious pathogens. This can refer to increased expression of HLA-molecules (Conti-Fine et al, 1997), aberrant expression of HLA molecules, presentation of antigens that are normally invisible for the immune system. These phenomena are frequently seen as a component of normal immune reactions (hence another important implication of infectious agents in the pathogenesis) or autoimmune inflammatory reactions.

It is a well known fact that stimulation with inflammatory cytokines causes an increase in expression of MHC molecules. This refers both to professional APCs (macrophages, B-lymphocytes, dendritic cells) and most other cell lines (in the latter case, expression of HLA I is increased, making the cells vulnerable to autoreactive CD8+ cytotoxic lymphocytes). Inflammatory signaling also stimulates aberrant expression of MHC, causing expression of HLA II by endothelial cells, fibroblasts and other cell lines that normally only express HLA I and don't function as antigen-presenting cells. Such aberrant expression of HLA molecules may lead to presentation of antigen determinants of the self that were previously unknown to the immune system.

Presentation of normally invisible antigens may occur as a result of breakdown of specific blood-brain barriers of "immunologically privileged" organs. This mechanism plays an important role in the pathogenesis of autoimmune uveitis, multiple sclerosis, etc.

4.4. Presentation of altered self-antigens. Epitope spreading

Disclosure of cryptic antigenic epitopes is an important mechanism in the progression of autoimmune diseases (Lehmann et al., 1997). Normal conformation of the body's proteins makes some epitopes invisible to antigen-recognizing receptors of the immune system. Conformation of peptides prevents those epitopes from being recognized by lymphoid cells. However, that also means that lymphocyte clones specific to those antigens do not get eliminated effectively during antigen-independent differentiation. Disclosure of those epitopes which may take place as a result of changes in protein conformation that result from immune inflammation may open up these epitopes for effective immune response. Those new targets for autoimmune reaction may have significantly higher affinity to antigen-recognizing receptors in comparison to the original ones. Clinically such an event is frequently associated with the disease taking rapidly progressive course, for example, with multiple sclerosis reaching secondary progressive type. The described phenomenon is known as epitope spreading – a process that is tightly associated with autoimmune diseases progression.

5. Conception of PIFAS as applied to explaining pathogenesis of autoimmune insulin-dependent diabetes mellitus

5.1. Introduction

Insulin-dependent diabetes mellitus (IDDM) is a chronic autoimmune disorder that results from autoimmune destruction of insulin-producing pancreatic beta cells. In IDDM, the autoimmune process is steadily progressive, inevitably leading to total destruction of Langerhans islet beta-cells and ceasing of production of insulin. Clinical manifestation of the disease, presented by symptoms of insulin deficiency, takes place quite late into the autoimmune inflammatory process, when about 90% of islet cells have been destroyed (Epstein, 1994). Such a gap between the status of the autoimmune process and clinical symptoms makes immunosuppressive therapy ineffective in most patients: although application of such therapy can low the intensity of immune inflammation or in some cases cause a relapse of the immune inflammation, patient almost always becomes insulin-dependant anyway. This is largely due to lack of functional reserves in the population of beta-cells at the time of the diagnosis. Early detection of the autoimmune process in IDDM and identification of risk factors for the disease would greatly broaden the grounds for pathogenetic therapy, but this problem has yet to be effectively solved.

Pathogenesis of IDDM includes following stages.

1. Genetic predisposition,

2. Primary immune response aimed at the mimicking infectious pathogen.

3. Latent autoimmune insulitis.

4. Asymptomatic impairment of beta-cell function (impairment of oral glucose tolerance).

5. Clinical manifestation of the disease.

Diagnostic markers vary for those stages: in the first stage, only markers of genetic predisposition can be detected (and used to calculate the risk of disease), while in the third stage it is possible to detect markers of autoimmune inflammation. In the manifesting stages of the full-term clinical illness canonical (routine) clinical diagnostic protocols would become possible and fruitful. It is evident that the key stage of pathogenesis in which the autoimmune process becomes irreversible and acquires self-progressive course is the third stage. An important task is diagnosing the disease at this stage, when there is room for pathogenetic therapy aimed at quenching immune inflammation.

5.2. Role of genetic factors in pathogenesis of IDDM

Important peculiarity of T1D pathogenesis is genetic predisposition that conditions the development of the disease. MHC (major histocompartibility complex) often elicits autoimmune responses by predetermining the inadequate behavior of immunocompetent cells. MHC represents a large family of genes encoding molecules of three major HLA (human leukocyte antigen) classes.

HLA class I

The HLA class I compartment contains both diabetoprotective genotypes and highly associative genes. HLA class I initiate and potentiate autoimmune destruction of beta cells. The diabetogenic alleles of MHC class I genes display age-related features. For example, HLA-E*0101 is predominant in patients in whom T1D developed during the first 10 years of life, while HLA-E*0103 is found in children under 10. (Kordonouri et al, 2010)

HLA class II

HLA class II constitute a family of genes which encode glycoproteins with an Ig-like structure and are predominantly localized on the APCs (antigen presenting cells) surface. Their functional role covers the presentation of antigen peptides to CD4 (+) T helper cells type I. Several autoimmune diseases (including T1D) are supported by promoting effects of HLA class II Ags. (Murdock et al., 2004).

HLA class III

The contribution of HLA class III to background predisposition of T1D is far fewer (compared to HLA classes I and II) but there are several HLA class III genes manifesting a diagnostically significant association with T1D. As an overall trend, HLA classes II and III provoke diabetes at the highest levels of the odds ratio, while the effect of HLA class I on T1D is much less expressed. (Lipponen et al., 2010).

Non-MHC genes also may play a prominent role in the development of autoimmune diseases.

There is quite a vast repertoire of non-MHC genes with a multitude of SNPs (single nucleotide polymorphism) that determine the attacks at some structural components of the pancreas or directly at insulin. Under certain conditions, e.g., under negative impacts of environmental factors these genes are "switched on" giving rise to immune disorders.

An immense variety of genes responsible for susceptibility to T1D are known, but their functional capabilities are either obscure or poorly investigated. Some genes whose role in etiology and pathogenesis of T1D leaves no doubt are described below.

TNFAIP3

Tumor necrosis factor, alpha-induced protein 3 is inhibitor of TNF-induced apoptosis. This gene realizes miscellaneous functions to provide protection of beta cells from programmed cell death, inactivation of NF-kappa B signals, prevention of inflammatory lesions of pancreatic cells, deceleration or delayed recruitment of immunocompetent cells into target organs, and so on. Mutations in this gene represent the most common mechanism of disregulation and disorganization of immune reactions resulting in autoimmunity. (Petrone et al., 2008)

INS

INS (insulin) gene is a key participant in the synthesis of insulin molecules. Proinsulin molecules are formed during transcription of INS. Mutations in INS are manifested as insulinopathies, e.g., enhanced production of "odd" insulin with impaired amino acid sequences and atypical conversion of proinsulin into insulin. The latter abnormality is unrelated to T1D; however, any change in the amino acid sequence may lead to immune failure and secretion of autoAbs. (Pociot et al., 2002)

ERBB3

ERBB3 (Erythroblastic Leukemia Viral Oncogene Homolog) modulates the presentation of Ags and increases the risk of T1D. Mutations in ERBB3 lead to immunoregulatory collapses coupled with continuous emergence of autoreactive cells.

IL2RA

It regulates immune and inflammatory responses, exerts negative control over cell proliferation and favors differentiation of T cells. In addition, IL2RA (interleukin-2 receptor-alpha) controls apoptosis via a positive feedback mechanism.

Mutation in IL2RA predetermine the susceptibility to T1D by interfering with the transcription and/or splicing of mRNA. In this way, IL2 and IL2RA exert genetic control over protein expression in different cell subpopulations.

IFIH1

Interferon induced with helicase C domain 1(IFIH1) gene is involved in innate immune defense against viruses. Upon interaction with intracellular dsRNA(double-stranded RNA) produced during viral replication, triggers a transduction cascade involving MAVS/IPS1, which results in the activation of NF-kappa-B, IRF3 and IRF7 and the induction of the expression of antiviral cytokines such as IFN-beta and RANTES (CCL5). IFIH1 is directly involved in the destruction of Langerhans islets due to pooling and mobilization of autoreactive cells in response to viral invasion. This circumstance aggravates immune dissonance and promotes self-restructuring of targeted organs by provoking persistent deficiency of the pancreas and accelerating insulin failure.

CD226 (rs763361) SNPs regulate the activity of certain cells involved in immune mechanisms mediating beta cell destruction.

5.3. Pathology of IDDM

Morphologic substrate of the disease is autoimmune insulitis, The characteristic feature of insulitis in patients with IDDM is complete lack of beta cells. Other types of cells in the Langerhans islets remain intact. The inflammatory infiltrate consists mostly of CD8+ cells with some other lymphocytes, macrophages and plasmocytes. Beta-cells of the islets demonstrate increased expression of HLA I, while the APCs and endothelial cells show increased expression of HLA II. This is a characteristic feature of immune inflammation with cell-mediated immune response.

The key factor in beta-cells destruction is thought to be CD8+-cells-mediated cytotoxycity. However, CD4+ cells are also crucial for pathogenesis, since blocking their proliferation in mice hampers the disease progress. This is quite logical, since, CD8+ cells activation requires participation of CD4+ cells. Furthermore, it seems that apart from cell-mediated cytotoxicity, another mechanism playing just as important role in the disease progression is inflammatory cytokine production by macrophages and CD4+ cells. Cytokines that have been implicated in the pathogenesis of IDDM are interleukin-1 (IL-1) and interferon-alpha (Fabris et al., 1998, Waguri et al., 1994). There have been reports of patients developing fulminant IDDM in the course of interferon-alpha therapy (Fabris et al., 1998). These and other cytokines contribute to inflammatory response and promote CD8+ cells activity. IL-1 causes increased NO production in beta cells which leads to excessive synthesis of free radicals. Beta-cells are quite sensitive to damage caused by free radicals, which makes them especially vulnerable to inflammatory responses. This data shows that even non-specific inflammation can cause beta-cell destruction (and become the foundation for specific autoimmune response to emerge). Apart from creating a condition of increased susceptibility to specific immune reaction against beta-cells, inflammatory status by itself may cause beta-cells destruction, as well as serve as a mechanism of stimulation of the immune system with altered antigens of the destroyed cells.

Autoantibodies present in IDDM include:

- GAD(Glutamic acid decarboxylase) 65 and GAD67 autoantibodies to glutamate decarboxylase (an enzyme that catalyzes the conversion of glutamic acid into γ-aminobutyric acid and CO2;
- IA-2(insulinoma antigen 2) autoantibodies to membrane-bound proteins IA-2 and IA-2β;
- ICA (islet cell antibody) autoantibodies to a heterogeneous cluster of antigens expressed in beta cells;
- ZnT8 autoantibodies to a member of the zinc transporter protein family;
- IAA - autoantibodies to insulin.

Serving as markers of the autoimmune inflammatory process, these antibodies can be present before clinical onset of the disease, and can be used for detecting IDDM at latent stages. The ICA autoantibodies, reacting with cytoplasmic antigens of islet cells, are found in IDDM patients in 0.5 % of normal subjects and in 70-80 % of patients with newly diagnosed IDDM. Those oligoclonal antibodies react with a variety of antigens. One of those is pancreatic enzyme glutamate decarboxylase. Presence of ICA autoantibodies in healthy subjects increases the risk for future development of the disease. The risk is lower for the patients with ICA autoantibodies that react with glutamate decarboxylase than for those who have antibodies specific for other targets. The link is age-dependent, which is attributed to the risk of autoimmune IDDM being higher in younger people. The disease also takes more rapid course in younger patients, with less time passing between clinical onset and complete loss of insulin production.

The anti-insulin antibodies are found in about 50% of patients with newly diagnosed IDDM. Those antibodies may also originate from insulin administration, which is a case in patients receiving non-human insulin, and interferes with efficiency of treatment. However, in IDDM anti-insulin antibodies may represent autoimmune reaction to own tissues, before any insulin administration. They can be used in combination with islet-cell cytoplasmic autoantibodies for prediction of IDDM development. Combined use of both autoantibodies greatly increases diagnostic value of the test.

In vitro, mononuclear cells of patients with IDDM proliferate in response to glutamate decarboxylase. This reaction can be detected earlier than diagnostically significant levels of anti-glutamate decarboxylase Abs. So, in vitro reaction of mononuclear cells with glutamate decarboxylase is considered to be one of the earliest markers of autoimmunity against beta-cells.

5.4. Role of infection in the pathogenesis of IDDM

One of the conceptions proposed to explain the pathogenesis of IDDM is the conception of molecular mimicry. Pathogens having antigen determinants homological to those of beta-cells include Coxacie virus (common epitopes with glutamate decarboxylase – an enzyme characteristic for beta-cells), mumps virus and Chlamidia pneumoniae. There are several mechanisms that allow viral infection to contribute to pathogenesis. In case of rubella virus and cytomegalovirus, there is evidence of direct induction of autoimmunity. Infection with those agents is associated with presence of autoantibodies in newly diagnosed patients with IDDM. Also, cytomegalovirus has been shown to induce production of antibodies to 38 kDa protein of the islet cells (Yoon et al., 1990). Those antibodies are frequently detected in patients with IDDM. However, as of now there is little reliable data on amino acid sequences homology between proteins of rubella virus and cytomegalovirus and islet cell antigens.

Another way infectious pathogens can contribute to pathogenesis of IDDM is through direct cytolytic effect on islet cells. An example is Coxsackie B virus, which mediates immune-independent cytolysis of beta-cells (Andreoletti et al., 1998). Coxsackie B virus infection has been shown to be a risk factor for IDDM (Andreoletti et al., 1998), and homology has been shown between viral protein 2C and islet cell antigen GAD 65 (Huang et al., 2011). Cytolytic effect even further amplifies the contribution of this agent to pathogenesis, as antigen release from beta-cells and non-specific inflammatory response greatly facilitate the conditions for autoimmune reaction.

6. Conception of PIFAS as applicated to explaining pathogenesis of multiple sclerosis

6.1. Introduction

Multiple sclerosis (MS) is a tissue-specific autoimmune disease, characterized by immune inflammation in the central nervous system (CNS) and chronic processes of demyelization. In MS, the primary targets of immune response are myelin antigens, with the myelin basic protein (MBP) usually described as the main target. Degradation of myelin impairs conductive function of neurons and causes specific symptoms of the disease. The disease develops in genetically predisposed individuals as a result of cross-reactivity of the immune system to exogenous pathogenetic agents. According to PIFAS conception, the following stages can be described in pathogenesis of MS:

1. Genetic predisposition.
2. Induction of immune response to antigens of myelin in genetically predisposed individuals, mediated by infectious processes in the CNS or by other factors.
3. Latent autoimmune inflammation in the CNS.
4. Latent impairment of neurological functions.
5. Manifestation of the disease in the form of clinically independent syndrome (CIS) or primary progressive multiple sclerosis.

6.2. Genetic factors in pathogenesis of multiple sclerosis

For developing genetic markers of increased susceptibility to MS, three groups of genes are usually studied: HLA genes, cytokine genes (IRF8, TNFa, CD6) and genes taking part in metabolism of myelin (MBP, CTLA1). (Dujmovic, 2011). Among genetic risk factors for MS, human leukocyte antigen (HLA)-class II alleles, specifically the HLA DR and DQ loci, are the best studied. It is currently thought that susceptibility to MS is defined not by individual alleles, but rather by their interaction (conception of epistasis – interaction between certain alleles of HLA). Lincoln and colleagues reported epistasis among 3 HLA-class II alleles (DRB1, DQA1, and DQB1) in 2 independent Canadian cohorts. For example, HLADQ1*0102 increased MS risk when combined with HLADRB1*1501, thereby implicating the HLA-DQ molecule in susceptibility to MS. Some alleles of HLA seem to reduce the risk of MS, an example being HLA-DRB1*01 (Fernandez-Morera et al., 2008, Isobe et al., 2010). In De Luca's study, HLA-DRB1*01 has been shown to be notably underrepresented in patients with malignant cases of MS in comparison to those with benign cases (DeLuca et al., 2007), implicating its role in determining the severity of the disease.

http://dx.doi.org/10.5772/53597

Prognostically, some HLA alleles correlate with higher incidence of neutralizing Abs to IFN b (HLA-DRB1*0408) (Caminero et al., 2011).

TNFRSF1A (TNFa) gene mutations also play a role in genetic predisposition to MS. A correlation has been found between MS and another autoimmune disease - TNF receptor-associated periodic syndrome. The latter is firmly associated with TNFRSF1A mutations (IMSGC, 2011). Also, a link has been shown between MS and variants of several other cytokines, most notably IR8 and CD6 (Yoon et al., 1989).

6.3. Clinical classification of multiple sclerosis. Natural history of multiple sclerosis

The first manifestation of MS is termed as clinical isolated syndrome – CIS. Diagnosis of MS can be maintained after two distinct exacerbations of the disease, diagnosed clinically or instrumentally – by MRI. Extensive data shows that about 80% of patients with CIS that have changes in their MRI develop MS in 20 years. However, disease modifying treatment can in certain cases prolong latent stages of the disease. Research of biomarkers determining risk of progression to MS in the groups of risk is, therefore, of much importance. One of such markers is Protein 14-3-3, which is thought to act as a chaperone in neurons and oligodendrocytes. Protein 14-3-3 is a sensitive marker of damage to neural tissue, and it gas been shown to be an independent factor in predicting conversion of CIS to MS.

An important moment in pathogenesis of MS is loss of protective function of the blood-brain barrier (BBB). Normally, low permeability of BBB makes the CNS immunologically privileged, preventing immune response to its antigens. However, in MS this protective function of the BBB is lost as a result of primary inflammatory response to infection or other factors leading to damage to neurons and glial cells. Immunoregulatory defects including reduced levels of regulatory T cells (Tr1, Th2, Th3) in MS patients allow myelin-reactive Th1-cells to extravasate, cross the blood brain barrier (BBB) and enter the CNS. This barrier is not normally accessible to T-cells, unless it is affected by a virus, which reduces the strength of the junctions forming the barrier. Within the CNS, myelin-reactive Th1-cells interact with microglia (localized APCs) presented antigens and secret inflammatory cytokines (IL-2, IF gamma, TNFalpha) which initiate inflammatory cascades. Mononuclear phagocytes, T-cells and microglia containing the RANTES (CCL5) (regulated on activation, normal T-cell expressed and secreted) receptor CCR5 and T-cells containing the interferon-gamma-inducible protein of 10 kDa (IP-10) (CXCL10); monokine induced by interferon-gamma (Mig) (CXCL9) receptor CXCR3 are targeted to the inflammation, demyelination sites by the RANTES and IP-10/Mig chemokines, respectively.

An important mechanism mediating lymphoid cells migration in inflammatory conditions increased expression of integrins, such as VLA-4. Interacting with ICAM receptor of endothelial cells, VLA-4 plays an important role in the process of lymphocytes passing the BBB. That makes VLA-4 one of potential targets for MS therapy. Immunomodulatory therapy with interferon-beta also affects BBB permeability, reducing migration of CD8+-lymphocytes.

Increased permeability of BBB allows antigen-specific lymphocytes and antibodies to reach the CNS. However, clinically the disease may remain silent for some time: as it is common with autoimmune diseases, MS is characterized with extended latent stage (third stage according to the conception of PIFAS). The silent autoimmune process can be identified by presence of specific markers of the disease.

Clinically MS is categorized as either primary progressive MS (PPMS) (15% of cases at onset) or relapsing-remitting MS (RRMS). The latter can evolve into secondary progressive MS (SPMS), which takes place in about 65% of patients who presented with RRMS. Morphologically progressive forms of the disease are characterized by diffuse inflammatory changes in the CNS, while in RRRS inflammatory changes are local (Leech et al., 2007). Even healthy-looking white matter of patients with progressive forms of MS shows increased permeability of the BBB, and this may be an evidence of diffuse inflammatory process in those forms of the disease (DeStefano et al., 2001). Research of factors affecting clinical course of the disease is of much importance. Disease evolution to secondary progressive variant may be mediated by changes of the immune response, as well as by changes in target tissues. One of the mechanisms involved in disease progression is transportation of the antigens to cervical lymph nodes, with activation of new antigen-specific T-cells and expansion of antigen repertoire. This doesn't explain, however, why evolution to secondary-progressive variant is seen only in certain subjects. The key role in this process is given to a previously discussed factor - epitope spreading, taking place as a result of changes in conformation of myelin leading to opening of previously inaccessible epitopes. Those epitopes may show higher affinity ro antigen-binding sequences of autoantibodies and autoreactive TCRs. Epitope spreading is accompanied by changes in biomarker profiles, with occurrence of new antibody types. This may be seen before clinical signs of secondary progressive MS. Another factor that might play a role in MS transformation to secondary progressive type is degree of excitability of neurons (Kutzelnigg et al., 2005). There is data that the CSF of patients with RRMS inhibits activity of Na+-canals of neurons, which allows to presume it might show an in vivo effect of reducing excitability of neurons. This might reduce the degree of neuronal damage and serve as a "protective" factor preventing the development of SPMS.

An independent hypothesis of MS progression explains the development of SPMS as a naturally determined result of continuous disease progression (DeStefano et al., 2001). After damage to CNS reaches a certain threshold, a break of compensation occurs after which further disease progression results in equivalent progression of functional disability. Before this point, the clinical symptoms don,t fully reflect the severity of autoimmune process. This hypothesis explains low efficiency of disease-modifying treatment at the stage of SPMS. In the light of such point of view, RRMS should be viewed as a state of partial compensation preceding manifestation of the disease in the form of SPMS.

6.4. Pathology of multiple sclerosis. Role of infection in pathogenesis of multiple sclerosis

The characteristic morphological feature of relapsing-remitting MS are MS lesions disseminated in location and age. Typically, the plaques are located in the white matter of the CNS.

http://dx.doi.org/10.5772/53597

The most frequent locations of the plaques are periventricular white matter, optic nerve and the spinal cord. Another demyelization process can also usually be detected, affecting individual nerve fibers in the spinal cord. Even areas that are not affected by demyelization process show abnormalities that some researchers believe may contribute to the pathogenesis of progressive forms of the disease. MS plaques can be detected by functional diagnostics, and their localization correlates with clinical findings. Acute MS plaques show signs of immune inflammation and degradation of myelin. The mechanisms active in MS plaques are not completely understood. It is clear that damage to myelin, glial and neural cells is mediated by classic immune effector mechanisms: cell-mediated cytotoxity and antibody production. Cerebrospinal fluid and MS lesions of the patients show high levels of cytotoxyc CD8+ cells specific to MBP, and neural and glial cells have been shown to increase production of MHC I molecules in conditions of immune inflammation, becoming targets for CD8+ cytotoxyc activity. How those mechanisms act together is, as of yet, unclear. Recent results of have shed some light on this problem. They have described four morphological types of inflammation in MS plaques (Luchinetti et al., 2000). Three of these mechanisms are typical for RRMS, and the fourth type is characteristic for PPRS.

1. Demyelination associated with T-cell and macrophages-mediated inflammation.

2. Demyelination associated with T-cell and macrophages-mediated inflammation with extensive antibody deposition in tissues and in glial cells. This pattern seems to be the most common, and is associated with morphological signs of remyelination.

3. Demyelination associated with an infiltrate of T-lymphocytes and activation of macrophages and microglia.

4. Demyelination associated with infiltration with T-cells. This pattern is found in PPRS and is characteristic for this type of the disease.

This shows heterogenic nature of effector mechanisms active in MS. Authors of the study hypothesize that different pathological patterns can represent different pathogenetic pathways of the disease which may be associated with different prognosis and respond to treatment.

In chronic plaques, the inflammatory process becomes inactive. Activated inflammatory cells leave central areas of the plaque, while in the periphery, they retain their activity for some time. During relapses of the disease, reactivation of some chronic plaques can follow. This is accompanied by an increase in permeability of the BBB and by migration of macrophages and antigen-specific T-cells.

The inflammatory process in MS plaques is accompanied by axonal degeneration. Acute axonal degeneration can be morphologically detected by presence of axonal "ovoids". Later on, ovoids disappear, and morphological picture starts pointing at Wallerian degeneration. Axonal damage in MS is thought to be irreversible, and to be responsible for chronic disability in MS patients. It has been shown that markers of neurodegeneration correlate well with state of functional disability.

As with IDDM, it is yet unclear (Anderson et al., 2009) whether the disease is initiated by cross-reactivity of the immune system to MBP, or the primary event is morphological damage to the cells caused by infection or other factors. The immune initiation conception is the more widely accepted one. It is supported by events of experimental transfer of MS to laboratory animals by one of the following ways: a) immunizing the animals with antigens of myelin b) transplantating antigen-specific CD4+ cells. The latter experiments have become the basis for viewing CD4+ cells as a key factor in disease initiation (as opposed to IDDM, where CD8+ lymphocytes seem to be the key mediator of pathogenetic events, although they are supported by CD4+ Th1-cells). In accordance with these views, blood of patients with MS contains increased numbers of CD4++ cells specific to MBP.

The neural initiated conception views alteration of glial cells caused by chronic infection as the initiating mechanism of the disease. While the speculation of the infectious factor being the main etiological agent would seem too awkward, there is enough evidence to consider some viruses persisting in the CNS as a factor initiating immune response. Cells of microglia have been shown to raise expression of MHC molecules and inflammatory cytokines in conditions of tissue injury and viral infection. They are able to serve as APCs, playing an important role in primary recruitment of lymphocytes specific to antigens of myelin.

That is quite logical, seeing as antigen mimicry is believed to play quite an important role in the pathogenesis of MS. MS is believed to initiate in genetically susceptible hosts, when common microbes that contain protein sequences cross-reactive with self-myelin antigens activate antigen presenting cells (APC) in the blood. The most studied as a MS risk factor is Epstein-Barr virus infection. In Ascherio et al study, all 100% of patients with MS were infected by EBV (Rudick, 2001). Frequency of MS in patients that had infectious mononucleosis is higher than in general population. It has been shown that BCRs of B-lymphocytes active towards MBP show homology with antibodies specific to EBV latent membrane protein 1 (LMP1) (Gabibov et al., 2011). However, evidence for correlation between DNA load and frequency of MS remain conflicting, as well as that for similarity of geographic patterns of EBV infection and MS. In contrary, antiEBV antibodies seem to be a perfect risk marker, as their level in serum strongly correlates to frequency of MS (Andreoletti et al., 1998). This means that latent EBV infection seems to be the most significant risk factor. The key role is thought to belong to patterns of EBV genes expression in latent state. Changes in methylation of the viral DNA might result in increase in production of certain proteins involved in autoimmune response (Niller et al., 2011). Other viruses that show high expression in tissues of MS patients are HHV-6 and HERV. Increase of expression of those agents might contribute to disease pathogenesis by augmenting the inflammatory response against oligodendrocytes.

Another agent thought to be involved in MS pathogenesis is Acinetobacter. There is statistically significant increase of anti-Acinetobacter antibodies in the serum of patients with MS. There is also correlation between distribution of Acinetobacter sinusitis and MS. Also, DNA sequences of Acinetobacter show homology with sequence of myelin.

Current data suggest that infectious triggers are most likely ubiquitous, i.e., highly prevalent in the general population, and that they require a permissive genetic trait which predisposes for MS development.

As the disease progresses, the protective function of the BBB becomes chronically impaired. Morphological investigation of tissues of patients with secondary progressive MS shows formation of lymphoid follicle-like structures in the meninges. Those follicles are hypothesized to be the place of production of autoantibodies specific to various antigens of CNS. Those include previously discussed anti-neurofilament antibodies.

Pathogenetic role of autoantibodies in MS remains unclear. While some researchers claim that autoantibodies in MS just serve as a "witness" of pathological process mediated by other mechanisms (such as cell-mediated cytotoxycity), there is data (Lincoln et al., 2010) showing that some antibody types may play a role in the disease progression through modifying normal antigens of myelin and provoking specific immune response. This refers to catalytic antibodies (abzymes) with proteolytic activity (antibody proteases). The typical mechanism of catalysis for these antibodies is nucleophilic catalysis. Recently abzyme-dependent catalytic degradation of an autoantigen, MBP (myelin basic protein), was associated with the course of the neurodegenerative disease MS and its rodent model, experimental autoimmune encephalomyelitis (EAE). Autoantibody-mediated degradation of MBP was shown to be site specific, with cleavage sites localized to the immunodominant epitopes of the protein. These findings were supported by studies from others. Interestingly, this reaction was inhibited in vitro by glatiramer acetate (Copaxone), an established treatment for MS. (Belogurov et al., 2008)

6.5. Prediction and prognosis: changes in the proteome characteristic for multiple sclerosis

Main diagnostic criteria for MS are based on dissemination of clinical, instrumental, laboratory findings. The three clinical stages of MS are preclinical phase, phase of immune inflammation and degenerative stage. In the preclinical phase there are no morphological changes, but biomarkers of immune inflammation might already be found, although at low titers. At this stage, abs to the "mimic" epitopes of microbial pathogens are found, supporting the view that the disease is triggered by reaction of the immune system to such epitopes. The process becomes self-supporting after immune respond shifts towards determinants of the CNS. Preclinical diagnostics of MS aims at discovering autoantibodies before morphological and/or clinical manifestation of the disease.

Markers of the autoimmune process in MS can be divided into two main categories: markers of immune inflammation and markers of neurodegenerative processes. Biological fluids used for sampling include blood serum and the cerebrospinal fluid (CSF). Advantages of using blood serum include higher availability of the material, lower risk of the procedure and economical advanteges. However, proteome of blood serum is less selective to pathology of the central nervous system than that of the CSF. Certain markers are difficult to detect, and there are technical problems associated with high-abundance proteins of the blood serum. These have to be removed from the sample in order to reach diagnostically applicable levels of sensitivity and specifity. CSF is much more convenient in terms of sample preparation, sensitivity and specifity. However, obvious reasons prevent widely using it for screening, expecially in healthy individuals.

Non-specific markers of immune inflammation include oligoclonal IgG bands, light Ig chains, chromogranin A, clusrerin, CC3.

Markers specific to autoimmune processes taking place in MS are autoantibodies to myelin basic protein (anti-MBP) and to myelin oligodendrocyte protein (anti-MOG). Antibodies found in MS patients include anti-myelin basic protein antibodies, antiganglioside antibodies, anti-myelin oligodendrocyte glycoprotein antibodies (Yoon et al., 1990). Anti-MBP antibodies are the most common markers used for preclinical diagnostics. To raise the specifity of the method, selective reactivity of autoantibodies to certain MBP fragments can be measured. It should be noted that anti-MBP antibodies are also found in some healthy people.

Antiganglioside (AGM)-antibodies are found in patients with various neurological disorders and are not specific for MS. However, they can be used for prognostic purposes. There ere several subtypes of anti-AGM antibodies. Presence of several common AGM-antibodies as opposed to typical AGM-1 antibodies reflects high degree of disease progression. Clinically this correlates with secondary-progressive form of MS and bad prognosis.

Myelin oligodendrocyte protein is a superficial component of myelin. In animal models, this protein has been shown to be quite vulnerable to both cell and humoral immune response. It is thought to be one of the primary targets in initiation of MS. Antibodies to this protein might offer a promising perspective for preclinical diagnostics of MS. MOG is the most interesting candidate B-cell autoantigen in MS. Because of its location it is an ideal target for antibody-mediated demyelination. Anti-MOG antibodies are indeed able to cause myelin destruction in EAE models, while other antibodies against major myelin proteins such as MBP or PLP, which are both not located on the myelin surface, do not cause myelin destruction on their own. Anti-MOG Abs mediate a characteristic vesicular transformation of compact myelin in acutely demyelinated lesions that also has been documented in human MS lesions strongly suggesting a role of anti-MOGAbs in MS. The B-cell response to MOG is enhanced in MS also supporting the pathogenic importance of anti-MOG Abs.

Antiganglioside antibodies (anti-GM) are more of prognostic value, as there is a correlation between anti-GM antibody type and clinical type of the disease (primary progressive, back-and-remitting, secondary progressive).

Prognostic use of antibodies is based on the fact that correlation can be made between types of main determinants and antibodies and prognosis/ clinical stage of the disease. In the course of the disease, autoantibodies cause changes in myelin structure, which leads to formation of new, more immunogenic epitopes, and changes in autoantibodies specter. Clinically this is accompanied by transformation of MS into secondary-progressive form. While the disease progresses, immune inflammation becomes less specific, with initiation of immune response to various determinants of the CNS as opposed to primary response which affects just the components of myelin.

It is necessary to note, however, that markers of immune inflammation do not show exact correlation with degree of axonal damage, although changes in antibody profiles can be useful in predicting evolution to secondary progressive clinical type. That is why markers of neurodegeneration are just as important.

Markers of neurodegeneration are components of structures altered during the clinical attack of MS. The body fluid that reflects their level most accurately is the CNF. However, it is often inconvenient to use CSF, making it necessary to use blood as the more accessible material, although its proteome doesn,t reflect proteome of the CNS as accurate as CSF does.

One of such markers is NF-L – the light chain of neurofilaments constituting cytoskeleton of axons. NF-l is raised in a number of neurodegenerative diseases, reflecting axonal damage. There is also correlation between NF-L levels and exacerbation of the disease, and an increase in NF-L levels has been detected in patients with CIS prior to manifestation of MS. (3 years). In patients with MS it is also not uncommon to detect antibodies against neurofilaments – anti-nerofilament antibodies.The best studied marker is the main target of autoimmune reactions in MS – myelin basic protein (MBP). MBP is is one of the most abundant proteins of myelin, and is present in both central and peripheral nervous system. High levels of MBP have been shown to correlate with upcoming relapses of MS, as well as with the disease attaining the progressive clinical type. In combination with anti-MBP and anti-MOG antibodies, detection of fragments of MBP can be used for predicting relapses in the course of the disease (Huang et al., 2011). Another prognostic marker is acidic calcium-binding protein – a component of axons damaged during the course of the disease. Tau-protein – a cytoskeleton protein involved in formation of microtubules, is another marker of neurodegeneration. Changes in phosphorilation of the protein lead to impairment of axonal transport, and to formation of insoluble neurotoxic aggregates. In patients with MS, levels of abnormally phosphorilated tau-protein have a tendency to rise with time (Lincoln et al., 2009).

7. Conclusion

The pathogenesis of autoimmune diseases is a complex process, with both genetic and environmental factors playing equally important role. In genetically predisposed organisms, the key event promoting the start of autoimmune response is often infection, usually with a viral pathogen. There is a variety of specific patterns by which infections can contribute to autoimmunity. Those patterns were analyzed in the light of fundamental conceptions of autoimmunity. Also, models of infectious pathogens inducing autoimmune processes were discussed on the base of two autoimmune conditions: IDDM and MS, both of which seem to fit the introduced model.

Author details

S. A. Krynskiy[1*], A. V. Kostyakov[1], D. S. Kostyushev[1], D. A. Gnatenko[1] and S. V. Suchkov[1,2,3]

*Address all correspondence to: srgkr002@gmail.com

1 I.M. Sechenov The First Moscow State Medical University, Moscow, Russia

2 Moscow State Medical and Dental University, Moscow, Russia

3 National Research Center,Kurchatov Institute, Russia

References

[1] J. M. Anderson, R. Patani, R. Reynolds et al., "Evidence for abnormal tau phosphorylation in early aggressive multiple sclerosis," Acta Neuropathologica 2009; vol. 117, no. 5, pp. 583–589.

[2] Andréoletti L, Hober D, Hober-Vandenberghe C, Fajardy I, Belaich S, Lambert V, Vantyghem MC, Lefebvre J, Wattre P. Coxsackie B virus infection and beta cell autoantibodies in newly diagnosed IDDM adult patients. Clin Diagn Virol. 1998 Apr; 9(2-3):125-33.

[3] Caminero A, Comabella M, Montalban X. Role of tumour necrosis factor (TNF)-α and TNFRSF1A R92Q mutation in the pathogenesis of TNF receptor-associated periodic syndrome and multiple sclerosis. Clin Exp Immunol. 2011; 166(3):338-45.

[4] Cherepakhina NE, Shogenov ZS, Elbeik T, Akhmedilova KA, Agirov MM, Tabaksoeva ZhA, Ogneva EA, Matsuura E, Mukhin NA, Shoenfeld Y, Pal'tsev MA, Suchkov SV. Post-infectious clinical-immunological syndrome and its place in clinical practice. Ter Arkh. 2009;81(12):71-8.

[5] Conti-Fine BM. et al. Myasthenia Gravis: The Immunobiology of an Autoimmune Disease. 1st ed. R. G. Landes, Austin, TX, 1997.

[6] Irena Dujmovic. Cerebrospinal Fluid and Blood Biomarkers of Neuroaxonal Damage in Multiple Sclerosis. Multiple Sclerosis International 2011; Article ID 767083.

[7] DeLuca GC, Ramagopalan SV, Herrera BM, Dyment DA, Lincoln MR, Montpetit A, Pugliatti M, Barnardo MC, Risch NJ, Sadovnick AD, Chao M, Sotgiu S, Hudson TJ, Ebers GC. An extremes of outcome strategy provides evidence that multiple sclerosis severity is determined by alleles at the HLA-DRB1 locus. Proc Natl Acad Sci U S A. 2007; 104(52):20896-901.

[8] Franklin H. Epstein. The Pathogenesis of Insulin-Dependent Diabetes Mellitus. N Engl J Med 1994; 331: 1428-1436.

[9] Fabris P, Betterle C, Greggio NA, Zanchetta R, Bosi E, Biasin MR, de Lalla F. Insulin-dependent diabetes mellitus during alpha-interferon therapy for chronic viral hepatitis. J Hepatol. 1998; 28(3):514-7.

[10] Fang-Ping Huang. Autoimmune Disorders - Current Concepts and Advances from Bedside to Mechanistic Insights. InTech 2011; ISBN 978-953-307-653-9.

[11] Fernandez-Morera JL, Rodriguez-Rodero S, Tunon A, Martinez-Borra J, Vidal-Castineira JR, Lopez-Vazquez A, Rodrigo L, Rodrigo P, González S, Lahoz CH, Lopez-Larrea C. Genetic influence of the nonclassical major histocompatibility complex class I molecule MICB in multiple sclerosis susceptibility. Tissue Antigens. 2008 Jul; 72(1):54-9.

[12] Foy T. et al. Immune regulation by CD40 and its ligand gp39. Immune regulation by CD40 and its ligand gp39. Annu. Rev. Immunol. 1996; 14: 591–617.

[13] Gabibov AG, Belogurov AA Jr, Lomakin YA, Zakharova MY, Avakyan ME, Dubrovskaya VV, Smirnov IV, Ivanov AS, Molnar AA, Gurtsevitch VE, Diduk SV, Smirnova KV, Avalle B, Sharanova SN, Tramontano A, Friboulet A, Boyko AN, Ponomarenko NA, Tikunova NV. Combinatorial antibody library from multiple sclerosis patients reveals antibodies that cross-react with myelin basic protein and EBV antigen. FASEB J. 2011 Dec;25(12):4211-21. Epub 2011 Aug 22.

[14] Gajanan Sherbet. Bacterial Infections and the Pathogenesis of Autoimmune Conditions. BJMP 2009; :2(1): 6-13.

[15] hristopher C. Goodnow et al. Pathogenesis of Autoimmune Disease. Cell 2007; 1: 25-35.

[16] International Multiple Sclerosis Genetics Consortium. The genetic association of variants in CD6, TNFRSF1A and IRF8 to multiple sclerosis: a multicenter case-control study. PLoS One. 2011 Apr 28;6(4): e18813.

[17] Isobe N, Matsushita T, Yamasaki R, Ramagopalan SV, Kawano Y, Nishimura Y, Ebers GC, Kira J. Influence of HLA-DRB1 alleles on the susceptibility and resistance to multiple sclerosis in Japanese patients with respect to anti-aquaporin 4 antibody status. Mult Scler. 2010 (2):147-55.

[18] Kordonouri O. et al. Genetic risk markers related to diabetes-associated auto-Abs in young patients with type 1 diabetes in berlin, Germany. Experimental and clinical endocrinology and diabetes 2010; 116 (4): 245-249.

[19] Kutzelnigg A, Lucchinetti CF, Stadelmann C, et al. Cortical demyelination and diff use white matter injury in multiple sclerosis. Brain 2005; 128: 2705–12.

[20] Leech S, Kirk J, Plumb J, McQuaid S. Persistent endothelial abnormalities and blood-brain barrier leak in primary and secondary progressive multiple sclerosis. Neuropathol Appl Neurobiol 2007; 33: 86–98.

[21] Lees Murdock, D.J. et al. DNA damage and cytotoxicity in pancreatic beta-cells expressing human CYP2E1. Biochemical pharmacology 2004; Vol.68, No.3 ISSN 523-30.

[22] Lehmann PV et al. Spreading of T-cell autoimmunity to cryptic determinants of an autoantigen.Nature 1997; 358: 155–157.

[23] Lincoln MR, Ramagopalan SV, Chao MJ, Herrera BM, Deluca GC, Orton SM, Dyment DA, Sadovnick AD, Ebers GC. Epistasis among HLA-DRB1, HLA-DQA1, and HLA-DQB1 loci determines multiple sclerosis susceptibility. Proc Natl Acad Sci U S A. 2009 May 5;106(18):7542-7. Epub 2009 Apr 20.

[24] Lipponen K. et al. Effect of HLA class I and class II alleles on progression from autoantibody positivity to overt type 1 diabetes in children with risk-associated class II genotypes. Diabetes 2010; Vol.59, No.12, ISSN 3253-6

[25] Lucchinetti C., Bruck W., Parisi J., et al. Heterogenity of multiple sclerosis lesions: implications for the pathogenesis of demyelination. Ann Neurol 2000; 47:707-717.

[26] Niller HH, Wolf H, Ay E, Minarovits J. Epigenetic dysregulation of epstein-barr virus latency and development of autoimmune disease. Adv Exp Med Biol. 2011;711:82-102.

[27] Petrone, A.; Spoletini, M.; Zampetti, S.; Capizzi, M.; Zavarella, S.; Osborn, J.; Pozzilli, P. & Buzzetti, R. et al. The PTPN22 1858T gene variant in type 1 diabetes is associated with reduced residual beta-cell function and worse metabolic control. Diabetes Care 2008; Vol.31, No.6 (June 2008) ISSN 214-8

[28] Pociot F. and McDermott M. F. Genetics of type 1 diabetes mellitus. Genes and Immunity 2002; 3: 235–249.

[29] Richard A. Rudick Evolving Concepts in the Pathogenesis of Multiple Sclerosis and Their Therapeutic Implications. J Neuroophthalmol 2001; 21(4):279-283.

[30] N. De Stefano, S. Narayanan, G. S. Francis et al., "Evidence of axonal damage in the early stages of multiple sclerosis and its relevance to disability," Archives of Neurology 2001; vol. 58, no. 1, pp. 65–70.

[31] Yoon JW. The role of viruses and environmental factors in the induction of diabetes. Curr Top Microbiol Immunol. 1990;164:95-123.

[32] Yoon JW, Ihm SH, Kim KW. Viruses as a triggering factor of type 1 diabetes and genetic markers related to the susceptibility to the virus-associated diabetes. Diabetes Res Clin Pract. 1989; 7 Suppl 1:S47-58.

[33] Waguri M, Hanafusa T, Itoh N, Imagawa A, Miyagawa J, Kawata S, Kono N, Kuwajima M, Matsuzawa Y. Occurrence of IDDM during interferon therapy for chronic viral hepatitis. Diabetes Res Clin Pract. 1994; 1:33-6.

[34] Wan Y.et al. Regulatory T-cell functions are subverted and converted owing to attenuated Foxp3 expression. Nature 2007; 445: 766–770.

Chapter 10

Chronic Fatigue Syndrome/Myalgic Encephalomyelitis and Parallels with Autoimmune Disorders

Ekua W. Brenu, Lotti Tajouri, Kevin J. Ashton,
Donald R. Staines and Sonya M. Marshall-Gradisnik

Additional information is available at the end of the chapter

http://dx.doi.org/10.5772/53440

1. Introduction

Autoimmune disorders are known to affect a substantial number of people worldwide and in some cases may be fatal. They occur in the presence of unregulated inflammatory responses including failure in self-tolerance. Some unexplained disorders with immune compromises may demonstrate certain characteristics that suggest an autoimmune disorder including Chronic Fatigue Syndrome/Myalgic Encephalomyelitis (CFS/ME). CFS/ME remains an unsolved disorder with multiple symptoms and no single causative factor. These symptoms may include but are not limited to incapacitating fatigue, weakened short term memory or attentiveness, sore throat, tender cervical or axillary lymph nodes, muscle pain, severe headaches, impaired sleep and postexertional malaise. To date succinct and concise mechanisms that underlie this disorder have not yet being identified although, many hypotheses have been put forward. CFS/ME often occurs as a consequence of a post-infectious episode accompanied by compromises in the immune, endocrine and nervous systems. The sequences of these events have not being clearly identified. Importantly, immune deterioration in CFS/ME is related to heightened or suppressed cell function, differential gene expression, equivocal levels of immune cell numbers and protein secretion promoting adverse inflammatory activation. Both innate and adaptive immune system perturbations persist in CFS/ME. These characteristics are in many respects similar to mechanisms of disease in autoimmune disorders suggesting that the changes in immune response may develop from cellular and molecular changes in immune cells and proteins. We propose here that as the mechanism of CFS/ME may involve certain immunological factors that have been shown to be compromised in other autoimmune diseases, CFS/ME may in some cases have an autoimmune component or perhaps the symptoms of CFS/ME are hallmarks of a novel autoimmune disorder yet to be identified.

2. Characteristics of CFS/ME

CFS/ME belongs to a class of unexplained disorders whose causal factor(s) remains to be proven. The prevalence rate of CFS/ME worldwide is 0.4-4% with a female to male ratio of 6:1 (Lorusso et al., 2009). A predominant characteristic of patients with this disorder is persistent debilitating fatigue. Apart from the debilitating and unrelenting fatigue, patients may also experience other symptoms which may include sore throat, headaches, post exertional malaise etc (Fukuda et al., 1994). A diagnosis of CFS/ME is affirmed if these symptoms have persisted for at least 6 months. To assist with correct diagnosis of CFS/ME patients, various diagnostic tools have been developed. Currently, most researchers prefer to use two definition criteria, the CDC and the Canadian definition, for assessing their patients.

Occurrences of disparities in immunological, neurological, endocrinological, cardiac and metabolic function have been reported among CFS/ME patients (Klimas et al., 2012). Although, these observations highlight the extent of physiological damage associated with CFS/ME, the findings are most often not consistent across studies thus posing doubt as to whether these reported disparities are associated with CFS/ME. Nonetheless, alterations in immunological function are the most consistent data associated with CFS/ME (Klimas et al., 2012). Important among them is the observation that CFS/ME patients have a significant decrease in cytotoxic activity (Brenu et al., 2010; Brenu et al., 2011; Fletcher et al., 2010; Klimas et al., 1990; Maher et al., 2005). Other factors such as cytokines also vary in CFS/ME patients in comparison to non-CFS individuals (Patarca, 2001). Thus considerable evidence exists to suggest that CFS/ME is an immune dysfunction disorder and therefore it may share homology with some autoimmune disorders.

Autoimmune disorders arise as a consequence of increased creation of pathological antibodies against self-antigens, in other words the body assumes a diseased state and therefore generates antibodies to attack self-cells and molecules. The result of this over active immune system is tissue damage and inflammation. Tissue damage may develop from elevations in antibody or cellular processes. Autoimmune disorders can either be systemic or organ specific, exemplified by the presence of autoantibodies, autoreactivity to autoantigens, loss in B cell tolerance, alterations in regulatory T cells (Treg) function, changes in T cell repertoire, genetic abnormalities or environmental agents (Davidson and Diamond, 2001). In most autoimmune diseases including Multiple Sclerosis (MS), autoimmune Rheumatoid Arthritis (RA) Systemic Lupus Erythematosus (SLE), and Autoimmune Diabetes (AID), disparities in immune cells such as neutrophils, Natural Killer (NK), T and B cells have been reported. Perturbations in the normal function of these cells are contributory factors to the mechanism of these diseases. Incidentally, these cells have also being described in CFS/ME. Hence, the purpose of this chapter is to describe the findings related to the above mentioned cells in autoimmune disorders and relate these to CFS/ME. At present, a mechanism for CFS/ME remains to be identified. Exploring such parallels between CFS/ME and other autoimmune disorders may highlight components of the CFS/ME mechanism that may suggest an autoimmune profile and may serve as a platform for further research.

CFS/ME is known to affect both the innate and adaptive immune system. To date despite the numerous findings on the immune system there is still no definitive informative description on the extent and nature of damage to the immune system. However, the research on the innate and adaptive immune system has identified important irregularities in patients with CFS/ME.

3. The CFS/ME immune system

3.1. Innate immunity in CFS

The innate immune system comprises of cells such as neutrophils, monocytes, dendritic cells and NK cells. Using phagocytosis and cytotoxic activity these cells are able to elicit and effectively eliminate pathogens that invade the immune system. Most innate immune cells act as antigen presenting cells and also produce a variety of cytokines that are important in activation, proliferation and development of other immune cells. In CFS/ME, immune cell numbers and cytokines have been investigated and there is evidence suggesting equivocal levels of innate immune cells and reduced functional capacity of most immune cells including neutrophils and NK cells (Brenu et al., 2010; Brenu et al., 2011; Klimas et al., 1990; Maher et al., 2005). Neutrophils are phagocytic cells that mediate immune response against bacteria and other microbes while NK cells are responsible for early response against viral pathogens and tumour cells. NK cells release lytic proteins such as perforin and granzymes that effectively lyse these pathogens thereby preventing infections. In the presence of a compromised immune system involving a decrease in cytotoxic activity, these cells are not able to effectively clear viral pathogens. Reduced cytotoxic activity may in most cases increase susceptibility to viral infections among patients with CFS/ME. Similarly, alterations in the availability of lytic proteins, perforin and granzymes, among CFS/ME patients, may also affect the rate of cytotoxicity in NK cells in response to pathogen infiltration (Brenu et al., 2011; Klimas et al., 2012; Maher et al., 2005). Polymorphism in the NK cell receptors importantly the Killer-cell immunoglobulin-like receptors (KIR) family of receptors may also contribute to the reduced NK activity (Pasi et al., 2011). Compromises to neutrophil function in some CFS /ME patients affect their ability to lyse or clear bacterial pathogens owing to the lack of oxidative phosphorylation (Brenu et al., 2010). A similar mechanism may also exist among the monocyte/macrophages although, this remains to be determined. These findings highlight an inability of the immune cells in CFS/ME patients to eliminate viral, microbial and bacterial pathogens.

During infection there is an immediate immune response involving the release of cytokines such as interleukin (IL)-1α and β, IL-6, interferon (IFN)-α and tumour necrosis factor (TNF)-α by dendritic cells and monocytes (Borish and Steinke, 2003). The release of these cytokines stimulates the production of cell adhesion molecules and chemotactic molecules that recruit innate immune cells to the sites of infection. There is currently no apparent consistency in the cytokine profile in CFS/ME, however, deficiencies in these cytokines may affect immune function at the innate level. Importantly, these proteins are responsible for recruiting adaptive immune cells and initiating adaptive immune cell responses.

3.2. Adaptive immunity in CFS/ME

The cells of the adaptive immune system include B and T cells. T cells can be sub-grouped in to cluster differentiation (CD)4^{+} and CD8^{+}T cells as they recognise peptides with MHCII and MHCI molecules respectively. CD4^{+}T cells can be further subdivided into the T helper (Th) 1, 2, 17 and regulatory T cells (Tregs). CD8^{+}T cells are the main cytotoxic cells in the adaptive immune system while CD4^{+}T cells are producers of cytokines either pro or anti-inflammatory cytokines. The B cells are important for producing antibodies of various classes. Compared to the innate immune system, initialization of the adaptive immune response is a much slower immune response. Presentation of antigenic peptides via the MHC class I and II complex is an important step in the induction of adaptive immune response in particular T cell related responses (Visvanathan and Lewin, 2006).

The role of B cells in CFS/ME remains to be expounded. However, there are suggestions that in CFS/ME these cells produce equivocal levels of antibodies against various antigens contributing to the persistence of symptoms over long periods of time. Thus in CFS/ME, B cells may be impaired allowing infections to persist in the absence of efficient memory cells to exterminate pathological antigens. Alternatively B cell responses may be aberrantly self-reactive. T cell investigations in CFS/ME have mostly focused on cytokines and cytotoxic activity. Although, only few studies have directly investigated the status of CD8^{+}T cells (Brenu et al., 2011), direct investigations of CD4^{+}T cells are yet to be undertaken in CFS/ME. Shifts in cytokines causing either a predominant anti- or pro-inflammatory immune profile occur in some cases of CFS/ME confirming perturbations in cytokines (Patarca, 2001). Other CD4^{+}T cell proteins such as FOXP3 are elevated in CFS/ME which may signal an over reactive Treg profile (Brenu et al., 2011). A potential over reactive Treg profile may affect the function of other immune cells and this may be important in understanding the CFS/ME immune profile.

4. Cells, cellular process and proteins in autoimmune diseases

4.1. Neutrophils in autoimmune diseases

Neutrophils are innate immune cells derived from common myeloid progenitor cells in the bone marrow (Eyles et al., 2006). Neutrophils are important in defending the body against antimicrobial pathogens in the presence of various receptor recognition pathways. Activated neutrophils contain factors that are released into the phagosome during pathogen infiltration these include azurophilic, explicit or secondary, gelatinase granules and secretory vesicles (Nathan, 2006). Derivatives of these neutrophil compartments are discharged via degranulatioin causing destruction of microbes, modifications in cytokines, chelation of microbial nutrients and heightened sensitivity to inflammatory response (Nathan, 2006). Reactive oxygen species are also generated via oxidative phosphorylation in the neutrophil phagolysosome to ensure effective clearance of pathogens.

Neutrophil function is altered in autoimmune diseases such as AID, MS, RA and SLE (Nemeth and Mocsai, 2012). In RA, considerably high levels of neutrophils are present in the synovial fluid of the diseased joints and cartilage interface (Mohr et al., 1981). These neutrophils are highly active and may be responsible for the release of IL-1β or IL-8 into the synovial fluid thus causing inflammation in the joint (Edwards and Hallett, 1997). Autoantibody mediated RA can be induced by neutrophils through the production of LFA-1, C5aR and FcγR which are essential for the migration of autoantibodies into the joint (Binstadt et al., 2006). This was confirmed by the observation that removal of neutrophils from the joint terminated the amassing of autoantibodies in the joint (Wipke et al., 2004). Highly reactive neutrophils in RA synovial fluid generate unwarranted amounts of reactive oxygen species (Cedergren et al., 2007).

IFN-α and neutrophils are among the key mediators of immune dysfunction in SLE patients. IFN-α is highly prevalent in the circulation of patients with SLE (Decker, 2011; Lindau et al., 2011). Neutrophil traps have been proposed to cause significant activation of dendritic cells while neutrophil antimicrobial peptide, LL37, in circulating DNA also stimulates plasmacytoid dendritic cells which sequentially release IFN-α (Lande et al., 2011). Neutrophil extracellular traps (NET) are formed during netosis (a form of neutrophil death) and this is responsible for the death of microbes under normal immune conditions (Warde, 2011). However, in SLE, impairments in NETs, may be attributed to DNase I inhibitors such as G-actin or mutations in the DNase I enzyme (Bosch, 2011; Yasutomo et al., 2001). Persistency of microbe infiltration and tissue damage in SLE results from weakened neutrophil phagocytosis, thus, suggesting an increased rate of infection and a failure to recognise pathogens for destruction (de la Fuente et al., 2001). Oxidative burst may also be reduced in SLE demonstrating a failure in complete clearance of pathogens (Marzocchi-Machado et al., 2002). The presence of reactive oxygen species is protective especially in AID as it prevents the destruction of β cells (Chen et al., 2008).

Neutrophils in mice model of AID are able to permeate the pancreas due to stimulatory signals from FasL facilitating entry of the neutrophil into the islets (Savinov et al., 2003). In humans, impairments in neutrophil oxidative burst have been confirmed in AID (Marhoffer et al., 1993). Additionally, the expression of certain receptors on the cell surfaces of neutrophils such as CD11b and CD18 are increased suggesting increased activity of these cells as confirmed in mice models of AID (Grykiel et al., 2001). Deterioration in neutrophil function increases the likelihood of pathogenesis and prevalence of infections. The presence of high incidence of TNF receptors such as sp55 and sp75 is indicative of substantial neutrophil priming in MS patients in particular those with RRMS (Ziaber et al., 1999). (Naegele et al., 2012). This may be related to increased neutrophil oxidative burst in RRMS (Ferretti et al., 2006). Similarly most MS patients demonstrates increased amounts of NETs in the serum and this is indicative of a severe pathological episode (Logters et al., 2009). Other abnormalities of neutrophils in MS include heightened levels of IL-8, TLR2, degranulation, impediment in apoptosis (Naegele et al., 2012).

In CFS/ME, neutrophils have been reported to be highly susceptible to apoptosis in the presence of increased incidence of TNFR1 (tumor necrosis factor receptor 1) and TGFβ1 (Transforming growth factor beta 1) (Kennedy et al., 2004). Deregulation in neutrophil function may however arise as a consequence of decreases in oxidative phosphorylation while recognition of pathogen by neutrophils remains unaffected (Brenu et al., 2010). Although, neutrophil related cytokines have not been formally associated with increasing levels of neutrophils, low levels of IL-8 have been observed in CFS/ME patients (Fletcher et al., 2009).

4.2. Natural killer cells in autoimmune diseases

NK cells are primarily responsible for the lysis and destruction of viral infected and tumour cells and they also produce an array of cytokines (Caligiuri, 2008; Vivier et al., 2008). They are distinguished from other lymphocytes by the expression of CD56 (Neural Cell Adhesion Molecule) and CD16 (Fragment Crystallisation Gamma Receptor III (FcγRIII)) surface molecules (Farag et al., 2002). Thus NK cells can be classified into two main subtypes, $CD56^{dim}CD16^{positive}$ and $CD56^{bright}CD16^{negative}$ NK cells which are highly cytotoxic and producers of cytokines respectively (Caligiuri, 2008; Farag et al., 2002). NK cells execute cell death or cytotoxicity against other infected cells via granule independent and dependant pathways. The granule dependant pathways require lytic granules, perforin and granzymes, for cytotoxicity (Bryceson et al., 2006).

NK cells have been found to be decreased in some autoimmune diseases including SLE and RA (Schleinitz et al., 2010). Reduced numbers in NK cells are normally correlated with a decrease in cytotoxic activity (Park et al., 2009; Yabuhara et al., 1996). In AID NK cells have been noticed in pancreatic islets thus they may be involved in obliterating pancreatic beta cells (Willcox et al., 2009). IFN-γ producing NK cells are densely populated in the synovial fluids of the inflamed joint (Aramaki et al., 2009; Dalbeth and Callan, 2002). The presence of high levels NK cells especially the CD56 phenotype can influence prolonged joint inflammation as they foster the prevalence of monocyte derived dendritic cells in the inflamed joint (Zhang et al., 2007). These cells encourage pro-inflammatory immune response by increasing the generation of Th1 cells and cytokines in the joint. NK cells can also influence macrophages to become lethal contributing to abnormal immune responses (Nedvetzki et al., 2007). In some autoimmune disorders variations in KIR genes are associated with disease presentation. A reduced expression of inhibitory KIRs occurs in type 1 diabetes (van der Slik et al., 2007), while the expression of certain genotype combinations increases susceptibility to certain autoimmune diseases including psoriatic arthritis (2DS1/2DS2 and HLA-Cw), systemic sclerosis ($2DS2^+$/2DL2- and $2DS1^+$/2DS2-) and SLE ($2DS^+$/2DS2-) (Momot et al., 2004; Pellett et al., 2007). Similarly, polymorphism in the FcγRIIIa in SLE affects antibody dependent cellular cytotoxicity (ADCC) thus suggesting a role of CD16 subsets of NK cells as a potential contributory factor to atypical NK function (Jonsen et al., 2007). NK cell activity is reduced in MS, however, this may fluctuate as the disease progresses (Benczur et al., 1980; Kastrukoff et al., 1998). Similarly, the levels of NK cells in MS are significantly reduced in comparison to non-MS patients (Munschauer et al., 1995). Experimental models of MS, EAE, have demonstrated that removal of NK cells substantially worsens the disease while restoration of NK cell numbers decreased the MS symptoms (Zhang et al., 1997). Components of cytotoxic function such as TRAIL and perforin may be affected in MS contributing to the decreases in cytotoxic activity (Hilliard et al., 2001).

NK cells in the tissues of some autoimmune diseases have similar characteristics to those in the periphery (Park et al., 2009). The morphology of NK cells in tissues of CFS/ME patients is unknown. In CFS/ME patients, genetic variability has been shown in the KIR alleles, increased levels of KIR3DS1 and a lack of KIR2DS5 with an absence of HLA-Bw4Ile80 on KIRS3DS1 and KIR3DL1 in CFS/ME patients is possibly associated with the reduced activity and ineffectiveness of NK cells to clear pathogens (Pasi et al., 2011).The importance of NK cells in both immune and physiological function is highly prolific as their interactions with both immune and non-immune cells are vital for disease clearance and health. Hence, interaction between NK cells and dendritic cells regulates the production of immature dendritic cells, maturation of dendritic cells and the proliferation of NK cells (Della Bella et al., 2003).

4.3. B cells and autoimmune diseases

B cells are fundamental cells of the adaptive immune system, they can be categorised into plasma B cells, B effector 1, B effector 2 and regulatory B cells (Mauri, 2010). B cells act as antigen presenting cells and are the main source of an array of immunoglobulins (Jonsen et al., 2007). The source of most autoantibodies in most autoimmune diseases is from the B cell (Stevenson and Natvig, 1999) hence, B cells are pathogenic (Edwards et al., 1999). Autoantibodies can exacerbate autoimmune states by activating autoreactive T cell reactions, however, under normal immune conditions they are responsible for the removal of dead cells and reducing autoantigens (Shlomchik et al., 2001). Additionally, pro-inflammatory cytokines such as TNF-α, IFN-γ and IL-12 and anti-inflammatory cytokines IL-4 and IL-13 are secreted by B effector 1 and 2 cells respectively (Harris et al., 2000). In humans three important B cell tolerance check points have been described including central, peripheral and an undefined check point. The central check point is described as the point of substantial decrease in self-reactive and poly reactive B cells in immature B cells, the peripheral check point is the point of obliterating auto-reactive B cells and the final check point denotes a considerable decline in auto-reactive B cells in naïve and IgM memory B cells (Pillai et al., 2011). Alterations in these check points contribute to autoimmunity (Menard et al., 2011; Samuels et al., 2005b). Another type of B cell, regulatory B cells (Bregs), has been shown to contribute to autoimmunity. The exact source of these Bregs remains to be determined however, they have been characterised as B cells with high expression of CD1d and predominant secretors of IL-10 (Yanaba et al., 2008). In mice models of autoimmunity, these cells may be responsible for the induction of Foxp3 Tregs, suppression of inflammation, and induction of Th1 and Th17 $CD4^{+}T$ cells (Carter et al., 2011). In humans Bregs can be distinguished from other cells via the expression of $CD19^{+}CD24^{hi}CD38^{hi}$ with high levels of CD1d, $CD5^{+}$ and IL-10 (Blair et al., 2010; Sims et al., 2005). In many autoimmune diseases, these cells are ineffectual when compared to those from healthy participants.

In SLE, the presence of autoantibodies suggests a disruption in B cell central tolerance (Yurasov et al., 2005). Similarly, gene rearrangement and alterations in somatic hypermutation occurring during the development of memory B cells are frequently imprecise thus encouraging the development of autoantibodies (Cappione et al., 2005). Peripheral tolerance may be impaired as a consequence of mutations in the VH gene rearrangement for anti-DNA antibodies (Zhang et al., 2008). A high level of plasma B cells with excessive levels of HLA-DR is associated with SLE confirming defects in B cell negative selection (Odendahl et al., 2005). The existence of additional abnormal memory cells in SLE such as $CD27^{+}$B cells and CD27-/IgD-B (Dorner et al., 2009), may strongly influence immune function by suppressing immune activation (Tiller et al., 2007). Memory B cells in SLE are therefore class switched and highly activated thus they respond to stimulation from IL-21, IL-10, BAFF, BCR and TLR ligands (Jacobi et al., 2008).

The precise mechanism of B cells in RA is not clearly understood however, B cell therapies have shown that depletion of B cells effectively reduces the severity of RA (Menard et al., 2011). Nonetheless, a plausible cause for the pathogenesis of B cells in RA may be attributed to flaws in early B cell development (Meffre and Wardemann, 2008; van Vollenhoven, 2009). Defective selection during VDJ recombination in the bone marrow and in the periphery facilitates the existence of autoreactive B cells overriding the selection criteria at the tolerance check points (Samuels et al., 2005a). In RA, a predominant cytokine that provokes the existence of severe inflammatory responses is the TNF-α, TNF-α alters the predominance of naïve and memory B cells however, following anti-TNF-α therapies adequate levels of memory B cells and naïve B cells were restored (Anolik et al., 2008; Menard et al., 2011; Souto-Carneiro et al., 2009).

B cells with characteristic $CD19^{+}CD27^{+}$CD38-CD138- and $CD19^{+}CD38^{+}CD138^{+}$ (plasmablasts) markers and others with a short life are found in the cerebrospinal fluid (CSF) of MS patients with progressive symptoms (Cepok et al., 2001; Cepok et al., 2005; Pascual et al., 1994). These CSF related B cells are largely responsible for inflammatory reactions in MS (Kuenz et al., 2008). Peripheral B cells are characterised by the expression of $CD19^{+}CD27^{-}$ and these are mostly naïve B cells (Cepok et al., 2005; Corcione et al., 2004). IgG molecules with oligoclonal patterns are abundant in the synovial fluid and these cells stimulate complement activation (Silverman and Carson, 2003). The pathogenesis of B cells in MS ensues from high levels of chemokine such as CXCL13 in active lesions sites, CSF and intrameningeal follicles (Franciotta et al., 2008). CXCL13 is regulated by B cells during the formation of lymphoid organogenesis resulting in the formation of ectopic lymphoid tissues (Barone et al., 2008). Dyregulation of B cells permits the survival of certain viruses such as EBV which has been linked to the central nervous system (CNS) infection in MS (Opsahl and Kennedy, 2007). In such cases the presence of EBV infected B cells promotes the persistence of EBV in the brain (Buljevac et al., 2005).

B cells are the principal source of autoantibodies in AID, these cells are also implicated as pancreatic regulators (Marino and Cosentino, 2011). Similar to MS depletion of B cells can be effective in reversing the symptoms of autoimmune diabetes. The presence of B cells results in the destruction of the β cells thus their deletion prolongs the life of the β cells (Xiu et al.,

http://dx.doi.org/10.5772/53440

2008). Different subsets of B cells have been found in AID, in comparison to the non-AID individuals these cell numbers deviate from the norm (Marino et al., 2008; Noorchashm et al., 1999; Tian et al., 2006).

In CFS/ME an in-depth study into the various subsets of B cells remains to be described. This may be important in deciphering the concept of compromised immune mechanisms in CFS/ME. In some studies depletion of B cells in patients with CFS/ME led to a substantial improvement in CFS/ME (Fluge et al., 2011; Fluge and Mella, 2009). Improvement in health following B cell depletion has been noticed in cases of MS and RA this presupposes that in CFS/ME there may be a possible defect in the B cell tolerance check point thus increasing the likelihood for errors during positive selection and rearrangement of the VDJ recombination repertoire. Therefore, only cells that are required for the formation of auto reactive B cells may be selected. Hence, depletion of these B cells may effectively improve the health status of the CFS/ME patients. This has not being confirmed however, future studies may be important in identifying the exact role of B cells in CFS/ME patients. Additionally, B cells and T cells interact with each other to assist in mutual activation. Thus, interference in the normal function of these cells may affect the responses that are communicated to the T cell and possibly initiate the presence of autoreactive T cells. B cell memory is a highly important mechanism for regulating subsequent infections and immune responses, in MS, failure in this mechanism has severe consequences on the CNS function as EBV infected B cells have been known to thrive in MS. Nonetheless, changes in the formation of B cell memory suggests a possible genetic predisposition and these need to be investigated in CFS/ME.

4.4. Regulatory T cells and autoimmune diseases

Regulatory T cells (Tregs) of the immune system can be grouped in to $CD8^+$ Tregs or $CD4^+$Tregs. However, for the purposes of this chapter the focus will be on the $CD4^+$Tregs which have received much attention in autoimmune diseases currently being reviewed in relation to CFS. IL-3, IL-4, IL-7, IL-15, TGF-β and CD28 are important for the development, proliferation and thrive of Treg cells (Josefowicz et al., 2012). Treg profiles in a number of autoimmune disorders maybe perturbed resulting in hypo or hyperactive state in suppression. Deficiencies in Treg suppressive function may ensue from a lack in the expression of certain surface molecules such as CD39, CD95, cytotoxic T lymphocyte antigen 4 (CTLA4) and lymphocyte activation gene 3 (LAG3) (Sakaguchi et al., 2010; Schmetterer et al., 2012; Schmidt et al., 2012). Most autoimmune diseases are characterised by decreases in the function of Tregs with equivocal levels of Tregs in the tissues and periphery (Buckner, 2010).

Most of the studies on Tregs in autoimmune disorders were performed using mice models of increased susceptibility to autoimmune diseases. The state of Tregs in humans is not fully known and animal models have highlighted some important aspects of Treg function in autoimmune disorders. For example in AID, Treg cells and Foxp3 expression Tregs from NOD mice are more likely to be decreased (Clough et al., 2008; D'Alise et al., 2008; You et al., 2005). Incidentally, some patients with AID demonstrate a significant decrease in peripheral $CD4^+CD25^+$Tregs while others have shown no difference in $CD4^+CD25^+$, $CD4^+CD25^{hi}$, $CD4^+FOXP3^+CD45RO^+$, $CD4^+FOXP3^+CD45RA^+$ Treg cells or FOXP3 when compared with non-diabetics (Putnam et al., 2009). Nonetheless, it is thought that discrepancies in Treg function in AID patients may be as a consequence of poor IL-2 function (Bluestone et al., 2008). In the periphery, IL-2 has been shown to be a necessary factor in the survival and maintenance of Tregs while CD28 is important for Treg proliferation (Fontenot and Rudensky, 2004). In mice deficient in CD28, the lack of Tregs led to the progression of autoimmune diabetes, however, adoptive transfer of Tregs into the NOD mice confers protection against AID thus indicating that the presence of Tregs is necessary to guard against diabetes (Salomon et al., 2000).

The mouse model of MS, EAE, has confirmed an involvement of Tregs in the pathogenesis of MS, in these mice depletion of Tregs is a hallmark of EAE (Kohm et al., 2003). In CNS of highly developed MS patients the ability of Tregs to regulate inflammatory processes is impaired (Venken et al., 2008a; Venken et al., 2008b). Reduced FOXP3 expressing Treg cells in MS is more common in patients with relapsing remitting MS (Huang and Elferink, 2005; Venken et al., 2006) and treatment with IFN-β normalized the Tregs levels as it caused an increase in the number of $CD4^+CD25^+$Foxp3 Tregs (Chen et al., 2012). Similarly, $CD39^+$Tregs are reduced in patients with relapsing-remitting MS (Borsellino et al., 2007). These cells are necessary for the abrogation of Th17 cells in MS patients hence a reduction in these cells promote inflammatory reaction related to IL-17 (Fletcher et al., 2009). In the CNS however, Treg cells are elevated in the CSF (Feger et al., 2007). Defective Tregs cells in MS is characterised by an inability of these cells to suppress the proliferation and production of cytokines such as IFN-γ by Th1 cells (Costantino et al., 2008). It has been suggested that this may be linked to decreases in subsets of Tregs such as the $CD4^+CD25^{hi}$ Tregs (Costantino et al., 2008). Similarly in MS patients IL-10 production by the Tr1 subset of Tregs is dysfunctional (Astier et al., 2006). MS patients may present with decreased $CD127^+FOXP3^+$ Tregs (Costantino et al., 2008). Although, levels or numbers of Tregs are more likely to differ between patients, there are consistent irregularities in the suppressive capacity of these cells in MS. A hypo-suppressive Treg state transpires in the presence of decreases in IL-10 (Martinez-Forero et al., 2008).

In SLE, equivocal evidence exists for the changes in the levels of Tregs this may be related to inaccuracies in the methodology. Natural Tregs and FOXP3 Tregs in SLE have been shown to be decreased in number (Crispin et al., 2003; Lee et al., 2008; Lee et al., 2006; Miyara et al., 2005). Peripheral $CD4^+CD25^{hi}$ Tregs in SLE are reduced and this correlates with a substantial insufficiency in function and an increased expression of CD69 and CD71 (Bonelli et al., 2008). In the active form of SLE, Tregs are less suppressive and show an inability to produce efficient cytokines the opposite occurs in the dormant SLE (Valencia et al., 2007). Impairment in Treg function may occur as a result of IFN-α producing APCs, CD95 apoptosis and diminishing levels of IL-2 (Katsiari and Tsokos, 2006). Similarly, the observation of defective $CD4^+CD25^+$ Tregs or a reduced number of these cells in the lymph nodes and other areas may be due to susceptibility to Fas related apoptosis (Okamoto et al., 2011). TGF-β is necessary for the peripheral generation of $CD4^+CD25^+$Tregs incidentally their reduction may be linked to reduced levels of these cytokines in the serum in particular in patients with active SLE (Xing et al., 2012).

Treg numbers in peripheral circulation of patients with RA are also inconsistent (Boissier et al., 2009). In the synovial fluid there are uniformities in the data describing the presence of Tregs which generally tends to be high in RA patients (Cao et al., 2003), however these Tregs may not be able to effectively suppress the generation of anti-inflammatory IFN-γ and TNF-α (Leipe et al., 2005). Similarly, CTLA4 signalling in Tregs is ineffective in RA (Fiocco et al., 2008). Other factors may influence the ability of Tregs to confer suppression in the synovial fluid, mainly, the presence of macrophages in the joint resulting in excessive levels of TNF-α, IL-6 and IL-7. Synovial fluids enriched in these cytokines have an altered Treg suppressive function (Pasare and Medzhitov, 2003). High levels of FOXP3 Tregs have been found in the inflamed synovial fluid compared to the peripheral blood in RA (Jiao et al., 2007).

RA is the only disease where an apparent increase in FOXP3 expressing Tregs has been confirmed, this is consistent with what we have found in our CFS/ME patients where FOXP3 expression was higher in the periphery (Brenu et al., 2011). In CFS/ME inflamed sites may appear in the periphery and the CNS thus explaining the presence of high levels of FOXP3 in the periphery. Incidentally, the exact function of these cells in the CFS/ME patients is yet to be determined. In MS, Tregs may remain unchanged while their suppressive function on other cells and cytokine proliferation in particular the pro-inflammatory cytokines is dysfunctional. A similar mechanism may occur in CFS/ME thus likely contributing to the pathogenesis of this disease.

4.5. Immune related proteins in autoimmune diseases

Cytokines and chemokines are soluble proteins with an involvement in inflammatory reactions as they can either be pro or anti-inflammatory or both. They can also be cytotoxic to certain cells and tissues. $CD4^{+}$T cells are the predominant producers of both anti and pro-inflammatory cytokines. Th1 cells produce IL-2 and IFN-γ and are therefore pro-inflammatory while Th2 cells are anti-inflammatory as they produce IL-4, IL-5, IL-10 and IL-13 (Zhou et al., 2009). The pathogenesis of most autoimmune diseases incorporates changes in these inflammatory molecules with augmented levels of these cytokines observed in the periphery and in certain tissues. For example diseases such as RA, SLE and MS are characterised by a predominant Th1 immune profile.

IL-23, IL-17 and IL-27 are the most dominant cytokines in RA as they are necessary for inflammation in the joints (IL-23), osteoclastogenesis formation (IL-17) and activation of pro-inflammatory reactions due to a diminished amount of IL-27 (Baek et al., 2012). The mechanism of cytokine production during RA and other autoimmune diseases may rely heavily on a number of factors such as disease onset, severity, inflammatory state and source of cytokines. RA patients with severe cases of inflammation are known to have high mRNA levels of STAT1 and its associated genes suggesting that disease severity affects the pattern of cytokines in RA (Gordon et al., 2012). RA patients with an early incidence of synovitis express high levels of IL-1, IL-2, IL-4, IL-13 and IL-15 while premature RA results in substantial quantities of IL-2, IL-4, IL-13, and IL-17 in the synovial fluid (Arend, 2001; McInnes and Schett, 2007; Raza et al., 2005). Characteristically high levels of TNF-α, IL-1β, IL-6, IL-13 and IL-15 are found in the serum (Yilmaz et al., 2001). The profile of cytokines in

RA suggests a shift towards a predominant anti-inflammatory response as a consequence of elevated levels of Th2 derived cytokines IL-4 and IL-13 (Wong et al., 2000). Other cytokines including anti-inflammatory IL-10 and IL-20, and pleiotropic IL-7 may be implicated in the pathogenesis of RA (Katsikis et al., 1994; Kunz and Ibrahim, 2009).

Insulitis lesions in AID provoke inflammatory responses and the recruitment of T cells and islet-infiltrating macrophages (Eizirik et al., 2009). These cells produce cytokines that affect insulin levels in patients (Rabinovitch, 2003; Rabinovitch and Suarez-Pinzon, 2003). Suppression of insulin synthesis, secretion and destruction of β and α cells occurs in the presence of cytokines such as IL-1, IFN-γ, TNF-α and TNF-β (Mandrup-Poulsen et al., 1990; Rabinovitch et al., 1993). β cells may indirectly stimulate autoreactive T cells via the production of IFN-α during stress while T cells may stimulate IFN-γ which in turn penetrate the islets and cause their destruction (Chakrabarti et al., 1996; Stewart et al., 1993). Similarly increase in the expression of MHCI and Fas increases the likelihood for the destruction of β cells by $CD8^{+}T$ cells (Itoh et al., 1993). In serum samples, high levels of Th1 related cytokines have been observed in autoimmune diabetes with no changes in the levels of Th2 cytokines. Contrarily, Th2 cytokines have been shown to be decreased in other patients following activation of peripheral blood mononuclear cells (Kallmann et al., 1997; Rapoport et al., 1998). The levels of cytokines in autoimmune diabetes are discordant across studies and this may be related to factors such as disease severity, and the source of the cytokines.

In MS, cytokines are responsible for the oligodendrocyte cell death, axonal degeneration and neuronal impairments (Bjartmar and Trapp, 2003; Bjartmar et al., 2003; Lucchinetti et al., 2000; Wujek et al., 2002). The most prominent cytokine in MS is IFN-γ which is elevated both in MS and in the experimental condition, EAE (Ferber et al., 1996). In EAE mice IFN-γ is usually expressed in the CNS during the initial manifestations of MS and increases progressively with disease causing advancement in demyelination (Begolka et al., 1998; Issazadeh et al., 1995). In the absence of IFN-γ, EAE is not obliterated as there is evidence to suggest an increase in severity in mice depleted of IFN-γ (Hassani et al., 1999). Although, IFN-γ may have a deleterious role in EAE it may be necessary for the regulation of other inflammatory activities, deletion of certain components of IFN-γ such as STAT4 prevents the occurrence of EAE (Chitnis et al., 2001). Different classes of MS may differ in their cytokine pattern, for example, IFN-γ and IL-10 are elevated in RP and SP but not in PP MS patients (Balashov et al., 2000). The presence of TNF-α in the CNS of EAE mice is an indication of severe infiltration and inflammation in the spinal cord and oligodendrocyte cell death (Selmaj and Raine, 1988).

A number of cytokines have been implicated in the pathogenesis of SLE including IL-6, TNF-α, IFN-γ, IL-2, IL-21 and IL-17. Serum levels of IL-6 are elevated in SLE patients this is linked to the presence of hyperactive B cells and a high incidence of autoantibodies (Linker-Israeli et al., 1991; Tackey et al., 2004). Similarly CSF levels are higher in SLE patients compared to non-SLE individuals (Alcocer-Varela et al., 1992). The presence of abnormal levels of IL-6 in SLE can have systemic effects as IL-6 is a highly inflammatory cytokine. IFN-γ mRNA and serum levels are known to be increased in SLE suggesting an increase in IgG (Csiszar et al., 2000). Similarly, susceptibility to SLE is linked to polymorphism in the IL-21 and its receptor, and in the serum increased secretions of IL-21 are noticed (Sawalha et al., 2008). IL-17 secretions by cells in the plasma and serum are also noted to be increased in SLE (Crispin et al., 2008; Wong et al., 2008; Yang et al., 2009). Elevations in pro-inflammatory cytokines in SLE are important indicators of significant inflammations. Deficiencies in IL-2 occur in SLE and this is possibly linked to over activation of B and T cells (Ohl and Tenbrock, 2011). Importantly IL-2 is a necessary factory in the Treg development and function and increased levels of IL-17 (Brandenburg et al., 2008; Laurence et al., 2007).

In CFS/ME, the cytokine profiles differ from one study to another and this may be due to other factors such as age of onset and severity or cell and tissue specific cytokines. However, it is most likely that the cytokine pattern in CFS/ME resembles that of the above described autoimmune diseases where the cytokines implicated are mainly IL-2, IL-4, IL-10, IFN-γ and TNF-α. An in-depth examination of these cytokines is necessary for establishing a definitive mechanism for CFS/ME. Governance of pro-inflammatory over anti-inflammatory or vice versa has been reported in CFS/ME (Patarca et al., 2001) and this has been observed in RA and MS hence, it is possible that in RA and MS the inflammatory status of cytokines is attributed to the diseases.

5. Therapy

Currently there are no definitive therapeutic drugs for CFS/ME although current trials with rituximab may be effective in reducing the symptoms of CFS/ME. Other strategies such as cognitive behavioural therapies have being used in CFS/ME. The present immune dysfunction in CFS/ME shares similarities with certain disorders where significant improvement has been observed following administration of certain drugs. Hence, CFS/ME patients may benefit to some extent from similar therapies.

Glatiramer acetate has been shown to be effective in dampening the atypical immune response in MS (Arnon et al., 2009). Significant improvement in NK cell cytotoxic activity and cytokine secretion occur following glatiramer acetate intake in MS patients (Schrempf et al., 2007). Similarly, the use of phosphodiesterase inhibitors may be important in modulating Treg function in CFS/ME patients. These inhibitors are known to enhance the presence of cAMP resulting in the induction of cytokines that regulate the immune response (Folcik et al., 1999). B cell depletion therapies in CFS/ME may likely be essential as patients administered with substances such as Rituximab demonstrate significant improvement in health (Levesque et al., 2008). Although the cause of CFS/ME remains to be determined there are suggestions that CFS/ME may arise following viral infections. Therefore, failure to effectively clear the viral infections and subsequent infections in CFS/ME may arise as a consequence of low levels or abnormal memory cells. Rapamycin an inhibitor of mTOR may be essential in promoting the presence of memory cells in CFS/ME, in particular, the memory T cells (Araki et al., 2010).

The exact role of these drugs in CFS/ME has not being investigated and whether these treatment strategies may be useful in CFS/ME remains to be determined. It may be necessary to administer some of these drugs in combinations to ensure effective improvement in immune related responses.

6. Conclusion

CFS/ME shares certain parallels with a number of autoimmune diseases as described above, these similarities include decreases in oxidative phosphorylation, reduced NK cytotoxic activity, defects in B cells and equivocal levels of cytokines. NK cytotoxic activity is the most common immunological impairment in CFS/ME and the aforementioned autoimmune disorders. Although, disease presentation in each case is dissimilar to CFS/ME there are certain characteristics that seem to be present in CFS/ME and in each of the autoimmune diseases described above.

It is evident that most autoimmune diseases demonstrate equivocal levels of immune cell numbers however, in terms of the functional profile of most cells there is consistent confirmation for alterations in the activation or functional capacity of immune cells. The differences in relation to different cell numbers and phenotypes may be related to the severity or the stage of the disease, therefore, patients in the latent phases may differ in the relative numbers of immune cells in comparison to those in the early stages of the disease. Additionally, in the active state, most autoimmune diseases are characterised by high number of abnormal cells and relatively low levels of normal cells in comparison to the inactive state. Although, in CFS/ME these observations remain to be confirmed, it is thought that fluctuations in cell numbers may occur during periods of less severe symptoms that is, a substantial increase in wellness and periods of worsening symptoms. Thus, in these instances the production and generation of immune cells may differ while a substantial decrease in function still persists. Incidentally, in CFS/ME lymphocyte phenotypes have not been successfully associated with the disease presentation and this is also true of most autoimmune diseases where changes in the levels of lymphocyte phenotypes did not explain the decrease or increase in function. These findings therefore suggest that with regards to autoimmune diseases a standard assessment of leukocyte phenotypes may not necessarily explain the mechanism.

Importantly, almost all autoimmune diseases have an association with reduced cytotoxic activity and decreases in neutrophil function. Suggesting that CFS/ME may have a potential to be described as autoimmune, as this is the only consistent immunological abnormality associated with CFS/ME. A loss or a reduced function in NK cells seems to occur both in the periphery and tissues. Tissue specific NK activity has not being reported in CFS/ME however, it may be interesting to investigate NK function in other tissues and to determine whether a similar profile is observed as in other immune diseases. Nonetheless the findings from immune function in CFS/ME including reduced NK cell cytotoxic activity, low lymphocyte response to mitogenic stimulation and deficits in immunoglobulins are indicative of immune deficiency. Treg function and FOXP3 expression patterns in CFS/ME are consistent with some RA patients, however Treg suppression is more often decreased in autoimmune diseases. A plausible explanation for these differences relates to the observation that Treg function is inextricably linked to cAMP metabolism and compromise of neuropeptides such as vasoactive neuropeptide function in some tissues. This may produce impaired cAMP synthesis. Hence, Treg function may be increased to compensate, as they are known that cAMP is directly transferred from Tregs to other cells. Nonetheless, further validatory studies are required to confirm these observations that we have observed in previous studies.

It is important to note that despite the inconsistencies in these autoimmune diseases mentioned above they all have a well established mechanism of action. However, in CFS/ME a mechanism for disease presentation is unknown. This is the biggest confounding factor in the study of CFS/ME, hence, it is very difficult to understand the nature of the disease and propose logical conclusions to explain the disease presentation and symptom profile.

Author details

Ekua W. Brenu[1,2], Lotti Tajouri[3], Kevin J. Ashton[3], Donald R. Staines[1,4] and Sonya M. Marshall-Gradisnik[1,2]

1 National Center for Neuroimmunology and Emerging Diseases, Griffith University, Gold Coast, Queensland, Australia

2 School of Medical Science, Griffith Health Institute, Griffith University, Gold Coast Campus, Gold Coast, QLD, Australia

3 Faculty of Health Science and Medicine, Bond University, Robina, Queensland, Australia

4 Queensland Health, Gold Coast Public Health Unit, Robina, Queensland, Australia

References

[1] Alcocer-Varela, J., Aleman-Hoey, D. and Alarcon-Segovia, D., 1992. Interleukin-1 and interleukin-6 activities are increased in the cerebrospinal fluid of patients with CNS lupus erythematosus and correlate with local late T-cell activation markers. Lupus. 1, 111-7.

[2] Anolik, J.H., Ravikumar, R., Barnard, J., Owen, T., Almudevar, A., Milner, E.C., Miller, C.H., Dutcher, P.O., Hadley, J.A. and Sanz, I., 2008. Cutting edge: anti-tumor necrosis factor therapy in rheumatoid arthritis inhibits memory B lymphocytes via effects on lymphoid germinal centers and follicular dendritic cell networks. Journal of immunology. 180, 688-92.

[3] Araki, K., Youngblood, B. and Ahmed, R. 2010. The role of mTOR in memory CD8 T-cell differentiation. Immunological reviews. 235, 234-43.

[4] Aramaki, T., Ida, H., Izumi, Y., Fujikawa, K., Huang, M., Arima, K., Tamai, M., Kamachi, M., Nakamura, H., Kawakami, A., Origuchi, T., Matsuoka, N. and Eguchi, K., 2009. A significantly impaired natural killer cell activity due to a low activity on a per-cell basis in rheumatoid arthritis. Modern rheumatology / the Japan Rheumatism Association. 19, 245-52.

[5] Arend, W.P., 2001. Physiology of cytokine pathways in rheumatoid arthritis. Arthritis and rheumatism. 45, 101-6.

[6] Arnon, R., Aharoni, R. 2009. Neuroprotection and neurogeneration in MS and its animal model EAE effected by glatiramer acetate. Journal of Neural Transmission. 116, 1443-1449.

[7] Astier, A.L., Meiffren, G., Freeman, S. and Hafler, D.A., 2006. Alterations in CD46-mediated Tr1 regulatory T cells in patients with multiple sclerosis. The Journal of clinical investigation. 116, 3252-7.

[8] Baek, S.H., Lee, S.G., Park, Y.E., Kim, G.T., Kim, C.D. and Park, S.Y., 2012. Increased synovial expression of IL-27 by IL-17 in rheumatoid arthritis. Inflammation research : official journal of the European Histamine Research Society ... [et al.].

[9] Balashov, K.E., Comabella, M., Ohashi, T., Khoury, S.J. and Weiner, H.L., 2000. Defective regulation of IFNgamma and IL-12 by endogenous IL-10 in progressive MS. Neurology. 55, 192-8.

[10] Barone, F., Bombardieri, M., Rosado, M.M., Morgan, P.R., Challacombe, S.J., De Vita, S., Carsetti, R., Spencer, J., Valesini, G. and Pitzalis, C., 2008. CXCL13, CCL21, and CXCL12 expression in salivary glands of patients with Sjogren's syndrome and MALT lymphoma: association with reactive and malignant areas of lymphoid organization. Journal of immunology. 180, 5130-40.

[11] Begolka, W.S., Vanderlugt, C.L., Rahbe, S.M. and Miller, S.D., 1998. Differential expression of inflammatory cytokines parallels progression of central nervous system pathology in two clinically distinct models of multiple sclerosis. Journal of immunology. 161, 4437-46.

[12] Benczur, M., Petranyl, G.G., Palffy, G., Varga, M., Talas, M., Kotsy, B., Foldes, I. and Hollan, S.R., 1980. Dysfunction of natural killer cells in multiple sclerosis: a possible pathogenetic factor. Clinical and experimental immunology. 39, 657-62.

[13] Binstadt, B.A., Patel, P.R., Alencar, H., Nigrovic, P.A., Lee, D.M., Mahmood, U., Weissleder, R., Mathis, D. and Benoist, C., 2006. Particularities of the vasculature can promote the organ specificity of autoimmune attack. Nature immunology. 7, 284-92.

[14] Bjartmar, C. and Trapp, B.D., 2003. Axonal degeneration and progressive neurologic disability in multiple sclerosis. Neurotox Res. 5, 157-64.

[15] Bjartmar, C., Wujek, J.R. and Trapp, B.D., 2003. Axonal loss in the pathology of MS: consequences for understanding the progressive phase of the disease. Journal of the neurological sciences. 206, 165-71.

[16] Blair, P.A., Norena, L.Y., Flores-Borja, F., Rawlings, D.J., Isenberg, D.A., Ehrenstein, M.R. and Mauri, C., 2010. CD19(+)CD24(hi)CD38(hi) B cells exhibit regulatory capacity in healthy individuals but are functionally impaired in systemic Lupus Erythematosus patients. Immunity. 32, 129-40.

[17] Bluestone, J.A., Tang, Q. and Sedwick, C.E., 2008. T regulatory cells in autoimmune diabetes: past challenges, future prospects. Journal of clinical immunology. 28, 677-84.

[18] Boissier, M.C., Assier, E., Biton, J., Denys, A., Falgarone, G. and Bessis, N., 2009. Regulatory T cells (Treg) in rheumatoid arthritis. Joint Bone Spine. 76, 10-4.

[19] Bonelli, M., von Dalwigk, K., Savitskaya, A., Smolen, J.S. and Scheinecker, C., 2008. Foxp3 expression in CD4+ T cells of patients with systemic lupus erythematosus: a comparative phenotypic analysis. Annals of the rheumatic diseases. 67, 664-71.

[20] Borish, L.C. and Steinke, J.W., 2003. 2. Cytokines and chemokines. The Journal of allergy and clinical immunology. 111, S460-75.

[21] Borsellino, G., Kleinewietfeld, M., Di Mitri, D., Sternjak, A., Diamantini, A., Giometto, R., Hopner, S., Centonze, D., Bernardi, G., Dell'Acqua, M.L., Rossini, P.M., Battistini, L., Rotzschke, O. and Falk, K., 2007. Expression of ectonucleotidase CD39 by Foxp3+ Treg cells: hydrolysis of extracellular ATP and immune suppression. Blood. 110, 1225-32.

[22] Bosch, X., 2011. Systemic lupus erythematosus and the neutrophil. The New England journal of medicine. 365, 758-60.

[23] Brandenburg, S., Takahashi, T., de la Rosa, M., Janke, M., Karsten, G., Muzzulini, T., Orinska, Z., Bulfone-Paus, S. and Scheffold, A., 2008. IL-2 induces in vivo suppression by CD4(+)CD25(+)Foxp3(+) regulatory T cells. European journal of immunology. 38, 1643-53.

[24] Brenu, E.W., Staines, D.R., Baskurt, O.K., Ashton, K.J., Ramos, S.B., Christy, R.M. and Marshall-Gradisnik, S.M., 2010. Immune and hemorheological changes in chronic fatigue syndrome. Journal of translational medicine. 8, 1.

[25] Brenu, E.W., van Driel, M.L., Staines, D.R., Ashton, K.J., Ramos, S.B., Keane, J., Klimas, N.G. and Marshall-Gradisnik, S.M., 2011. Immunological abnormalities as potential biomarkers in Chronic Fatigue Syndrome/Myalgic Encephalomyelitis. Journal of translational medicine. 9, 81.

[26] Bryceson, Y.T., March, M.E., Ljunggren, H.G. and Long, E.O., 2006. Activation, coactivation, and costimulation of resting human natural killer cells. Immunological reviews. 214, 73-91.

[27] Buckner, J.H., 2010. Mechanisms of impaired regulation by CD4(+)CD25(+)FOXP3(+) regulatory T cells in human autoimmune diseases. Nature reviews. Immunology. 10, 849-59.

[28] Buljevac, D., van Doornum, G.J., Flach, H.Z., Groen, J., Osterhaus, A.D., Hop, W., van Doorn, P.A., van der Meche, F.G. and Hintzen, R.Q., 2005. Epstein-Barr virus and disease activity in multiple sclerosis. Journal of neurology, neurosurgery, and psychiatry. 76, 1377-81.

[29] Caligiuri, M.A., 2008. Human natural killer cells. Blood. 112, 461-9.

[30] Cao, D., Malmstrom, V., Baecher-Allan, C., Hafler, D., Klareskog, L. and Trollmo, C., 2003. Isolation and functional characterization of regulatory CD25brightCD4+ T cells from the target organ of patients with rheumatoid arthritis. European journal of immunology. 33, 215-23.

[31] Cappione, A., 3rd, Anolik, J.H., Pugh-Bernard, A., Barnard, J., Dutcher, P., Silverman, G. and Sanz, I., 2005. Germinal center exclusion of autoreactive B cells is defective in human systemic lupus erythematosus. The Journal of clinical investigation. 115, 3205-16.

[32] Carter, N.A., Vasconcellos, R., Rosser, E.C., Tulone, C., Munoz-Suano, A., Kamanaka, M., Ehrenstein, M.R., Flavell, R.A. and Mauri, C., 2011. Mice lacking endogenous IL-10-producing regulatory B cells develop exacerbated disease and present with an increased frequency of Th1/Th17 but a decrease in regulatory T cells. Journal of immunology. 186, 5569-79.

[33] Cedergren, J., Forslund, T., Sundqvist, T. and Skogh, T., 2007. Intracellular oxidative activation in synovial fluid neutrophils from patients with rheumatoid arthritis but not from other arthritis patients. The Journal of rheumatology. 34, 2162-70.

[34] Cepok, S., Jacobsen, M., Schock, S., Omer, B., Jaekel, S., Boddeker, I., Oertel, W.H., Sommer, N. and Hemmer, B., 2001. Patterns of cerebrospinal fluid pathology correlate with disease progression in multiple sclerosis. Brain : a journal of neurology. 124, 2169-76.

[35] Cepok, S., Rosche, B., Grummel, V., Vogel, F., Zhou, D., Sayn, J., Sommer, N., Hartung, H.P. and Hemmer, B., 2005. Short-lived plasma blasts are the main B cell effector subset during the course of multiple sclerosis. Brain : a journal of neurology. 128, 1667-76.

[36] Chakrabarti, D., Huang, X., Beck, J., Henrich, J., McFarland, N., James, R.F. and Stewart, T.A., 1996. Control of islet intercellular adhesion molecule-1 expression by interferon-alpha and hypoxia. Diabetes. 45, 1336-43.

[37] Chen, J., Gusdon, A.M., Thayer, T.C. and Mathews, C.E., 2008. Role of increased ROS dissipation in prevention of T1D. Annals of the New York Academy of Sciences. 1150, 157-66.

[38] Chen, M., Chen, G., Deng, S., Liu, X., Hutton, G.J. and Hong, J., 2012. IFN-beta induces the proliferation of CD4+CD25+Foxp3+ regulatory T cells through upregulation of GITRL on dendritic cells in the treatment of multiple sclerosis. Journal of neuroimmunology. 242, 39-46.

[39] Chitnis, T., Najafian, N., Benou, C., Salama, A.D., Grusby, M.J., Sayegh, M.H. and Khoury, S.J., 2001. Effect of targeted disruption of STAT4 and STAT6 on the induction of experimental autoimmune encephalomyelitis. The Journal of clinical investigation. 108, 739-47.

[40] Clough, L.E., Wang, C.J., Schmidt, E.M., Booth, G., Hou, T.Z., Ryan, G.A. and Walker, L.S., 2008. Release from regulatory T cell-mediated suppression during the onset of tissue-specific autoimmunity is associated with elevated IL-21. Journal of immunology. 180, 5393-401.

[41] Corcione, A., Arduino, N., Ferretti, E., Raffaghello, L., Roncella, S., Rossi, D., Fedeli, F., Ottonello, L., Trentin, L., Dallegri, F., Semenzato, G. and Pistoia, V., 2004. CCL19 and CXCL12 trigger in vitro chemotaxis of human mantle cell lymphoma B cells. Clinical cancer research : an official journal of the American Association for Cancer Research. 10, 964-71.

[42] Costantino, C.M., Baecher-Allan, C. and Hafler, D.A., 2008. Multiple sclerosis and regulatory T cells. Journal of clinical immunology. 28, 697-706.

[43] Crispin, J.C., Martinez, A. and Alcocer-Varela, J., 2003. Quantification of regulatory T cells in patients with systemic lupus erythematosus. Journal of autoimmunity. 21, 273-6.

[44] Crispin, J.C., Oukka, M., Bayliss, G., Cohen, R.A., Van Beek, C.A., Stillman, I.E., Kyttaris, V.C., Juang, Y.T. and Tsokos, G.C., 2008. Expanded double negative T cells in patients with systemic lupus erythematosus produce IL-17 and infiltrate the kidneys. Journal of immunology. 181, 8761-6.

[45] Csiszar, A., Nagy, G., Gergely, P., Pozsonyi, T. and Pocsik, E., 2000. Increased interferon-gamma (IFN-gamma), IL-10 and decreased IL-4 mRNA expression in peripheral blood mononuclear cells (PBMC) from patients with systemic lupus erythematosus (SLE). Clinical and experimental immunology. 122, 464-70.

[46] D'Alise, A.M., Auyeung, V., Feuerer, M., Nishio, J., Fontenot, J., Benoist, C. and Mathis, D., 2008. The defect in T-cell regulation in NOD mice is an effect on the T-cell effectors. Proceedings of the National Academy of Sciences of the United States of America. 105, 19857-62.

[47] Dalbeth, N. and Callan, M.F., 2002. A subset of natural killer cells is greatly expanded within inflamed joints. Arthritis and rheumatism. 46, 1763-72.

[48] Davidson, A. and Diamond, B., 2001. Autoimmune diseases. The New England journal of medicine. 345, 340-50.

[49] de la Fuente, H., Richaud-Patin, Y., Jakez-Ocampo, J., Gonzalez-Amaro, R. and Llorente, L., 2001. Innate immune mechanisms in the pathogenesis of systemic lupus erythematosus (SLE). Immunology letters. 77, 175-80.

[50] Decker, P., 2011. Neutrophils and interferon-alpha-producing cells: who produces interferon in lupus? Arthritis research & therapy. 13, 118.

[51] Della Bella, S., Gennaro, M., Vaccari, M., Ferraris, C., Nicola, S., Riva, A., Clerici, M., Greco, M. and Villa, M.L., 2003. Altered maturation of peripheral blood dendritic cells in patients with breast cancer. British journal of cancer. 89, 1463-72.

[52] Dorner, T., Jacobi, A.M. and Lipsky, P.E., 2009. B cells in autoimmunity. Arthritis research & therapy. 11, 247.

[53] Edwards, J.C., Cambridge, G. and Abrahams, V.M., 1999. Do self-perpetuating B lymphocytes drive human autoimmune disease? Immunology. 97, 188-96.

[54] Edwards, S.W. and Hallett, M.B., 1997. Seeing the wood for the trees: the forgotten role of neutrophils in rheumatoid arthritis. Immunology today. 18, 320-4.

[55] Eizirik, D.L., Colli, M.L. and Ortis, F., 2009. The role of inflammation in insulitis and beta-cell loss in type 1 diabetes. Nat Rev Endocrinol. 5, 219-26.

[56] Eyles, J.L., Roberts, A.W., Metcalf, D. and Wicks, I.P., 2006. Granulocyte colony-stimulating factor and neutrophils--forgotten mediators of inflammatory disease. Nature clinical practice. Rheumatology. 2, 500-10.

[57] Farag, S.S., Fehniger, T., Ruggeri, L., Velardi, A. and Caligiuri, M.A., 2002. Natural killer cells: biology and application in stem-cell transplantation. Cytotherapy. 4, 445-6.

[58] Feger, U., Luther, C., Poeschel, S., Melms, A., Tolosa, E. and Wiendl, H., 2007. Increased frequency of CD4+ CD25+ regulatory T cells in the cerebrospinal fluid but not in the blood of multiple sclerosis patients. Clinical and experimental immunology. 147, 412-8.

[59] Ferber, I.A., Brocke, S., Taylor-Edwards, C., Ridgway, W., Dinisco, C., Steinman, L., Dalton, D. and Fathman, C.G., 1996. Mice with a disrupted IFN-gamma gene are susceptible to the induction of experimental autoimmune encephalomyelitis (EAE). Journal of immunology. 156, 5-7.

[60] Ferretti, G., Bacchetti, T., DiLudovico, F., Viti, B., Angeleri, V.A., Danni, M. and Provinciali, L., 2006. Intracellular oxidative activity and respiratory burst of leukocytes isolated from multiple sclerosis patients. Neurochemistry international. 48, 87-92.

[61] Fiocco, U., Sfriso, P., Oliviero, F., Pagnin, E., Scagliori, E., Campana, C., Dainese, S., Cozzi, L. and Punzi, L., 2008. Co-stimulatory modulation in rheumatoid arthritis: the role of (CTLA4-Ig) abatacept. Autoimmunity reviews. 8, 76-82.

[62] Fletcher, M.A., Zeng, X.R., Barnes, Z., Levis, S. and Klimas, N.G., 2009. Plasma cytokines in women with chronic fatigue syndrome. Journal of translational medicine. 7, 96.

[63] Fletcher, M.A., Zeng, X.R., Maher, K., Levis, S., Hurwitz, B., Antoni, M., Broderick, G. and Klimas, N.G., 2010. Biomarkers in chronic fatigue syndrome: evaluation of natural killer cell function and dipeptidyl peptidase IV/CD26. PloS one. 5, e10817.

[64] Fluge, O., Bruland, O., Risa, K., Storstein, A., Kristoffersen, E.K., Sapkota, D., Naess, H., Dahl, O., Nyland, H. and Mella, O., 2011. Benefit from B-lymphocyte depletion using the anti-CD20 antibody rituximab in chronic fatigue syndrome. A double-blind and placebo-controlled study. PloS one. 6, e26358.

[65] Fluge, O. and Mella, O., 2009. Clinical impact of B-cell depletion with the anti-CD20 antibody rituximab in chronic fatigue syndrome: a preliminary case series. BMC neurology. 9, 28.

[66] Folcik, V.A., Smith, T., O'Bryant, S., Kawczak, J.A., Zhu, B., Sakurai, H., Kajiwara, A., Staddon, J.M., Glabinski, A., Chernosky, A.L., Johnson, J.M., Tuohy, V.K., Rubin, L.L. and Ransohoff, R.M. Journal of Neuroimmunology. 97, 119-20.

[67] Fontenot, J.D. and Rudensky, A.Y., 2004. Molecular aspects of regulatory T cell development. Seminars in immunology. 16, 73-80.

[68] Franciotta, D., Salvetti, M., Lolli, F., Serafini, B. and Aloisi, F., 2008. B cells and multiple sclerosis. Lancet neurology. 7, 852-8.

[69] Fukuda, K., Straus, S.E., Hickie, I., Sharpe, M.C., Dobbins, J.G. and Komaroff, A., 1994. The chronic fatigue syndrome: a comprehensive approach to its definition and study. International Chronic Fatigue Syndrome Study Group. Annals of internal medicine. 121, 953-9.

[70] Gordon, R.A., Grigoriev, G., Lee, A., Kalliolias, G.D. and Ivashkiv, L.B., 2012. The IFN signature and STAT1 expression in RA synovial fluid macrophages are induced by TNFalpha and counter-regulated by synovial fluid microenvironment. Arthritis and rheumatism.

[71] Grykiel, K., Zozulinska, D., Kostrzewa, A., Wiktorowicz, K. and Wierusz-Wysocka, B., 2001. [Evaluation of expression of polymorphonuclear neutrophil surface receptors in patients with type 1 diabetes]. Pol Arch Med Wewn. 105, 377-81.

[72] Harris, D.P., Haynes, L., Sayles, P.C., Duso, D.K., Eaton, S.M., Lepak, N.M., Johnson, L.L., Swain, S.L. and Lund, F.E., 2000. Reciprocal regulation of polarized cytokine production by effector B and T cells. Nature immunology. 1, 475-82.

[73] Haskins, K., Bradley, B., Powers, K., Fadok, V., Flores, S., Ling, X., Pugazhenthi, S., Reusch, J. and Kench, J., 2003. Oxidative stress in type 1 diabetes. Annals of the New York Academy of Sciences. 1005, 43-54.

[74] Hassani, O., Loew, D., Van Dorsselaer, A., Papandreou, M.J., Sorokine, O., Rochat, H., Sampieri, F. and Mansuelle, P., 1999. Aah VI, a novel, N-glycosylated anti-insect toxin from Androctonus australis hector scorpion venom: isolation, characterisation, and glycan structure determination. FEBS letters. 443, 175-80.

[75] Hilliard, B., Wilmen, A., Seidel, C., Liu, T.S., Goke, R. and Chen, Y., 2001. Roles of TNF-related apoptosis-inducing ligand in experimental autoimmune encephalomyelitis. Journal of immunology. 166, 1314-9.

[76] Huang, G. and Elferink, C.J., 2005. Multiple mechanisms are involved in Ah receptor-mediated cell cycle arrest. Molecular pharmacology. 67, 88-96.

[77] Issazadeh, S., Ljungdahl, A., Hojeberg, B., Mustafa, M. and Olsson, T., 1995. Cytokine production in the central nervous system of Lewis rats with experimental autoimmune encephalomyelitis: dynamics of mRNA expression for interleukin-10, interleukin-12, cytolysin, tumor necrosis factor alpha and tumor necrosis factor beta. Journal of neuroimmunology. 61, 205-12.

[78] Itoh, N., Hanafusa, T., Miyazaki, A., Miyagawa, J., Yamagata, K., Yamamoto, K., Waguri, M., Imagawa, A., Tamura, S., Inada, M. and et al., 1993. Mononuclear cell infiltration and its relation to the expression of major histocompatibility complex antigens and adhesion molecules in pancreas biopsy specimens from newly diagnosed insulin-dependent diabetes mellitus patients. The Journal of clinical investigation. 92, 2313-22.

[79] Jacobi, A.M., Reiter, K., Mackay, M., Aranow, C., Hiepe, F., Radbruch, A., Hansen, A., Burmester, G.R., Diamond, B., Lipsky, P.E. and Dorner, T., 2008. Activated memory B cell subsets correlate with disease activity in systemic lupus erythematosus: delineation by expression of CD27, IgD, and CD95. Arthritis and rheumatism. 58, 1762-73.

[80] Jonsen, A., Gunnarsson, I., Gullstrand, B., Svenungsson, E., Bengtsson, A.A., Nived, O., Lundberg, I.E., Truedsson, L. and Sturfelt, G., 2007. Association between SLE nephritis and polymorphic variants of the CRP and FcgammaRIIIa genes. Rheumatology. 46, 1417-21.

[81] Josefowicz, S.Z., Lu, L.F. and Rudensky, A.Y., 2012. Regulatory T cells: mechanisms of differentiation and function. Annual review of immunology. 30, 531-64.

[82] Kallmann, B.A., Huther, M., Tubes, M., Feldkamp, J., Bertrams, J., Gries, F.A., Lampeter, E.F. and Kolb, H., 1997. Systemic bias of cytokine production toward cell-mediated immune regulation in IDDM and toward humoral immunity in Graves' disease. Diabetes. 46, 237-43.

[83] Kastrukoff, L.F., Morgan, N.G., Zecchini, D., White, R., Petkau, A.J., Satoh, J. and Paty, D.W., 1998. A role for natural killer cells in the immunopathogenesis of multiple sclerosis. Journal of neuroimmunology. 86, 123-33.

[84] Katsiari, C.G. and Tsokos, G.C., 2006. Transcriptional repression of interleukin-2 in human systemic lupus erythematosus. Autoimmunity reviews. 5, 118-21.

[85] Katsikis, P.D., Chu, C.Q., Brennan, F.M., Maini, R.N. and Feldmann, M., 1994. Immunoregulatory role of interleukin 10 in rheumatoid arthritis. The Journal of experimental medicine. 179, 1517-27.

[86] Kennedy, G., Spence, V., Underwood, C. and Belch, J.J., 2004. Increased neutrophil apoptosis in chronic fatigue syndrome. Journal of clinical pathology. 57, 891-3.

[87] Klimas, N.G., Broderick, G. and Fletcher, M.A., 2012. Biomarkers for chronic fatigue. Brain, behavior, and immunity.

[88] Klimas, N.G., Salvato, F.R., Morgan, R. and Fletcher, M.A., 1990. Immunologic abnormalities in chronic fatigue syndrome. Journal of clinical microbiology. 28, 1403-10.

[89] Kohm, A.P., Carpentier, P.A. and Miller, S.D., 2003. Regulation of experimental autoimmune encephalomyelitis (EAE) by CD4+CD25+ regulatory T cells. Novartis Foundation symposium. 252, 45-52; discussion 52-4, 106-14.

[90] Kuenz, B., Lutterotti, A., Ehling, R., Gneiss, C., Haemmerle, M., Rainer, C., Deisenhammer, F., Schocke, M., Berger, T. and Reindl, M., 2008. Cerebrospinal fluid B cells correlate with early brain inflammation in multiple sclerosis. PloS one. 3, e2559.

[91] Kunz, M. and Ibrahim, S.M., 2009. Cytokines and cytokine profiles in human autoimmune diseases and animal models of autoimmunity. Mediators of inflammation. 2009, 979258.

[92] Lande, R., Ganguly, D., Facchinetti, V., Frasca, L., Conrad, C., Gregorio, J., Meller, S., Chamilos, G., Sebasigari, R., Riccieri, V., Bassett, R., Amuro, H., Fukuhara, S., Ito, T., Liu, Y.J. and Gilliet, M., 2011. Neutrophils activate plasmacytoid dendritic cells by releasing self-DNA-peptide complexes in systemic lupus erythematosus. Science translational medicine. 3, 73ra19.

[93] Laurence, A., Tato, C.M., Davidson, T.S., Kanno, Y., Chen, Z., Yao, Z., Blank, R.B., Meylan, F., Siegel, R., Hennighausen, L., Shevach, E.M. and O'Shea J, J., 2007. Interleukin-2 signaling via STAT5 constrains T helper 17 cell generation. Immunity. 26, 371-81.

[94] Lee, H.Y., Hong, Y.K., Yun, H.J., Kim, Y.M., Kim, J.R. and Yoo, W.H., 2008. Altered frequency and migration capacity of CD4+CD25+ regulatory T cells in systemic lupus erythematosus. Rheumatology. 47, 789-94.

[95] Lee, J.H., Wang, L.C., Lin, Y.T., Yang, Y.H., Lin, D.T. and Chiang, B.L., 2006. Inverse correlation between CD4+ regulatory T-cell population and autoantibody levels in paediatric patients with systemic lupus erythematosus. Immunology. 117, 280-6.

[96] Leipe, J., Skapenko, A., Lipsky, P.E. and Schulze-Koops, H., 2005. Regulatory T cells in rheumatoid arthritis. Arthritis research & therapy. 7, 93.

[97] Levesque, M.C. and St Clair, E.W. B cell-directed therapies for autoimmune disease and correlates of disease response and relapse. Journal of Allergy and Clinical Immunology. 121, 13-21.

[98] Lindau, D., Ronnefarth, V., Erbacher, A., Rammensee, H.G. and Decker, P., 2011. Nucleosome-induced neutrophil activation occurs independently of TLR9 and endosomal acidification: implications for systemic lupus erythematosus. European journal of immunology. 41, 669-81.

[99] Linker-Israeli, M., Deans, R.J., Wallace, D.J., Prehn, J., Ozeri-Chen, T. and Klinenberg, J.R., 1991. Elevated levels of endogenous IL-6 in systemic lupus erythematosus. A putative role in pathogenesis. Journal of immunology. 147, 117-23.

[100] Logters, T., Margraf, S., Altrichter, J., Cinatl, J., Mitzner, S., Windolf, J. and Scholz, M., 2009. The clinical value of neutrophil extracellular traps. Medical microbiology and immunology. 198, 211-9.

[101] Lorusso, L., Mikhaylova, S.V., Capelli, E., Ferrari, D., Ngonga, G.K. and Ricevuti, G., 2009. Immunological aspects of chronic fatigue syndrome. Autoimmunity reviews. 8, 287-91.

[102] Lucchinetti, C., Bruck, W., Parisi, J., Scheithauer, B., Rodriguez, M. and Lassmann, H., 2000. Heterogeneity of multiple sclerosis lesions: implications for the pathogenesis of demyelination. Annals of neurology. 47, 707-17.

[103] Maher, K.J., Klimas, N.G. and Fletcher, M.A., 2005. Chronic fatigue syndrome is associated with diminished intracellular perforin. Clinical and experimental immunology. 142, 505-11.

[104] Mandrup-Poulsen, T., Helqvist, S., Wogensen, L.D., Molvig, J., Pociot, F., Johannesen, J. and Nerup, J., 1990. Cytokine and free radicals as effector molecules in the destruction of pancreatic beta cells. Curr Top Microbiol Immunol. 164, 169-93.

[105] Marhoffer, W., Stein, M., Schleinkofer, L. and Federlin, K., 1993. Evidence of ex vivo and in vitro impaired neutrophil oxidative burst and phagocytic capacity in type 1 diabetes mellitus. Diabetes research and clinical practice. 19, 183-8.

[106] Marino, E., Batten, M., Groom, J., Walters, S., Liuwantara, D., Mackay, F. and Grey, S.T., 2008. Marginal-zone B-cells of nonobese diabetic mice expand with diabetes onset, invade the pancreatic lymph nodes, and present autoantigen to diabetogenic T-cells. Diabetes. 57, 395-404.

[107] Marino, F. and Cosentino, M., 2011. Adrenergic modulation of immune cells: an update. Amino acids.

[108] Martinez-Forero, I., Garcia-Munoz, R., Martinez-Pasamar, S., Inoges, S., Lopez-Diaz de Cerio, A., Palacios, R., Sepulcre, J., Moreno, B., Gonzalez, Z., Fernandez-Diez, B., Melero, I., Bendandi, M. and Villoslada, P., 2008. IL-10 suppressor activity and ex vivo Tr1 cell function are impaired in multiple sclerosis. European journal of immunology. 38, 576-86.

[109] Marzocchi-Machado, C.M., Alves, C.M., Azzolini, A.E., Polizello, A.C., Carvalho, I.F. and Lucisano-Valim, Y.M., 2002. Fcgamma and complement receptors: expression, role and co-operation in mediating the oxidative burst and degranulation of neutrophils of Brazilian systemic lupus erythematosus patients. Lupus. 11, 240-8.

[110] Mauri, C., 2010. Regulation of immunity and autoimmunity by B cells. Current opinion in immunology. 22, 761-7.

[111] McInnes, I.B. and Schett, G., 2007. Cytokines in the pathogenesis of rheumatoid arthritis. Nature reviews. Immunology. 7, 429-42.

[112] Meffre, E. and Wardemann, H., 2008. B-cell tolerance checkpoints in health and autoimmunity. Current opinion in immunology. 20, 632-8.

[113] Menard, L., Samuels, J., Ng, Y.S. and Meffre, E., 2011. Inflammation-independent defective early B cell tolerance checkpoints in rheumatoid arthritis. Arthritis and rheumatism. 63, 1237-45.

[114] Miyara, M., Amoura, Z., Parizot, C., Badoual, C., Dorgham, K., Trad, S., Nochy, D., Debre, P., Piette, J.C. and Gorochov, G., 2005. Global natural regulatory T cell depletion in active systemic lupus erythematosus. Journal of immunology. 175, 8392-400.

[115] Mohr, W., Westerhellweg, H. and Wessinghage, D., 1981. Polymorphonuclear granulocytes in rheumatic tissue destruction. III. an electron microscopic study of PMNs at the pannus-cartilage junction in rheumatoid arthritis. Annals of the rheumatic diseases. 40, 396-9.

[116] Momot, T., Koch, S., Hunzelmann, N., Krieg, T., Ulbricht, K., Schmidt, R.E. and Witte, T., 2004. Association of killer cell immunoglobulin-like receptors with scleroderma. Arthritis and rheumatism. 50, 1561-5.

[117] Munschauer, F.E., Hartrich, L.A., Stewart, C.C. and Jacobs, L., 1995. Circulating natural killer cells but not cytotoxic T lymphocytes are reduced in patients with active relapsing multiple sclerosis and little clinical disability as compared to controls. Journal of neuroimmunology. 62, 177-81.

[118] Naegele, M., Tillack, K., Reinhardt, S., Schippling, S., Martin, R. and Sospedra, M., 2012. Neutrophils in multiple sclerosis are characterized by a primed phenotype. Journal of neuroimmunology. 242, 60-71.

[119] Nathan, C., 2006. Neutrophils and immunity: challenges and opportunities. Nature reviews. Immunology. 6, 173-82.

[120] Nedvetzki, S., Sowinski, S., Eagle, R.A., Harris, J., Vely, F., Pende, D., Trowsdale, J., Vivier, E., Gordon, S. and Davis, D.M., 2007. Reciprocal regulation of human natural killer cells and macrophages associated with distinct immune synapses. Blood. 109, 3776-85.

[121] Nemeth, T. and Mocsai, A., 2012. The role of neutrophils in autoimmune diseases. Immunology letters. 143, 9-19.

[122] Noorchashm, H., Moore, D.J., Lieu, Y.K., Noorchashm, N., Schlachterman, A., Song, H.K., Barker, C.F. and Naji, A., 1999. Contribution of the innate immune system to autoimmune diabetes: a role for the CR1/CR2 complement receptors. Cellular immunology. 195, 75-9.

[123] Odendahl, M., Mei, H., Hoyer, B.F., Jacobi, A.M., Hansen, A., Muehlinghaus, G., Berek, C., Hiepe, F., Manz, R., Radbruch, A. and Dorner, T., 2005. Generation of migra-

tory antigen-specific plasma blasts and mobilization of resident plasma cells in a secondary immune response. Blood. 105, 1614-21.

[124] Ohl, K. and Tenbrock, K., 2011. Inflammatory cytokines in systemic lupus erythematosus. Journal of biomedicine & biotechnology. 2011, 432595.

[125] Okamoto, A., Fujio, K., Okamura, T. and Yamamoto, K., 2011. Regulatory T-cell-associated cytokines in systemic lupus erythematosus. Journal of biomedicine & biotechnology. 2011, 463412.

[126] Opsahl, M.L. and Kennedy, P.G., 2007. An attempt to investigate the presence of Epstein Barr virus in multiple sclerosis and normal control brain tissue. Journal of neurology. 254, 425-30.

[127] Park, Y.W., Kee, S.J., Cho, Y.N., Lee, E.H., Lee, H.Y., Kim, E.M., Shin, M.H., Park, J.J., Kim, T.J., Lee, S.S., Yoo, D.H. and Kang, H.S., 2009. Impaired differentiation and cytotoxicity of natural killer cells in systemic lupus erythematosus. Arthritis and rheumatism. 60, 1753-63.

[128] Pasare, C. and Medzhitov, R., 2003. Toll pathway-dependent blockade of CD4+CD25+ T cell-mediated suppression by dendritic cells. Science. 299, 1033-6.

[129] Pascual, M.L., Muino-Blanco, T., Cebrian-Perez, J.A. and Lopez-Perez, M.J., 1994. Acquisition of viable-like surface properties of sperm cells by adsorption of seminal plasma proteins revealed by centrifugal countercurrent distribution. Biology of the cell / under the auspices of the European Cell Biology Organization. 82, 75-8.

[130] Pasi, A., Bozzini, S., Carlo-Stella, N., Martinetti, M., Bombardieri, S., De Silvestri, A., Salvaneschi, L. and Cuccia, M., 2011. Excess of activating killer cell immunoglobulin-like receptors and lack of HLA-Bw4 ligands: a twoedged weapon in chronic fatigue syndrome. Molecular medicine reports. 4, 535-40.

[131] Patarca, R., 2001. Cytokines and chronic fatigue syndrome. Annals of the New York Academy of Sciences. 933, 185-200.

[132] Pellett, F., Siannis, F., Vukin, I., Lee, P., Urowitz, M.B. and Gladman, D.D., 2007. KIRs and autoimmune disease: studies in systemic lupus erythematosus and scleroderma. Tissue antigens. 69 Suppl 1, 106-8.

[133] Pillai, S., Mattoo, H. and Cariappa, A., 2011. B cells and autoimmunity. Current opinion in immunology. 23, 721-31.

[134] Rabinovitch, A., 2003. Immunoregulation by cytokines in autoimmune diabetes. Advances in experimental medicine and biology. 520, 159-93.

[135] Rabinovitch, A. and Suarez-Pinzon, W.L., 2003. Role of cytokines in the pathogenesis of autoimmune diabetes mellitus. Rev Endocr Metab Disord. 4, 291-9.

[136] Rabinovitch, A., Suarez, W.L. and Power, R.F., 1993. Lazaroid antioxidant reduces incidence of diabetes and insulitis in nonobese diabetic mice. J Lab Clin Med. 121, 603-7.

[137] Rapoport, M.J., Mor, A., Vardi, P., Ramot, Y., Winker, R., Hindi, A. and Bistritzer, T., 1998. Decreased secretion of Th2 cytokines precedes Up-regulated and delayed secretion of Th1 cytokines in activated peripheral blood mononuclear cells from patients with insulin-dependent diabetes mellitus. Journal of autoimmunity. 11, 635-42.

[138] Raza, K., Falciani, F., Curnow, S.J., Ross, E.J., Lee, C.Y., Akbar, A.N., Lord, J.M., Gordon, C., Buckley, C.D. and Salmon, M., 2005. Early rheumatoid arthritis is characterized by a distinct and transient synovial fluid cytokine profile of T cell and stromal cell origin. Arthritis research & therapy. 7, R784-95.

[139] Sakaguchi, S., Miyara, M., Costantino, C.M. and Hafler, D.A., 2010. FOXP3+ regulatory T cells in the human immune system. Nature reviews. Immunology. 10, 490-500.

[140] Salomon, B., Lenschow, D.J., Rhee, L., Ashourian, N., Singh, B., Sharpe, A. and Bluestone, J.A., 2000. B7/CD28 costimulation is essential for the homeostasis of the CD4+CD25+ immunoregulatory T cells that control autoimmune diabetes. Immunity. 12, 431-40.

[141] Samuels, J., Ng, Y.S., Coupillaud, C., Paget, D. and Meffre, E., 2005a. Human B cell tolerance and its failure in rheumatoid arthritis. Annals of the New York Academy of Sciences. 1062, 116-26.

[142] Samuels, J., Ng, Y.S., Coupillaud, C., Paget, D. and Meffre, E., 2005b. Impaired early B cell tolerance in patients with rheumatoid arthritis. The Journal of experimental medicine. 201, 1659-67.

[143] Savinov, A.Y., Tcherepanov, A., Green, E.A., Flavell, R.A. and Chervonsky, A.V., 2003. Contribution of Fas to diabetes development. Proceedings of the National Academy of Sciences of the United States of America. 100, 628-32.

[144] Sawalha, A.H., Kaufman, K.M., Kelly, J.A., Adler, A.J., Aberle, T., Kilpatrick, J., Wakeland, E.K., Li, Q.Z., Wandstrat, A.E., Karp, D.R., James, J.A., Merrill, J.T., Lipsky, P. and Harley, J.B., 2008. Genetic association of interleukin-21 polymorphisms with systemic lupus erythematosus. Annals of the rheumatic diseases. 67, 458-61.

[145] Schleinitz, N., Vely, F., Harle, J.R. and Vivier, E., 2010. Natural killer cells in human autoimmune diseases. Immunology. 131, 451-8.

[146] Schmetterer, K.G., Neunkirchner, A. and Pickl, W.F., 2012. Naturally occurring regulatory T cells: markers, mechanisms, and manipulation. FASEB journal : official publication of the Federation of American Societies for Experimental Biology. 26, 2253-76.

[147] Schmidt, A., Oberle, N. and Krammer, P.H., 2012. Molecular mechanisms of treg-mediated T cell suppression. Front Immunol. 3, 51.

[148] Schrempf, W. and Ziemssen, T. Glatiramer acetate: mechanisms of action in multiple sclerosis. Autoimmunity Reviews. 6, 469-475.

[149] Selmaj, K. and Raine, C.S., 1988. Tumor necrosis factor mediates myelin damage in organotypic cultures of nervous tissue. Annals of the New York Academy of Sciences. 540, 568-70.

[150] Shlomchik, M.J., Craft, J.E. and Mamula, M.J., 2001. From T to B and back again: positive feedback in systemic autoimmune disease. Nature reviews. Immunology. 1, 147-53.

[151] Silverman, G.J. and Carson, D.A., 2003. Roles of B cells in rheumatoid arthritis. Arthritis research & therapy. 5 Suppl 4, S1-6.

[152] Sims, G.P., Ettinger, R., Shirota, Y., Yarboro, C.H., Illei, G.G. and Lipsky, P.E., 2005. Identification and characterization of circulating human transitional B cells. Blood. 105, 4390-8.

[153] Souto-Carneiro, M.M., Mahadevan, V., Takada, K., Fritsch-Stork, R., Nanki, T., Brown, M., Fleisher, T.A., Wilson, M., Goldbach-Mansky, R. and Lipsky, P.E., 2009. Alterations in peripheral blood memory B cells in patients with active rheumatoid arthritis are dependent on the action of tumour necrosis factor. Arthritis research & therapy. 11, R84.

[154] Stevenson, F.K. and Natvig, J., 1999. Autoantibodies revealed: the role of B cells in autoimmune disease. Immunology today. 20, 296-8.

[155] Stewart, T.A., Hultgren, B., Huang, X., Pitts-Meek, S., Hully, J. and MacLachlan, N.J., 1993. Induction of type I diabetes by interferon-alpha in transgenic mice. Science. 260, 1942-6.

[156] Tackey, E., Lipsky, P.E. and Illei, G.G., 2004. Rationale for interleukin-6 blockade in systemic lupus erythematosus. Lupus. 13, 339-43.

[157] Tian, J., Zekzer, D., Lu, Y., Dang, H. and Kaufman, D.L., 2006. B cells are crucial for determinant spreading of T cell autoimmunity among beta cell antigens in diabetes-prone nonobese diabetic mice. Journal of immunology. 176, 2654-61.

[158] Tiller, T., Tsuiji, M., Yurasov, S., Velinzon, K., Nussenzweig, M.C. and Wardemann, H., 2007. Autoreactivity in human IgG+ memory B cells. Immunity. 26, 205-13.

[159] Valencia, X., Yarboro, C., Illei, G. and Lipsky, P.E., 2007. Deficient CD4+CD25high T regulatory cell function in patients with active systemic lupus erythematosus. Journal of immunology. 178, 2579-88.

[160] van der Slik, A.R., Alizadeh, B.Z., Koeleman, B.P., Roep, B.O. and Giphart, M.J., 2007. Modelling KIR-HLA genotype disparities in type 1 diabetes. Tissue antigens. 69 Suppl 1, 101-5.

[161] van Vollenhoven, R.F., 2009. How to dose infliximab in rheumatoid arthritis: new data on a serious issue. Annals of the rheumatic diseases. 68, 1237-9.

[162] Venken, K., Hellings, N., Broekmans, T., Hensen, K., Rummens, J.L. and Stinissen, P., 2008a. Natural naive CD4+CD25+CD127low regulatory T cell (Treg) development

and function are disturbed in multiple sclerosis patients: recovery of memory Treg homeostasis during disease progression. Journal of immunology. 180, 6411-20.

[163] Venken, K., Hellings, N., Hensen, K., Rummens, J.L., Medaer, R., D'Hooghe M, B., Dubois, B., Raus, J. and Stinissen, P., 2006. Secondary progressive in contrast to relapsing-remitting multiple sclerosis patients show a normal CD4+CD25+ regulatory T-cell function and FOXP3 expression. Journal of neuroscience research. 83, 1432-46.

[164] Venken, K., Hellings, N., Thewissen, M., Somers, V., Hensen, K., Rummens, J.L., Medaer, R., Hupperts, R. and Stinissen, P., 2008b. Compromised CD4+ CD25(high) regulatory T-cell function in patients with relapsing-remitting multiple sclerosis is correlated with a reduced frequency of FOXP3-positive cells and reduced FOXP3 expression at the single-cell level. Immunology. 123, 79-89.

[165] Visvanathan, K. and Lewin, S.R., 2006. Immunopathogenesis: role of innate and adaptive immune responses. Semin Liver Dis. 26, 104-15.

[166] Vivier, E., Tomasello, E., Baratin, M., Walzer, T. and Ugolini, S., 2008. Functions of natural killer cells. Nature immunology. 9, 503-10.

[167] Warde, N., 2011. Autoimmunity: the role of neutrophils in SLE: untangling the NET. Nature reviews. Rheumatology. 7, 252.

[168] Willcox, A., Richardson, S.J., Bone, A.J., Foulis, A.K. and Morgan, N.G., 2009. Analysis of islet inflammation in human type 1 diabetes. Clinical and experimental immunology. 155, 173-81.

[169] Wipke, B.T., Wang, Z., Nagengast, W., Reichert, D.E. and Allen, P.M., 2004. Staging the initiation of autoantibody-induced arthritis: a critical role for immune complexes. Journal of immunology. 172, 7694-702.

[170] Wong, C.K., Lit, L.C., Tam, L.S., Li, E.K., Wong, P.T. and Lam, C.W., 2008. Hyperproduction of IL-23 and IL-17 in patients with systemic lupus erythematosus: implications for Th17-mediated inflammation in auto-immunity. Clinical immunology. 127, 385-93.

[171] Wong, W.M., Vakis, S.A., Ayre, K.R., Ellwood, C.N., Howell, W.M., Tutt, A.L., Cawley, M.I. and Smith, J.L., 2000. Rheumatoid arthritis T cells produce Th1 cytokines in response to stimulation with a novel trispecific antibody directed against CD2, CD3, and CD28. Scandinavian journal of rheumatology. 29, 282-7.

[172] Wujek, J.R., Bjartmar, C., Richer, E., Ransohoff, R.M., Yu, M., Tuohy, V.K. and Trapp, B.D., 2002. Axon loss in the spinal cord determines permanent neurological disability in an animal model of multiple sclerosis. Journal of neuropathology and experimental neurology. 61, 23-32.

[173] Xing, Q., Su, H., Cui, J. and Wang, B., 2012. Role of Treg cells and TGF-beta1 in patients with systemic lupus erythematosus: a possible relation with lupus nephritis. Immunological investigations. 41, 15-27.

[174] Xiu, Y., Wong, C.P., Bouaziz, J.D., Hamaguchi, Y., Wang, Y., Pop, S.M., Tisch, R.M. and Tedder, T.F., 2008. B lymphocyte depletion by CD20 monoclonal antibody prevents diabetes in nonobese diabetic mice despite isotype-specific differences in Fc gamma R effector functions. Journal of immunology. 180, 2863-75.

[175] Yabuhara, A., Yang, F.C., Nakazawa, T., Iwasaki, Y., Mori, T., Koike, K., Kawai, H. and Komiyama, A., 1996. A killing defect of natural killer cells as an underlying immunologic abnormality in childhood systemic lupus erythematosus. The Journal of rheumatology. 23, 171-7.

[176] Yanaba, K., Bouaziz, J.D., Haas, K.M., Poe, J.C., Fujimoto, M. and Tedder, T.F., 2008. A regulatory B cell subset with a unique CD1dhiCD5+ phenotype controls T cell-dependent inflammatory responses. Immunity. 28, 639-50.

[177] Yang, J., Chu, Y., Yang, X., Gao, D., Zhu, L., Yang, X., Wan, L. and Li, M., 2009. Th17 and natural Treg cell population dynamics in systemic lupus erythematosus. Arthritis and rheumatism. 60, 1472-83.

[178] Yasutomo, K., Horiuchi, T., Kagami, S., Tsukamoto, H., Hashimura, C., Urushihara, M. and Kuroda, Y., 2001. Mutation of DNASE1 in people with systemic lupus erythematosus. Nature genetics. 28, 313-4.

[179] Yilmaz, M., Kendirli, S.G., Altintas, D., Bingol, G. and Antmen, B., 2001. Cytokine levels in serum of patients with juvenile rheumatoid arthritis. Clinical rheumatology. 20, 30-5.

[180] You, S., Belghith, M., Cobbold, S., Alyanakian, M.A., Gouarin, C., Barriot, S., Garcia, C., Waldmann, H., Bach, J.F. and Chatenoud, L., 2005. Autoimmune diabetes onset results from qualitative rather than quantitative age-dependent changes in pathogenic T-cells. Diabetes. 54, 1415-22.

[181] Yurasov, S., Wardemann, H., Hammersen, J., Tsuiji, M., Meffre, E., Pascual, V. and Nussenzweig, M.C., 2005. Defective B cell tolerance checkpoints in systemic lupus erythematosus. The Journal of experimental medicine. 201, 703-11.

[182] Zhang, A.L., Colmenero, P., Purath, U., Teixeira de Matos, C., Hueber, W., Klareskog, L., Tarner, I.H., Engleman, E.G. and Soderstrom, K., 2007. Natural killer cells trigger differentiation of monocytes into dendritic cells. Blood. 110, 2484-93.

[183] Zhang, B., Yamamura, T., Kondo, T., Fujiwara, M. and Tabira, T., 1997. Regulation of experimental autoimmune encephalomyelitis by natural killer (NK) cells. The Journal of experimental medicine. 186, 1677-87.

[184] Zhang, J., Jacobi, A.M., Wang, T. and Diamond, B., 2008. Pathogenic autoantibodies in systemic lupus erythematosus are derived from both self-reactive and non-self-reactive B cells. Molecular medicine. 14, 675-81.

[185] Zhou, L., Chong, M.M. and Littman, D.R., 2009. Plasticity of CD4+ T cell lineage differentiation. Immunity. 30, 646-55.

http://dx.doi.org/10.5772/53440

[186] Ziaber, J., Tchorzewski, H., Chmielewski, H., Baj, Z., Pasnik, J. and Kaczmarek, J., 1999. [TNF-alpha binding ability as a sign of peripheral blood neutrophils preactivation in the course of multiple sclerosis]. Neurol Neurochir Pol. 33, 789-96.

Chapter 11

Biomarkers of Inflammatory Arthritis and Proteomics

Opeyemi S. Ademowo, Lisa Staunton,
Oliver FitzGerald and Stephen R. Pennington

Additional information is available at the end of the chapter

http://dx.doi.org/10.5772/54218

1. Introduction

Autoimmune diseases are systemic and organ–specific inflammatory conditions involving a cell-mediated immune response against self tissues. Whilst it is known that they are characterized by autoantibodies in both the systemic fluid and tissues [1, 2], the detailed aetiology and pathogenesis of auto-immune diseases are still poorly understood [3, 4]. These types of diseases occur when self molecules, often unknown antigens (auto-antigens), are seen by the immune system as non-self and are thereby attacked immunologically by the production of autoantibodies against them. In this process, the immune system mistakenly reacts with the body's own cellular gears as if they were foreign antigens. The clinical presentations of autoimmune diseases vary with the disease course and delay in diagnosis as well as inappropriate therapy, increases tissue damage [3, 5].

Inflammatory arthritis (IA), an autoimmune disorder of the joint tissue, is characterised by influx of white blood cells in the joint fluid. The disease often progresses to articular destruction, joint ankylosis (stiffness of the joint) and functional disability [3]. IA is a chronic disease, persisting as it often does for a long time, and some forms of the condition are systemic affecting many tissues and organs other than the joint and skin. IA is a significant cause of disability in those over fifty-five years of age, and is among the leading conditions restricting an individual's capacity to work. The healthcare, socio- and pharmaco-economic challenges of IA are significant. The most important issues for healthcare include: i) recognition and establishing an early diagnosis for disease; ii) identification of patients who are likely to develop a worse prognosis; iii) predicting and selecting therapies to which patients will respond; and, iv) understanding the balance between limited healthcare resources and the expensive disease modifying anti-rheumatic drugs (DMARDs) [3].

There has been much excitement about the potential of the omics technologies to deliver novel biological markers (biomarkers) of sufficient discriminatory power that they could herald an era of personalised medicine [6]. Personalized medicine being a medical approach that customizes healthcare; tailoring decision to individual patients based on genetic, proteomic or other information. Accurate prediction is essential for personalized medicine to ensure that therapy is given to those individuals who are likely to develop worse prognosis [7]. More specifically, the application of proteomics (the study of proteins), has been suggested to hold special promise for the discovery of clinically useful biomarkers [6, 8]. Biomarkers are characteristics that can be measured or evaluated to indicate a normal biologic process, a patho-physiologic condition, or a pharmacologic response to therapy. Biomarkers are also defined as measurable variables of how a patient feels or functions. [9, 10]. Proteomics is extremely powerful for both biomarker discovery and for the investigation of biochemical processes involved in diseases. At its most straightforward, proteomics involves the comprehensive determination of protein expression levels and hence enables pathway determination of cellular processes [11]. Several proteomic approaches have been applied to the investigation of autoimmune disorders including (i) autoantigen and biomarker discovery by 2-dimensional gel electrophoresis (2-DE) based separation of proteins and subsequent protein identification by mass spectrometry; (ii) protein microarrays for the characterisation of antibody responses; (iii) reverse phase protein arrays to analyze protein phosphorylation (iv) antibody array technologies to profile cytokines and other biomolecules; and (v) flow cytometric analysis of phosphoproteins [2, 3].

Here we review the role of autoimmunity in IA with emphasis on disease aetiology, pathogenesis, existing biomarkers, assessment of disease activity, autoantibodies capable of predicting disease outcomes and latest therapies. We then outline the application of proteomics to the discovery of protein biomarkers in rheumatoid arthritis. The processes and challenges involved in validating potential biomarkers and developing them to laboratory tests of clinical utility are also summarised. Finally, we discuss some future directions in protein biomarker research in IA that may support personalised medicine for this autoimmune disease.

1.1. Inflammatory arthritis: An autoimmune disorder

Inflammatory arthritis is an autoimmune disease; it has the characteristic hallmark of activated immune cells that target self tissues. This auto-immunity is always as a result of complex interaction between genetic and environmental factors [3]. There are several forms of IA including rheumatoid arthritis (RA), psoriatic arthritis (PsA), juvenile idiopathic arthritis (JIA), ankylosing spondylitis (SpA) as well as the inflammatory form of osteoarthritis (OA). Cells involved in autoimmune IA include macrophages, T cells, B cells, fibroblasts, chondrocytes, and dendritic cells. It is known that the expression of key cytokines such as tumor necrosis factor alpha (TNF-α) and interleukin-6 (IL-6) drives the inflammatory and destructive processes. TNF-α is a pro-inflammatory cytokine that is associated with fever and some other symptoms such as pain, tenderness and swelling, in several inflammatory conditions and over recent years has been a major target of treatment for IA [12].

In this review, emphasis is placed on RA, the most common form of IA. With its course clinically unpredictable, RA is associated with synovial inflammation in which the synovium, a thin layer of tissue that lines the joint cavity, is the primary site of the cell-mediated inflammatory reaction [13]. RA has a very poor prognosis when compared to entheseal-based inflammatory conditions such as spondyloarthropathy where the entheses - the site where tendons, joint capsules or ligaments insert into bone – are inflamed [14]. RA is often characterised by chronic inflammation of the joint that has been infiltrated by activated mononuclear cells. Inflammation is usually accompanied with swelling, pain and the destruction of articular cartilage, which ultimately lead to functional impairment of the affected joint [5, 15]. RA can hence be classified as an heterogeneous disease due to its different forms of clinical manifestations, serological abnormalities, functional impairment and joint damage [16, 17]. It has been reported that early and aggressive treatment of RA can prevent cartilage damage [3]. Before the introduction of 'biologic' therapies, the direct and indirect costs incurred for medical, social care and loss of employment experienced by RA patients and society at large were estimated to be $98 million to $122 million per million population in developed countries [18, 19].

1.2. The aetiology / pathogenesis of rheumatoid arthritis

The synovial membrane is the thin layer that lines the joint. It produces synovial fluid, which nourishes and lubricates the joint. Two cell types characterise the synovial membrane: macrophage–like and fibroblast-like synoviocytes. Although the pathogenesis and the aetiology of RA remain unclear, it is sometimes associated with genetic and environmental factors. Environmental factors associated with RA include cigarette smoking, alcohol, some reproductive factors in women, bacterial products, viral components and some other diverse environmental stimuli [12, 20]; the genetic factors are linked to the class 11 major histocompatibility complex (MHC) region on chromosome 6 and an association with the non-MHC gene (PTPN22-a protein tyrosine phosphatase that regulates T cell activation). Additionally, predisposing genes such as the HLA-DR4 allele are reported to be prevalent [18, 21]. Innate immunity is a primitive pattern-recognition system that leads to rapid inflammatory responses. In RA, innate immunity has been implicated through the engagement of Fc receptors by immune complexes and perhaps Toll-like receptors (TLRs) by bacterial products. Antigen-driven T cell and B cell responses may also participate as a result of either xenoantigen reactivity or, more likely, responses directed at numerous autoantigens. Evidence of autoimmunity, including high serum levels of autoantibodies such as rheumatoid factor (an antibody against the Fc region of other antibodies) and anti-citrullinated peptide antibodies, can be present for many years before the onset of clinical arthritis [20]. In some patients, worse prognosis of RA has been linked to the presence of rheumatoid factor and anti-CCP (antibody against citrullinated epitopes on post-translationally modified proteins). The proliferation of synoviocytes as RA progresses leads to the invasion of the hyperplastic synovial tissue and is responsible for the destruction of the underlying bone and the articular cartilage [21]. Cytokines and chemokines play an essential role in the angiogenesis and pathogenesis of RA [22, 23]. The expression of cytokines such as tumour necrosis factor-α (TNFα), interleukin (IL)-1β, IL-6, IL-15 and IL-17 during new blood vessel formation (angiogenesis) and inflammatory cell infiltration drives the inflammatory and destructive processes of this disease [21, 23]. The clinical presentation of RA differs from other forms of arthropathies with its characteristic symmetric polyarticular joint inflammation and destruction as well as its extra-articular manifestation (rheumatoid nodules/vasculitis) and the presence of intracellular citrullinated proteins. The synovial membrane is affected in a number of ways which include architectural changes (neovascularisation, lymphocyte infiltration and thickening of the synovial lining layer) [23, 24]. Cardiovascular diseases, excess morbidity and mortality from myocardial infarction and allied disorders, high risk of lung diseases, coronary artery disease, lymphoma, infection as well as reduced life expectancy are associated with rheumatoid arthritis [16].

A model has suggested that in predisposed individuals, a stimulus or an infective agent binds to toll-like receptors on macrophages and peripheral dendritic cells; thereby triggering a rapid response from the innate immune system involving inflammatory mediators, cytokines, complements, neutrophils and natural killer cells. The migration of these cells to the joint leads to joint damage as a result of the actions of growth factors, proteases and activated osteoclasts. This damage is associated with the development of locally invasive pannus tissue [18]. The major joint destruction occurs at the pannus; this is the point at which the synovium meets the cartilage and the bone. The pannus is rich in macrophages and it is the major site at which irreversible tissue damage originates [25, 26]. The main cause of disability in RA is joint destruction that is characterised by progressive bone erosion [18]. As shown in Figure 1 below, infiltration of the joint by macrophages ultimately form the pannus that migrates into the bone leading to bone erosion. The inflamed joint compared to the normal joint is characterised by the influx of a number of inflammatory cells in the joint.

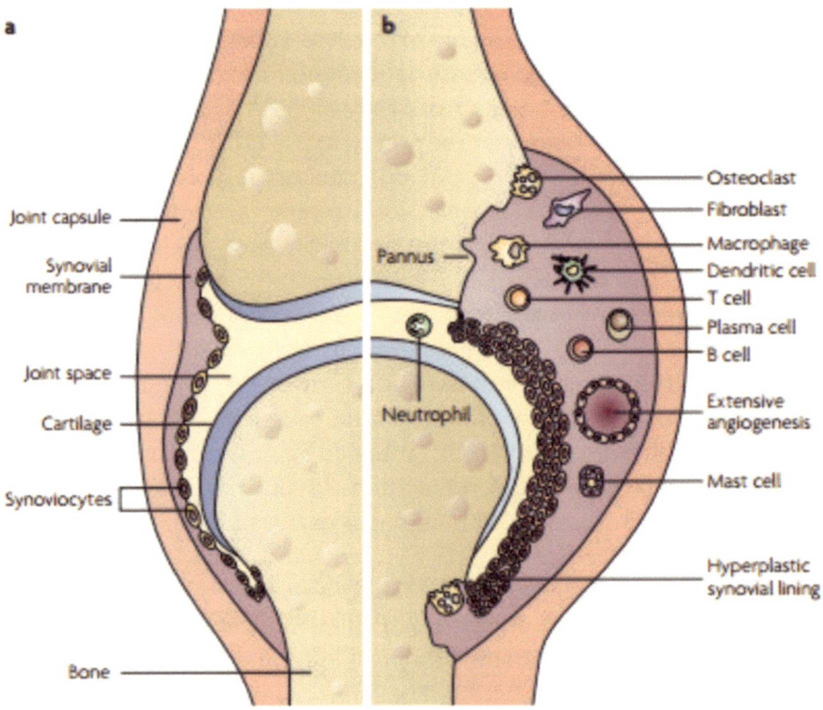

Figure 1. Normal healthy joint (a) and rheumatoid arthritic joint (b). [21]

In the healthy joint (a), a thin synovial membrane lines the non-weight-bearing aspects of the joint. While in the arthritic joint (b), the synovial membrane becomes hyperplastic and infiltrated by chronic inflammatory cells that develops into 'pannus', which migrates onto and into the articular cartilage and underlying bone causing bone erosion.

1.3. Current therapeutic targets and therapy in RA

Cytokine networks involving tumor necrosis factor, interleukin-6, and many other factors participate in disease perpetuation and can be targeted by therapeutic agents [20]. Disease-modifying antirheumatic drugs (DMARDs) have been used for decades to manage rheumatic diseases. Methotrexate is the most widely used disease DMARD. Other DMARDS include leflunomide, sulfasalazine, cyclosporine and hydroxy-chloroquine (20). However, in the past decade, biologic therapies such as fusion proteins and monoclonal antibodies have revolutionized the management of autoimmune IA. Biologics have provided more specific therapeutic interventions with less immunosuppression by targeting immune cells and key cytokines [21]. The biologicals neutralize the actions of cytokines and proteins through human or chimeric monoclonal antibodies or by using a recombinant-antagonist form of the cytokine receptor [14, 27]. Example of such biologicals is the TNF-α inhibitors. TNF-α being a key component in the cascade of cytokines induced in RA, is a target compound for treatment. To exert its effects, TNF-α bind to two receptors, the type 1 TNF receptor (p55) and the type 2 TNF receptor (p75), found on immune, inflammatory, and endothelial cells. TNF inhibitors were first licensed for clinical use in 1998; three have been approved for the treatment of RA. TNF inhibitors are introduced to patients with active disease who have not had a response to conventional DMARDs. Examples of the monoclonal antibodies include infliximab (Remicade), a chimeric human-murine IgG1 anti-TNF-α antibody administered intravenously. Infliximab is also cytotoxic for TNF-expressing cells; adalimumab (Humira) or certolizumab pegol (Cimzia). Humira is a recombinant humanized monoclonal anti-TNF-α antibody administered subcutaneously. There are also circulating receptor fusion proteins such as etanercept (Enbrel), a recombinant soluble p75 TNF- receptor fusion protein administered subcutaneously [18]. By inhibiting the action of TNF-α, the 'biologicals' reduce the signs and symptoms of inflammation and stop the progression of joint damage. Therapeutic response in RA is assessed by clinical disease activity score 28 (DAS28) or ACR (American College of Rheumatology) criteria, structural (sharp or Larsen scores) and or functional evaluation standards (HAQ score). Treatment efficacy is usually estimated by comparing these assessments before and after treatment [27].

1.4. Disease activity and progression in RA

The terms 'activity' and 'severity' are usually used to characterize RA. Disease activity in this sense refers to the degree of overall inflammation measured by considering factors that include acute phase reactants, tender/swollen joints, pain, general impact, grip, strength and functional disability. Disease severity on the other hand, is more complex as it refers to the outcome or result of RA. Disease severity is measured by assessing radiographic abnormalities, indirect and direct costs, work disability, mortality and social losses; generally elucidate the extent the disease has affected the patient and its effects. Severity explains the absolute social and physical damage resulting from RA as well as the rate at which the damage occurs [28, 29]. Informative characteristics for clinical outcomes can be broadly divided into prognostic or predictive biomarkers. Prognostic biomarkers show the expected clinical outcomes of patients such as progression or death. However, they do not inform the choice of therapy while predictive biomarkers would identify group of patients whose diseases are likely to be resistance or sensitive to therapy based on the biomarker status [30].

2. Assessment of disease activity and response criteria in RA

In practice today, the European League Against Rheumatism (EULAR) criteria are used to classify the disease activity in IA while the American College of Rheumatology (ACR) improvement criteria is the second method used for clinical evaluation of patients [31]. In RA, inflammatory activities cannot be measured using one single variable. The disease activity score (DAS) was developed to solve this problem [32]. DAS score provides important quantitative analysis in clinical research of RA and the score includes tender joint count, swollen joint count, C-reactive protein (CRP) or erythrocyte sedimentation rate (ESR) level and the general assessment of the patient's health measured on a visual analog scale. At baseline and follow up, responses to treatment are assessed as low, moderate or high disease activity. DAS is best defined by statistical methods which include multiple regression analysis and discriminant analysis [31, 33]. A low disease activity is indicated by a DAS score <3.2, a moderate disease activity is indicated by DAS score 3.2- 5.1 while a DAS score >5.1 indicates a high disease activity [34]. These criteria are being used by the EULAR to define good responders, moderate responders and non responders to treatment as shown in Table 1 below. Advantages of the DAS include the following: its content is more informative than single variables, its values can be interpreted clinically and it has a continuous scale with a Guassian (normal) distribution [32].

Disease Activity Level	Disease Activity Score (DAS 28) at Endpoint	DAS Improvement from Baseline		
		>1.2	>0.6≤1.2	≤0.6
'Low'	≤3.2	Good responce	Moderate responce	No responce
'Moderate'	>3.2≤5.1	Moderate	Moderate	None
'High'	>5.1	Moderate	None	None

Table 1. The EULAR response criteria [32]

http://dx.doi.org/10.5772/54218

The ACR improvement criteria are used in clinical trials for the evaluation of RA patients. It is also referred to as the core data set. It involves swollen joint count, tender joint count, acute phase reactants i.e. ESR/CRP and the general health assessment questionnaire (HAQ score). The questionnaire assesses the pain, disability, and overall health of the patient. The ACR measures improvement in percentage of the changes in the criteria scales used. 20%, 50% and 70% improvement in any 4-6 of the scale used is an indication that the patient meets the criteria [34].

2.1. Clinical and biological markers used in practice for RA

Clinically meaningful biomarkers may be based on proteins, genotypes, histology, metabolic patterns, or imaging techniques and they are ideal for early diagnosis, monitoring and prediction of therapeutic response. In a number of diseases and especially in RA, some patients do not respond to therapy at all and several others show diverse degrees of response. Therefore, biomarkers are urgently needed in the clinical setting (i) to select patients before treatment, (ii) to monitor the patients' response to the therapy as well as the disease activity, (iii) to classify patients into their different response categories (good responders, moderate responders and nonresponders) and (iv) to determine the OBD (optimal biological dose) for the drug [35-37].

Clinical markers are the physical symptoms or variables such as swollen joint count, tender joint count, pain assessment and radiological findings while biomarkers are molecular indicators of pathological processes as described earlier to assess diagnostic, prognostic and predictive features [38]. Biomarkers of RA can be broadly divided into two groups: Biomarkers of disease activity and biomarkers of joint damage.

Biomarkers of disease activity in RA are also referred to as 'momentary predictors' and include factors that change with time revealing the disease activity e.g. ESR and CRP [19]. Biomarkers of disease activity include cells, cytokines and acute phase reactants/ proteins. Cells involved in RA synovitis exhibit increased number of macrophages in the synovium. B-cell depletion and the serum level of proinflammatory cytokines (IL-6 being the most abundant cytokine) can give the reflection of active disease. High Composition of synovial tumour necrosis factor (TNF) is also a biomarker of RA. Serum amyloid A, an acute phase protein, blood sedimentation rate as well as the presence of rheumatoid factor (RF) also reflects disease activity; as this can be used to calculate the disease activity score 28 (DAS28 i.e. 28 joint counts) [5, 17]. CRP, an acute phase protein has been successful to some extent to monitor early stage disease and progression after the commencement of therapy. CRP can be alternatively measured by calculating ESR [21]. However, some other factors have been found to influence the levels of both ESR and CRP rendering these as non–specific markers; these factors include anemia, aging and the presence of immunoglobulin such as rheumatoid factor [9]. Studies have shown CRP as a marker of different inflammatory disease activity [39]. As momentary predictors reveal outcomes, they require re-sampling to boost the accuracy [28].

Biomarkers of joint damage in RA are also referred to as 'cumulative predictors' and their outcomes are variable and worsen with time. These include radiographic erosion and functional disability [28]. In RA, changes in bone and cartilage lead to joint damage. Spaces in the joint signify cartilage changes while erosion indicates bone destruction. Hence, either of these two changes can present a biomarker of RA joint destruction. Cartilage damage causes a change in the matrix composition of the cartilage thereby affecting the major proteins in cartilage: type 11 collagen (COL 2), aggrecan, and non-collagen and non-aggrecan proteins. The main structural protein in bone is the type 1 collagen and the non collagen protein in bone is the sialoprotein which is released during bone damage [17].

Some RA patients with active disease present with normal levels of some of these markers; this might be due in parts to genetics [40]. Due to lack of specificity, such markers might not be good for all RA patients; hence, a need for better biomarkers. The understanding derived from the disease biology has shifted the treatment strategy to targeted therapy. However, to develop, verify, validate and apply new and existing treatment successfully, there is a need to understand the difference and relationship between putative biomarker and treatment effect [30].

Notably, to date, there is no effective approach available to clinicians to predict which patient will respond to which therapy. For example, predicting which patients are likely to respond to TNF-α inhibitors would have significant value for the selection of patients whose condition warrants this high cost and 'high risk' treatment [41].Therefore, there is an urgent need for new and better biomarkers in IA to improve diagnosis, support emerging targeted therapies, monitor drug activity and evaluate therapeutic response [1, 3].

In RA, any indicator of inflammation could be a biomarker [5]. These may include genes or products of gene expression, a cytokine, autoantibody, some acute phase proteins, tissue degradation product or tissue abnormality observed immunohistochemically in synovial biopsy. Sources of these biomarkers may include the serum, synovial fluid, urine, cells (lymphocytes such as the peripheral blood mononuclear cells (PBMC)) and tissues taken from the inflamed synovium [17]. RA biomarkers effectively used in practice are acute phase reactants (CRP and ESR) as well as autoantibodies Such as rheumatoid factor (RF), anti citrullinated protein antibodies (ACPAs) and anti-nuclear antibodies (ANA). These autoantibodies are capable of predicting disease outcomes and are used as laboratory markers to classify and diagnose RA. Autoantibodies are dependent on the organ or tissue affected as well as the severity of the disease. [42-44]. Highlighted below are the markers used in clinical practice for the diagnosis and prognosis of RA:

- Rheumatoid factor (RF): These are antibodies against the Fc region of other antibodies [21]. This IgM isotype of the serologic indicator of RA is useful in determining the auto immune status of the disease but it is not very sensitive to the changes in the disease activity level or specific as it could be present in patients with chronic infections, other immune diseases or in the elderly. The main use of which is a prognostic marker [45, 46]. RF predicts disease severity but it is not a good marker for early diagnosis. It is not very sensitive and does not vary stoichiometrically with treatment [29].
- C-reactive protein (CRP): RA increases the level of an acute phase reactant, CRP. This is a typical marker of inflammation and it has an association with cardiovascular risk

[16]. CRP is a plasma protein used for drug dosage titration as well as clinical response assessment [47]. Although CRP is a widely used biomarker of RA, it lacks disease selectivity [48]. CRP correlates with disease activity but does not predict the severity of the disease [29].

- Erythrocyte sedimentation rate (ESR): This contributes highly to disease activity but it is not a sensitive parameter and it can be easily affected by external factors such as age, fibrinogen level, gender, hypergamma-globulinemia, anaemia and RF [48]. Like CRP, it does not predict the subsequent severity of the disease [29].

- Anti-citrullinated protein antibody (tested as anti-cyclic citrullinated peptide (Anti-CCP) antibody): Recently, anti-CCP antibody has been effectively used for the diagnosis of RA [43, 47]. ACPAs are circulating autoantibodies against citrullinated epitopes on post translationally modified proteins. Citrulline is a non standard amino acid that originates from the enzymatic modification of deiminated arginine residue [46]. The citrullination/modification of arginine by deimination occurs physiologically during inflammation, apoptosis or keratinization. These proteins can be found either in the sera or in the synovium of RA patients. The presence of citrullinated proteins are associated with a worse prognosis of RA[21]. ACPAs are markers of RA with a specificity of 95-98% and a sensitivity of 70-80% [49]. As a result of their excellent diagnostic value, they are a better alternative to RF and they are widely used for the diagnosis of RA [45, 46]. The presence of this autoantibody in the serum precedes the onset of the disease and also linked to the pathogenesis of the disease. The isotypes of this antibody includes IgA, IgG1, IgG2, IgG3, IgG4 and IgM [45, 49]. Anti-keratin antibodies (AKA) and anti-perinuclear factor (APF) are examples of members of ACPAs. An example of anticitrullinated antibodies that has been detected in the sera of RA patients is the antibody against citrullinated vimentin. Vimentin, a protein that plays vital biologic role in contraction, proliferation and migration has also been found to be highly expressed in RA [24]. The mutated form of this antibody was recently developed and it is known as anti-MCV antibody. The sensitivity of which is comparable to RF but no greater specificity [45, 46]. These antibodies alone or in combination with IL-6 have a high classification power for the establishment of RA [50]. These antibodies have recently predicted erosion. They are usually associated with high titre rheumatic factor; i.e≥50IU/ml. These antibodies and the presence of acute phase proteins are reliable to predict erosive RA. Anti-nuclear antibody (ANA) is also used for the diagnosis of arthritis and can be used to differentiate different forms of inflammatory arthritis [5].

2.2. Emerging potential biomarkers in RA

To demonstrate efficacy and define appropriate RA patients in clinical trials, the identification of easily measured, rugged, reliable markers of disease and the effects of drugs are critical and emerging [51]. Different research works are ongoing to reveal emerging and interesting biomarkers. During biomarker identification, attention needs to be paid to the selection of the biological matrix in which the particular biomarker level will be monitored keeping in mind the feasibility of sample collection from such matrix, the stability of analyte in such matrix, assay sensitivity requirement based on the anticipated biomarker level in such matrix as well as the relevance of the matrix to biology. Biomarkers that will be translatable from bench to bedside will have to be accessible with minimal invasive procedure. Plasma and serum are the most easily accessible body fluids. In addition to this however, there should be a link between the matrix and the originating tissue source for biomarkers measured in body fluids [52]. The synovial fluid is a good source of novel biomarkers for many arthritic diseases that involve joint inflammation [53]. However, any measure used as a biomarker has to be evaluated and validated to ensure that the laboratory test is accurate, specific, sensitive and reproducible. The emerging RA biomarkers may be used to subgroup, treat and monitor the treatment [17]. The focus here is on a group of protein biomarkers characterized by a known molecular structure or formula or heterogeneous proteins with or without posttranslational modifications and some cytokines. This does not include image measurement, cell type, count, activity, or behavioural models. Novel techniques are emerging to discover protein biomarkers of inflammatory arthritis [28, 29].

2.2.1. Emerging biomarkers from the serum

Emerging serum markers include circulating autoantibodies against citrullinated proteins. These have high selectivity and specificity for the early diagnosis of RA [54].

- Matrix metalloproteinase 1 (MMP-1) and tissue inhibitor of metalloproteinase 1 (TIMP-1): These are tissue destructive enzymes [21]. Murphy et al, found an association between elevated levels of MMP-1 in blood and synovial tissue of RA patients and formation of new erosion [55].

- Myeloid –related proteins/Pro-inflammatory cytokines: The innate immune system of the bone activates macrophages on recognition of invading microorganisms. This activation occurs by pathogen associated molecular patterns (PAMPs) and by reacting to tissue damage recognised as damage associated molecular patterns (DAMPs). Prominent proteins released by activated macrophages include calgranulins, myeloid related proteins MRP8 (S100A8) and MRP14 (S100A9). These S100 protein families are calcium binding proteins that induce pro-inflammatory responses in leucocytes and endothelial cells [56]. The pro-inflammatory cytokines include interleukins (IL-1β, IL-6, IL-15 and IL-17) and tumour necrosis factor-α (TNF-α) [5, 21]. A correlation exists between IL-6 and acute phase proteins; therefore IL-6 can be used to monitor disease activity in RA. However, due to its diurnal variability (variable concentrations in the morning and in the evening), it is not a reliable marker [48]. Macrophages are stimulated by inflammatory mediators such as interleukin (IL 1), tumour necrosis factor (TNF-α) or interferon (IFN) to secrete and up regulate myeloid- related proteins [56]. Serum amyloid protein A (SAA), is also an emerging biomarker of RA [57].

According to previous work from peripheral blood mononuclear cells, swiprosin 1, the ezrinmoesin binding protein EBP50, and non-muscle actin have been shown to be differentially expressed in RA. Additionally, GRP78 a glucose regulated protein and the heat shock protein HSP60 have been identified as major auto-antigens in RA., GRP78 has been suggest-

http://dx.doi.org/10.5772/54218

ed as an immunotherapeutic agent for the treatment of arthritis and targeting HSP60 is said to be beneficial for the treatment [5].

2.2.2. *Emerging biomarkers from the synovial fluid*

Calprotectin, a major leucocyte protein has been found in high concentration in the synovial fluid of RA patients. It is a calcium binding pro inflammatory S100 protein (S100A8/S100A9). It is also known as MRP-8/MRP14; calgranulin A/calgranulin B or cystic fibrosis antigen [58]. S100A8 (MRP-8/calgranulin A), S100A9 (MRP-14/calgranulin B) and S100A12 (calgranulin C) proteins have been found to be the most up-regulated proteins in the synovial fluid of RA patients. Although present in the serum of RA Patients, these proteins are predominant in their synovial fluid. RA can be diagnosed early by the serum expression of these proteins [24, 59]. In the synovial fluid and the synovial membrane of mononuclear cells, cytokines such as the IL-18 have been found to be highly expressed and it has also been found to contribute to inducing high levels of other monocytes such as the IL-6, TNF-α, IL-1β and the granulocyte-macrophage colony-stimulating factor (GM-CSF) [60]. Pro-inflammatory cytokines such as the IL-1 and TNF-α protein are also readily detectable in the synovial fluid. Other detected cytokines include the macrophage colony stimulating factor (M-CSF), leucocyte inhibitory factor (LIF), IL-6 and interferon α (IFNα) [26]. Studies on citrullinated proteins and autoantibodies in RA synovial fluid are ongoing and emerging; an example is the fibrinogen-derived endogenous citrullinated peptides [61].

2.2.3. *Emerging biomarkers from the bone and cartilage*

Abnormal and degraded cartilage in affected joint is one of the major clinical manifestations in RA. Collagens are markers of bone turnover/resorption. The synthesis and degradation products of metabolism of cartilage specific collagens and proteoglycans are released into the synovial fluid, serum and urine as by products. These biomarkers can be used to monitor the metabolism of the cartilage. The main collagen of the articular cartilage is the type 11 collagen (C11) and it is a major structural component of the tissue. It is excessively degraded in RA [60]. Cartilage oligomeric matrix protein (COMP) is another marker that has been shown to provide a measure of elevated cartilage degradation [62]. So pyridinoline and deoxypyridinolin (PYD, DPD) are also specific markers of bone resorption; these are cross-linking amino acids that strengthen collagen fibrils in the extracellular matrix. PYD and DPD are found in main fibril – forming collagen 1, 11 &111 of many tissues [63].

2.2.4. *Emerging biomarkers from the synovial membrane /tissue*

In RA, the synovial membrane of the affected joint is the most affected part and therefore it is the primary site of inflammation. The number of macrophages in tissue biopsies of RA patients has been identified to correlate with the degree of pain. A study into Tcell infiltration within the synovial membrane during the disease has shown that there is a correlation between an improvement in the clinical index of the disease activity and a decrease in Tcell infiltration. The clinical course of RA and the response to treatments has been found to correlate with the number of sublining macrophages in the tissue. However, the synovial membrane presently does not have a reliable marker for early detection of arthritis but useful for determining the prognosis of the disease [13]. The synovial biopsies from the synovial tissue are useful for diagnosis purposes as well as the evaluation of novel treatments [64]. Small chemoattractant cytokines known as chemokines play a role at the site of inflammation to accumulate inflammatory cells. The synovial tissue and fluid exhibits an increased concentration of some chemokines which includes the monocyte chemoattractant protein-4 (MCP-4/CCL13), the monokine induced by interferon-γ (Mig/CXCL9), pulmonary and activation-regulated chemokine (PARC/CCL18), the monocyte chemotactic protein 1 (MCP-1/CCL2), the stromal cell-derived factor-1 (SDF-1/CXCL12) and fractalkine (CXC3CL1). These chemokines and their receptors are important in the pathology of RA [22]. Studies on the synovial tissue are ongoing to discover better protein biomarkers from the synovial tissue. Although not yet validated for use in clinical practice, some proteins from the synovial tissue such as fibrinogen, annexin, fibronectin, vimentin, haptoglobin, S100A8, S100A10 and some others are under study for implications in RA. Proteome analysis of the synovial tissue is promising to give further understanding on the pathogenesis of joint diseases [65].

Although all the biomarkers listed above are good indicators of RA, factors such as the presence of other diseases like osteoporosis, some variations in gene composition and tissue content of some of the biomarkers as well as increased physical activities have been found to change biomarker concentration significantly [12]. Other factors affecting marker level in mediums includes the diurnal and day-to-day activity; the level of some markers has been shown to be higher in the morning compared to the evenings. It has been found that markers are more abundant in serum samples taken early in the morning before breakfast than the samples taken after eating. Variation has also been found to occur due to eating and calcium intake assay precision has also been affected by handling, collecting and storing samples/specimens inappropriately [63]. Better and novel biomarkers are being discovered using proteomic techniques and these are described in section 3. There are a number of ways that biomarker measurements can aid in the development and evaluation of novel treatments. Biomarkers provide information for dosing and minimize differences in inter individual response to treatment as the assessment of benefit and risk is the goal of developing all therapeutic interventions [39]. It has been suggested that proteins, being 'surrogates' for the dynamic biology in organisms, are the macromolecules of choice for biofluid biomarkers [51]. Hence, a range of proteomics techniques have been applied to the discovery of novel candidate protein biomarkers [66].

3. Proteins and proteomics techniques in biomarker discovery

Proteomics is the study of protein expression, structure and function directed towards the characterization of the entire protein complement of a cell, tissue or organism [67]. Proteome analysis supports the determination of protein expression levels and hence monitors cellular processes [11]. Protein expression analysis in biological samples is of utmost importance to identify and monitor biomarkers for the progression of RA and its therapeutic endpoint as well as providing insight into mechanisms of the disease [68]. Differentially expressed proteins and potential biomarkers of RA can be discovered using various proteomic techniques and has been applied to investigation the dynamic proteome of autoimmune diseases [66, 67, 69]. Once potential protein biomarkers have been identified, their development into diagnostic (or other) tests of clinical usefulness require significant effort and few if any biomarkers of clinical utility have emerged from proteomics. Reasons include significant limitations in the proteomics technologies used for biomarker discovery and challenges faced in their subsequent validation [70, 71].

One of the major issues to have emerged is the realisation that single protein biomarkers are unlikely to yield sufficient sensitivity and specificity. However, whilst there is much talk of multiplexed panels of markers, the application of appropriate statistical tests to the development of such a panel remains relatively poorly understood and applied. Furthermore, whilst much discovery of biomarkers has been undertaken on tissues and cells, an effective diagnostic assay may require measurement in a readily accessible patient sample such as serum or synovial fluid. Another major bottleneck has rested in the lack of opportunities or capabilities to continue the process of biomarker development to progressing them to clinical utility – a domain of translational research. The biomarker development is the step between biomarker discovery and confirmation [51]. Different strategies have been used in proteomics to identify various biomarkers of diseases. These proteomic strategies involve separation, analysis and detection of complex protein mixtures.

Historically gel-based proteomic techniques were the tool of choice to resolve complex protein mixtures followed by mass spectrometry (MS) to detect differences in protein expression patterns between normal and diseased samples. While gel-based proteomic techniques have lost favor within proteomic research groups due to its limitations, MS has remained at the forefront of proteomic biomarker discovery experiments coupled to more gel-free techniques.

3.1. Gel based proteomics

Pre-separation of target proteins is highly essential in proteomics and many proteomic techniques accomplishes this with the aid of one- or two-dimensional electrophoresis [72].

One-dimensional sodium dodecyl polyacrlamide gel electrophoresis (1D-SDS PAGE) is a gel-based method that involves separating proteins on a 1D- SDS Polyacrylamide gel whereby the proteins are separated solely based on molecular weight. The bands of the gel are excised and subjected to proteolytic digestion ready for analysis by MS. Identified proteins are used to provide a nonredundant list and the data from samples run in different gel lanes are compared. This is a good and powerful method for small or medium sized biomarker discovery studies [72].

Two-dimensional gel electrophoresis (2-DE) is used to separate complex protein mixtures based on their isoelectric points (pI) and molecular weights. 2-DE is one of the most powerful techniques for separating entire proteomes and was developed in 1975 by O'Farrell [73] and since has been developed further [74]. In the first dimension called isoelectric focusing (IEF), proteins are separated based on their (pI). Proteins are amphoteric substances and therefore can either be negatively or positively charged depending on the pH of their environment. During IEF proteins are separated along thin strips of polyacrylamide gel containing an immobilized pH gradient (IPG). As an electric current is applied to the IPG strip during IEF, proteins move through the strip until they reach their pI i.e. where they no longer have a net charge. In the second dimension the IPG strip is placed horizontally along the top of a large polyacrylamide gel and proteins are separated based on molecular weight whereby smaller proteins will move faster through the gel than larger ones [51, 67]. Proteins separated by 2-DE can then be visualized by a number of staining techniques. The individual gel 'spots' may be excised from the gel, digested with proteases and the resulting peptides analysed by MS [51]. However, accuracy and reproducibility are concerns in this type of experiments [75].

Two- dimensional in gel electrophoresis (2D-DIGE) is an improvement in the use of gel-based methods for protein quantitation and detection. It has the ability to co-detect several samples on the same 2DE gel, hence eliminating gel-to-gel variation [75]. In 2D-DIGE experiments, ester cyanine dyes are used to label proteins prior to 2-DE. The advantage of using these dyes is that they are size and charge matched and so ensure negligible shift during first and second dimensions. Each cyanine dye has different excitation emission spectra allowing different samples to be run within the same gel and allows the inclusion of an internal standard on each gel. 2-DIGE alleviates the pattern reproducibility problem but not the other problems associated with 2-DE [75].

In general, biomarker discovery experiments using gel-based methods have been difficult due to the inherent limitations of the methodologies. Firstly, the hydrophobic, insoluble nature of membrane and membrane associated proteins make them incompatible with the aqueous nature of the second dimension in 2-DE and so are significantly underrepresented in gel-based studies [51]. Invariably, due to the low dynamic range of the gel-method, the most abundant soluble proteins are best represented and detected in 2-DE studies. Even with advances in IEF and staining technologies 2-DE gels are notoriously difficult to reproduce [75].

Today, proteomic studies have moved away from gel-based techniques and now use gel-free proteomic techniques.

3.2. Mass spectrometry-based proteomics (gel free proteomics)

MS–based proteomics has been used for the global analysis of protein composition, modifications and dynamics and this involves three core experimental steps; (i) protein extraction which can be followed by sample fractionation (ii) enzymatic digestion and (iii) quantitative and qualitative analysis using MS [76]. For the analysis of complex protein mixtures, two MS based approaches are used; functional proteomics and expression proteomics. Functional proteomics also known as the top-down approach involves maintaining the native structure of the protein and gaining functional information on the protein. However, a major disadvantage of intact protein analysis is that it does not directly provide a sequence-based identification as there are a number of proteins with close given masses. Expression proteomics also known as the bottom-up approach involves the denaturation of proteins, and using subsequent MS analysis of resulting peptides to determine quantitative changes in the abundance of proteins under different conditions [77].

By definition, a MS consists of an ion source, a mass analyser that measures the mass-to-charge ratio (m/z) of the ionized analytes and a detector that registers the number of ions at each m/z value [77]. The primary methods of ionization in MS are electrospray ionisation (ESI), matrix-assisted laser desorption/ionisation (MALDI) or the surface-enhanced laser desorption ionisation (SELDI). Mass analysers could be the SELDI time-of-flight (often used for intact/whole protein analysis), MALDI time-of-flight, multiple stage quadrupole-time-of-flight or the quadrupole ion trap (often used for sequence-based identification) [58]. MS has solved the problem of identifying proteins resolved by 2D gel and other methods and has also been used to successfully analyse complex protein mixtures [58]. Data from Gel LC/MS often correlates with the data generated during protein assay development with the multiple reaction monitoring method (MRM) [51]. The main decision when carrying out gel- free based methods is whether to label proteins or not.

Protein labeling methods include; (i) SILAC-stable isotope labeling with amino acids in cell culture for metabolically labeled protein studies. In this technique, non-radioactive heavy isotopic forms of the amino acids are metabolically incorporated into the cellular proteins while cells are growing allowing the identification of cell surface proteins by MS [2], ii) ICAT-isotope coded affinity tag is used to label proteins after extraction from biological samples, (iii) iTRAQ-isotope tags for relative and absolute quantitation and (iv) TMT- tandem mass tag for studies involving peptides derived from proteolytically digested biosamples. Different peptides resulting from different samples are labeled with different tags or no tags. This allows different peptides from different samples to be mixed together for mass spectrometry assay. This proteomic technique is good for studies involving small number of samples up to eight that can be easily mixed together for analysis [51].

Label-free detection methods for biomarker discovery are simpler and faster [2]. Examples include label-free mass spectrometry (MS) and multi-dimensional liquid chromatography-Mass spectrometry (LC-MS). LC-MS is an analytical proteomic technique that measures the mass–to-charge (m/z) of peptide ions based on their motion in an electric or magnetic field. This technique is used to identify, characterize and quantify proteins based on the mono-isotopic mass of a peptide rather than the average mass of a peptide [67]. Quantitation is achieved by aligning the LC-MS data and carrying out statistical analysis across the samples. Differentially expressed peptides/protein are further analysed by MS for identification [51]. This method is good for large biosamples. Protein identification is dependent on the quality and quantity of fractionation. For more than two decades, reverse phase chromatography has been successfully used for peptide separations and it plays a key role in protein characterisation and identification. Routinely, peptide separation coupled on-line to tandem mass spectrometry equipped with electrospray ionisation has been used for peptide sequence analysis; this has been application and sample dependent [67]. Label free proteomics is a good method as it focuses on differential expression of proteins across groups. However, it has long time lines [51]. Examples of mass spectrometry techniques used to achieve this include the nanoflow liquid chromatography-tandem mass spectrometry (nanoLC-MS/MS) and matrix-assisted laser desorption/ionization time-of-flight mass spectrometry (MALDI-TOF MS) along with other techniques that involve immunocapture platforms of reverse phase protein assays [30].

3.3. Overview of RA biomarker discovery study using mass spectrometry

The main objective of a protein biomarker discovery study is to identify proteins whose levels are significantly altered in response to some state or conditions such as treatment, disease state, mutation, etc.[51]. This technique has also been found to give insight to different signaling pathways, has improved the discovery of new therapeutic targets, and has been used to indicate response to and the duration of treatment. The three major steps in the study of protein biomarkers are discovery, assay development and validation (testing) [51]. A biomarker discovery experiment produces a list of candidate biomarker; the presence and level of which must be eventually verified in the samples [78].

In RA, biomarker discovery requires identification and quantitation of proteins in the sera, synovial fluid/tissue of RA patients. These proteins exhibit diverse physico-chemical properties [79]. The biomarker discovery in RA using MS is promising to reveal biomarkers capable of predicting and/monitor disease activity, joint damage and therapeutic response in order to minimize expense and toxicity [17]. To accomplish this, early and better prognostic markers are required[13]. The steps involved in protein biomarker discovery experiment using proteomic techniques are as highlighted below.

- Sample collection and storage -This is the most crucial step in proteomics study. Quality samples are difficult to obtain and there are no means to test the quality of proteins in different samples. Suggestions include limiting the time of exposure of samples to room temperature, keeping samples frozen at -80°C as changes in protein are known to occur very quickly. Collection of serum or plasma from patients should also be carried out following standard operating procedures (SOP) for plasma collection [51].

- Sample preparation -This is the second crucial step in sample analysis. Sample preparation involves the disruption of cellular matrix as homogeneity of samples is essential; solubilization of proteins for example in detergents; fractionation of the complex protein mixture due to the diverse abundance of proteins in the mixture, depleting the most abundant proteins-albumin, IgG; protein digestion into peptides for MS analysis using trypsin; removal of nonprotein/nonpeptide molecules for some sample types such as the synovial fluid and urine. Methods of removing the interfering molecules include electrophoresis through polyacrylamide gel or solid phase extraction (SPE) [51].

- Sample assay -MS has been successfully used to analyse the differential patterns of protein and peptide expression in patient biospecimen. This is a high throughput approach used to assay for millions of peptides [30, 69]. Protein quantitation can be achieved by relative or absolute quantitation either by measuring the chromatogram peak area or spectral counting [51]. Potential biomarkers can be identified from differentially expressed proteins among different groups of samples from a proteomic discovery experiment with the aid of statistical analysis. The acquisition of knowledge on the function of the discovered potential biomarkers is the main goal of all proteomic research. This is achieved with the aid of external databases and the literature to know the involvement of each protein biomarker in different pathways and processes depending on the location of the protein in the cell [67].

- Statistical analysis - Different software tools are available for differential analysis of proteomic data. Usually the differential analysis between diseased/healthy materials, mutants/wild type species, treated/control samples is the best approach to study changes in protein expression levels. However, studies have shown that it is rare that proteins are either absent or present but they are in most cases up or down regulated in different samples. Hence, there is a need for a precise and confident analysis of the quantitative changes [67]. The type and amount of statistical analysis depend on the number of biological and technical replicates. Technical averages and variances are used to calculate the biological averages and variances. Analytical and technical variability and CV (coefficient of variation) should ideally be less than 10% while biological variation may be high [51]. Across groups, fold change calculations are done to identify differentially expressed proteins. Although, arbitrary cut-offs are used looking at the data and this is usually 1.5- or 2- folds change. For three or more biological replicates, pvalue (t-test) and/or false discovery rates (FDR) are calculated for the data analyses with cut-offs typically $p<0.05$ and FDR<20% considered significant respectively. Multivariate analysis such as hierarchical clustering, principal component analysis and other statistical programs are used for data analysis [51].

3.4. Verification and validation of protein biomarkers in RA

After the discovery phase of biomarkers using proteomic techniques, there is a need to confirm the biomarkers [51]. Verification is the paradigm shift from unbiased discovery experiments to targeted, hypothesis-driven methods [78]. It is necessary to reliably identify and reproducibly quantify a potential protein biomarker of interest over multiple samples before establishing its value as a protein biomarker [68]. There is a need to prove the functions of the potential biomarkers discovered by a second entirely independent analysis method. Western blotting and multiple reaction monitoring (MRM) methods are often used for this task [67]. LC-MS/MS using MRM is gaining acceptance as the primary analytical tool for quantitation of small molecule biomarkers in biological fluids. This is the quantitation of proteins using proteolytic digestion followed by MRM quantitation of unique peptides to the protein of interest [52]. Peptides with analytical or technical variance >20% are not suitable for a multiple reaction monitoring (MRM) assay [51]. A complete set of analytical samples with quality controls and standards are used for validation [52].

Analytical or technical validation is known as verification and this process confirms the assay performance characteristics as well as the required optimal conditions that will give reproducible and accurate data. The behaviour of a marker within and between populations gives the clinical and biological validation [30].

The procedures taking place after the development and optimization of bioanalytical procedures is known as validation. The word validation is broad and has been described as the process of linking a biomarker to clinical or behavioral endpoints [30]. These are aimed to show that the method is "fit for purpose"; and that the procedure is reproducible and reliable for its intended use. The fundamental parameters involved include accuracy, selectivity, sensitivity, stability, reproducibility, precision as well as effectiveness of results. [52, 55]. This process of reproducibly quantifying multiple proteins in complex backgrounds over large cohort of patients' specimen is highly important in biomarker research [80]. Without verification and validation of biomarkers, they cannot be used as drug response marker(s) in clinical practice [30].

There are two common types of assays developed to verify and validate the proteins of interest. These are the antibody-based assays and the MS-based assays. Both approaches can be complementary [51]. To develop the protein biomarkers discovered are some proteomic methods discussed below:

1. Antibody based assays - autoantigen microarrays for the characterisation of antibody responses, reverse phase protein array studies to analyze phosphoproteins, antibody array technologies to profile cytokines and other biomolecules (e.g western immunoblot assay, enzyme-linked immunosorbent assay –ELISA, platform specific assays such as luminex); flow cytometric analysis of phosphoproteins. However, each has their limitations. Antibody-based assays are highly sensitive, has medium to high specificity, low multiplexing capability (1-10 proteins), assay development is time consuming and expensive, and it has a low success rate as it is difficult to find a pair of antibodies with high specificity [51, 79, 80].

2. Mass spectrometry based assays- Peptide multiple reaction monitoring (MRM) assays have emerged as an alternative to affinity-based measurement of proteins [80]. This is a targeted proteomic method where the mass spectrometer is directed to monitor specific peptides for the proteins (biomarkers) of interest. This method involves a protein list and sample type for the assay, selection of unique peptides to the proteins of interest, selection of fragment ions of the peptide detectable by the mass spectrometer, tuning the mass spectrometer to look for the peptides and fragment ions in the samples (first for individual peptides and then multiplexed for multiple peptide/fragments ions for each protein), testing and selection of best peptides for the assay, as well as checking for technical, analytical and biological variability using different samples [51]. Quantitation is achieved in MRM assays from the peak areas of the fragment ions for each peptide. Results are refined to get the final list of peptides and product ions. The refined final list can then be used to test samples for absolute or relative quantitation comparing values across samples. For relative quantitation, a sample is chosen as the reference to which other samples are compared while absolute quantitation of protein concentration involves labeled and unlabeled standards for each peptides; calibration curves constructed from labeled peptide standards are used for peptide quantitation [51]. MRM has a high accuracy, high throughput, supports lower detection limits for peptides and supports the measurement of multiple

proteotypic peptides and efforts are ongoing to improve the development of MRM assay softwares, precision, accuracy and robustness [80]. MS based assays have a medium sensitivity, high specificity, high multiplexing capability (ability to quantify multiple proteins in parallel), takes a shorter period of time to develop assays compared to the antibody-based assays, has a high success rate and it is not as expensive as the antibody-based assay (cost- efficiency). It is highly reproducible across different instrument platforms and laboratories and has the potential to bridge the gap between generating candidate list and their clinical use [51, 80].

It has been predicted that the use of MRM protein assay will increase the number of validated medically important protein biomarkers. MRM can provide both relative and absolute quantitation of peptides like the antibody-based assay. MRM assays has three major advantages over the antibody based assay i) High specificity for the protein of interest or its isoform; ii)short time lines for assay development and iii) high multiplexing of the assay to include 25 proteins or more in a single assay [51].

The detection level of proteins using the MRM method depends greatly on the detection of the protein in a previous biomarker discovery experiment using the GeLC/MS or label free LC/MS/MS. Other proteins selected as potential biomarkers based on literature review or other experiments such as transcriptomics may likely exist in low abundance in the samples of interest. If need be, these protein can be boosted using different enrichment strategies[51].

Important to the development of a successful MRM protein assay is the detection of fragment ions that are well separated and sufficient data points obtained for each peak. In a typical MRM assay, the separation of peptides are based on the retention time in the liquid chromatography (LC) as well as their mass/charge (m/z) while the peak areas for the fragment ions for each peptide is used for the quantitative analysis [51].

Novel biomarkers discovered, verified and validated with proteomics are critical in the development of targeted compounds thereby directing rational treatment to patients. In many autoimmune diseases, studies are underway to define the inflammatory proteome, disease proteome, vascular proteome and other subsets of the pathologic environment. Potential biomarkers when verified and biologically validated are promising to lead to the selection of individuals most likely to benefit from treatment. MRM protein assay developed may be used routinely for testing biological samples [30, 51].

Using different proteomic techniques, a number of potential RA protein biomarkers are under study. These includes serum amyloid A [57]; S100 family of calcium binding proteins found to regulate joint inflammation and cartilage in arthritis [56] and many more as listed in Table 2. None of the available proteomic methods has emerged as the best for all proteins biomarker discovery studies. Each method has their pros and cons. The success of proteomic studies depend on sample quality, the technical variability of the method as well as the depth of protein analysis. The best platform for proteomic studies depends on factors such as the number of available samples, the timeline for completion of study and the funds available for the study [51].

Sample type	IA associated proteins	Sample preparation	Mass Spectrometry platform	References
Plasma	Actin, CRP, Calgranulin A, B and C (S100 family of calcium binding proteins – A4, A8, A9, A11, A12 and P)	Immunodepletion, GC and LC separation	2-dimensional LC/LC and MS/MS; ESI Triple Q/MRM	[29] [65]
Serum	Serotransferrin, Serum amyloid A, GAPDH, Alpha-1-antitrypsin, Citrullinated fibrinogen, Apolipoptotein A11, Vitamin D binding protein, C-reactive protein S100A8, S100A9, S100A12 and α-defensins	Acetone precipitation, 2DE, CIC/DIGE Immunodepletion +size exclusion chromatography (SEC) Immunoprecipitation+size exclusion chromatography (SEC)	LC MALDI TOF/TOF LC/ESI-MS/MS MALDI TOF-TOF LC ESI Triple Q/MRM SELDI-TOF-MS	SEE [81] [82] [83] [53] [84] [85] [57]
Synovial fluid	C-reactive protein, S100A8, S100A9, S100A12,S100A4,S100P, S100A11 Apolipoprotein A1 Cathepsin B Peptidyl prolyl isomerase Triose phosphate isomerise 14-3-3-protein alpha_beta Osteopontin Transgelin 2 Kininogen Vitamin K-dependent protein C α-defensins Citrullinated fibrinogen Calgranulin A, C (MRP 14 and MRP12)	Immunoprecipitation, Immunodepletion +size exclusion chromatography (SEC) Reverse HPLC fractionation Ultracentrifugation	LC ESI Q/TOF HPLC/LCQ ion trap LC MALDI TOF/TOF SELDI-TOF-MS LTQ-FT-ICR	[29] [85] [61] SEE [65] [29]

Sample type	IA associated proteins	Sample preparation	Mass Spectrometry platform	References
Synovial Tissue	Aldolase A, Annexin, Calcium-binding S100 proteins, Cathepsin D, CRP, ENOA, Ig κ-chain, MnSOD, NGAL, PRDX2, PRDX4, SOD2, TG2, TXNDC5	SCX, acetone precipitation	LC ESI ion trap/SRM MALDI-TOF MS	[29] [86] [87] [88]
Urine	Transferrin, Serum amyloid A,	1D gel, 2DE, Immunoprecipitatio n,	LC MALDI Triple Q/MRM	SEE [81]
Pannus tissue lysate	Citrullinated fibrinogen	1D GEL/ immunoprecipitatio n	LC ESI ion trap	[83]
Whole saliva	14-3-3 protein, apolipoprotein A, calgranulin A and B, E-FABP, GRP78/BiP, PRDX5	2D-DIGE	LC/MS/MS	[89]

E-FABP=Epidermal fatty acid binding protein, PRDX=Peroxiredoxin; GRP78/BiP=Glucose related protein precursor; TXNDC5=Thioredoxin domain-containing protein 5; MnSOD=Manganese superoxide dismutase; MRP = Myeloid related protein; CRP= C-reactive protein; SOD= Superoxide dismutase,GAPDH= Glyceraldehyde 3-phosphate dehydrogenase, ENOA= enolase, NGAL= d neutrophil gelatinase-associated lipocalin TG2= Tissue transglutaminase 2.

Table 2. A review on inflammatory arthritis associated proteins and mass spectrometry techniques used for identification. IEF=Ion exchange chromatography; 2D-DIGE=Two dimensional- differential in gel electrophoresis; ESI-MS=Electrospray ionisation mass spectrometry; 2-DE=Two dimensional gel electrophoresis; MALDI-TOF-MS=Matrix-assisted laser desorption ionisation time-of-flight mass spectrometry; SELDI-TOF-MS=Surface-enhanced laser desorption ionisation time-of-flight mass spectrometry; IP=Immunoprecipitation; ID=Immunodepletion; SEC=Size exclusion chromatography; LC=Liquid chromatography; HPLC=High performance liquid chromatography; MRM=Multiple reaction monitoring; LTQ-FT-ICR=Ion trap-Fourier Transform mass spectrometer.

3.5. Clinical utility of protein biomarkers in RA

The ultimate aim of RA treatment is to achieve and sustain remission but current targets include the suppression of disease activity, the improvement of functional ability and the slowing of joint damage [90]. Accurate measurement of disease activity can be used in therapy management as it should guide in ensuring that effective therapies are continued and ineffective ones discontinued [31]. Treatment response in RA is a measure of the suppression of inflammation solely with acute phase response indicators - CRP and ESR or in combination with clinical information. Prognostic factors that may affect response or no response to treatment include the presence of rheumatoid factor, rheumatoid nodules, HLA-DR4/sharp epitope and anti-cyclic citrullinated peptide antibodies although these cannot be used to predict response to therapy. Hence, there is a need for new biomarkers to predict response to therapy and to help in preventing long-term radiographic progression in patients [91]. Validation of new multiplex assay and technologies are essential before clinical applications [52].

A number of factors are responsible for the inability of lots of potential protein biomarkers reaching clinical utility. These factors have made the translation of biomarkers from bench to bedside difficult [51]. Decision making is one of the main factors for the utility of biomarkers hence, there is a need for all stakeholders in the decision to be involved in the biomarker development. Therefore, in addition to biologists, pharmacologists, medical practitioners in the appropriate fields, analytical experts are needed for the identification and quantification of potential biomarkers. They should all be involved in the analyses and optimal use of the data [92, 93]. With different biomarkers at different stages of validation, clinicians and researchers are finding it difficult to make a sense of it all [80].

3.6. Challenges /future of biomarkers and proteomics for inflammatory arthritis

Proteins are difficult molecules to monitor with the first technical issue being the insufficient depth of the current methods in regards to the broad range (12 orders of magnitude) of protein concentrations in biofluids. There are different orders of magnitudes for the dynamic range of most methods [51]. Another major limitation in translational research particularly in the validation step of protein biomarker include lack of reproducible, accurate and sensitive assays for most potential biomarker proteins described in the literature. However, MRM has been reported to allow reproducible protein quantification [80]. Technical variability is a key factor that affects the design of experiments in proteomics. The higher the technical variability, the higher the number of technical replicates that needs to be done and this is evaluated by comparing data from the replicates of the same sample. Comparing the data from the replicate samples, the correlation coefficient (R^2) calculated gives an indication on the technical variability. R^2 >0.9 is an indicator of low technical variability, R^2 between 0.8 and 0.9 is acceptable and $R^2 < 0.8$ is an indicator of high technical variability and a biological signal might be difficult with the high technical variability [51]. Multiplexing assays whereby multiple analytes are measured from the same sample is often used to fully understand the correlation between the biomarkers and the underlying biological pathways or to investigate the multiple potential biomarkers before deciding on the decision-making biomarker. Variability that may occur due to limited availability of samples or different separation methods can be minimized by multiplexing assays on an LC-MS/MS platform. Flow cytometry based technologies and planar–array technologies also have multiplexing options. There is a need to validate these new multiplex assay platforms before recommending them for clinical use [52]. In addition, most proteomic techniques are highly sophisticated to operate and have high demand for hands-on skills. Good operator knowledge and skill as well as the performance of the instrument are equally important. Therefore educative programs and tutorial are indispensable in proteomic societies [67].

http://dx.doi.org/10.5772/54218

The effect of combined therapy on response as well as the knowledge of predictive biomarkers of response is a potential emerging area in inflammatory arthritis, as this will promote personalised medicine. Future studies should aim at the knowledge and better understanding of the changes occurring in the synovial tissue prior to and upon administration of anti-TNF-α. In addition, futher studies on the identification of biomarkers that are down regulated by TNF-α inhibitors can be another useful therapeutic target.

4. Conclusions

The pace of discovery and development of protein biomarkers of IA is accelerating with the use of a range of proteomic techniques. Together, these have the opportunity to make a significant impact on the treatment of IA. However, the challenges associated with realising this potential as well as the progression of new biomarkers to clinical utility are significant.

Targeted therapy through the emerging proteomic technologies will help select patients who may be more likely to benefit from personalised medicine and this may bring about the clinical adoption of molecular proteomic stratification. Comprehensive proteomic profiling and trial-focused endpoint profiling will be critical for development of biomarkers and potential drug targets. Proteomics will also aid the understanding of the potential protein biomarker signaling pathways to define the preferred targets of molecular therapy. The discovery and validation of new biomarker signatures will broaden our understanding of the disease and may lead to development of new potential drugs for personalised medicine in IA.

Permission

Figure 1 adapted with permission from Nature Publishing Group. (License number-2981310304680)

Author details

Opeyemi S. Ademowo[1], Lisa Staunton[1], Oliver FitzGerald[1,2] and Stephen R. Pennington[1*]

*Address all correspondence to: Stephen.pennington@ucd.ie

1 UCD Conway Institute of Biomolecular and Biomedical Research, University College Dublin, Belfield Dublin, Ireland

2 Department of Rheumatology, St. Vincent's University Hospital, Dublin, Ireland

References

[1] Gibson D, Banha J, Penque D, Costa L, Conrads T, Cahill D, O'Brien J, Rooney M: Diagnostic and prognostic biomarker discovery strategies for autoimmune disorders. *Journal of Proteomics* 2009.

[2] Dasilva N, Diez P, Matarraz S, Gonzalez-Gonzalez M, Paradinas S, Orfao A, Fuentes M: Biomarker Discovery by Novel Sensors Based on Nanoproteomics Approaches. *Sensors* 2012, 12(2):2284-2308.

[3] Hueber W, Robinson W: Proteomic biomarkers for autoimmune disease. *Proteomics* 2006, 6(14):4100-4105.

[4] Karlson EW, Chibnik LB, Tworoger SS, Lee IM, Buring JE, Shadick NA, Manson JE, Costenbader KH: Biomarkers of inflammation and development of rheumatoid arthritis in women from two prospective cohort studies. *Arthritis Rheum* 2009, 60(3): 641-652.

[5] Schulz M, Dotzlaw H, Mikkat S, Eggert M, Neeck G: Proteomic analysis of peripheral blood mononuclear cells: selective protein processing observed in patients with rheumatoid arthritis. *J Proteome Res* 2007, 6(9):3752-3759.

[6] Sawyers C: The cancer biomarker problem. *Nature* 2008, 452(7187):548-552.

[7] Collins C, Purohit S, Podolsky R, Zhao H, Schatz D, Eckenrode S, Yang P, Hopkins D, Muir A, Hoffman M: The application of genomic and proteomic technologies in predictive, preventive and personalized medicine. *Vascular pharmacology* 2006, 45(5): 258-267.

[8] van Gool AJ, Henry B, Sprengers ED: From biomarker strategies to biomarker activities and back. *Drug discovery today*, 15(3-4):121-126.

[9] Curtis JR, van der Helm-van Mil A, Knevel R, Huizinga TW, Haney DJ, Shen Y, Ramanujan S, Cavet G, Centola M, Hesterberg LK: Validation of a novel multi-biomarker test to assess rheumatoid arthritis disease activity. *Arthritis Care & Research* 2012.

[10] De Vlam K, Gottlieb A, Fitzgerald O: Biological biomarkers in psoriatic disease. A review. *The Journal of Rheumatology* 2008, 35(7):1443.

[11] Sinz A, Bantscheff M, Mikkat S, Ringel B, Drynda S, Kekow J, Thiesen H, Glocker M: Mass spectrometric proteome analyses of synovial fluids and plasmas from patients suffering from rheumatoid arthritis and comparison to reactive arthritis or osteoarthritis. *Electrophoresis* 2002, 23(19):3445-3456.

[12] Nissen M, Gabay C, Scherer A, Finckh A: The effect of alcohol on radiographic progression in rheumatoid arthritis. *Arthritis & Rheumatism* 2010, 62(5):1265-1272.

[13] Humby F, Manzo A, Kirkham B, Pitzalis C: The synovial membrane as a prognostic tool in rheumatoid arthritis. *Autoimmunity Reviews* 2007, 6(4):248-252.

[14] McGonagle D, Gibbon W, Emery P: Classification of inflammatory arthritis by enthesitis. *The Lancet* 1998, 352(9134):1137-1140.

[15] Guang Ming Han, O'Neil- Andersen NJ, Zurier RB, Lawrence DA: $CD4^{+}$ and CD25 ^{high} T cell numbers are enriched in the peripheral blood of patients with rheumatoid arthritis. *Cellular Immunology* 2008, 253(1-2):92-101.

[16] Libby P: Role of inflammation in atherosclerosis associated with rheumatoid arthritis. *The American journal of medicine* 2008, 121(10S1):21-31.

[17] Smolen J, Aletaha D, Grisar J, Redlich K, Steiner G, Wagner O: The need for prognosticators in rheumatoid arthritis. Biological and clinical markers: where are we now? *Arthritis Research & Therapy* 2008, 10(3):208.

[18] Scott D, Kingsley G: Tumor necrosis factor inhibitors for rheumatoid arthritis. *New England Journal of Medicine* 2006, 355(7):704-712.

[19] Ingegnoli F, Fantini F, Favalli EG, Soldi A, Griffini S, Galbiati V, Meroni PL, Cugno M: Inflammatory and prothrombotic biomarkers in patients with rheumatoid arthritis: effects of tumor necrosis factor-alpha blockade. *J Autoimmun* 2008, 31(2):175-179.

[20] Firestein GS: Kelley's textbook of rheumatology: Saunders, Elsevier; 2008.

[21] Strand V, Kimberly R, Isaacs J: Biologic therapies in rheumatology: lessons learned, future directions. *Nature Reviews Drug Discovery* 2007, 6(1):75-92.

[22] Iwamoto T, Okamoto H, Toyama Y, Momohara S: Molecular aspects of rheumatoid arthritis: chemokines in the joints of patients. *FEBS J* 2008, 275:4448-4455.

[23] Page TH, Brown AC, Timms EM, Brennan FM, Ray KP, Foxwell BMJ: 116 Treatment with Non-steroidal Anti-inflammatory Drugs Increases TNF Production in Rheumatoid Arthritis. *Cytokine* 2007, 39(1):32-32.

[24] Tilleman K, Van Beneden K, Dhondt A, Hoffman I, De Keyser F, Veys E, Elewaut D, Deforce D: Chronically inflamed synovium from spondyloarthropathy and rheumatoid arthritis investigated by protein expression profiling followed by tandem mass spectrometry. *PROTEOMICS-Clinical Applications* 2005, 5(8):2247-2257.

[25] Kamijo S, Nakajima A, Kamata K, Kurosawa H, Yagita H, Okumura K: Involvement of TWEAK/Fn14 interaction in the synovial inflammation of RA. *Rheumatology* 2008, 47(4):442.

[26] Feldmann M, Brennan F, Maini R: Role of cytokines in rheumatoid arthritis. *Annual review of immunology* 1996, 14(1):397-440.

[27] Bansard C, LequerrÃ© T, Daveau M, Boyer O, Tron F, Salier JP, Vittecoq O, Le-LoÃ «t X: Can rheumatoid arthritis responsiveness to methotrexate and biologics be predicted? *Rheumatology* 2009, 48(9):1021-1028.

[28] Wolfe F: The Prognosis of Rheumatoid Arthritis: Assessment of Disease Activity and Disease Severity in the Clinic. *American Journal of Medicine* 1997, 103(6A):12S-18S.

[29] Liao H, Wu J, Kuhn E, Chin W, Chang B, Jones MD, O'Neil S, Clauser KR, Karl J, Hasler F: Use of mass spectrometry to identify protein biomarkers of disease severity in the synovial fluid and serum of patients with rheumatoid arthritis. *Arthritis & Rheumatism* 2004, 50(12):3792-3803.

[30] Lee J, Han JJ, Altwerger G, Kohn EC: Proteomics and biomarkers in clinical trials for drug development. *Journal of Proteomics* 2011, 74:2632-2641.

[31] Pincus T, Strand V, Koch G, Amara I, Crawford B, Wolfe F, Cohen S, Felson D: An index of the three core data set patient questionnaire measures distinguishes efficacy of active treatment from that of placebo as effectively as the American College of Rheumatology 20% response criteria (ACR20) or the Disease Activity Score (DAS) in a rheumatoid arthritis clinical trial. *Arthritis & Rheumatism* 2003, 48(3):625-630.

[32] Fransen J, van Riel P: The Disease Activity Score and the EULAR response criteria. *Rheumatic Disease Clinics of North America* 2009, 35(4):745-757.

[33] Van der Heijde D, Van't Hof M, Van Riel P, Van de Putte L: Development of a disease activity score based on judgment in clinical practice by rheumatologists. *The Journal of Rheumatology* 1993, 20(3):579.

[34] Wolfe F, Pincus T, O'Dell J: Evaluation and documentation of rheumatoid arthritis disease status in the clinic: which variables best predict change in therapy. *The Journal of Rheumatology* 2001, 28(7):1712.

[35] FitzGerald O, Winchester R: Psoriatic arthritis: from pathogenesis to therapy. *Arthritis Res Ther* 2009, 11(1):214.

[36] Bennett A, Peterson P, Zain A, Grumley J, Panayi G, Kirkham B: Adalimumab in clinical practice. Outcome in 70 rheumatoid arthritis patients, including comparison of patients with and without previous anti-TNF exposure. *Rheumatology* 2005, 44(8): 1026.

[37] Anderson NL, Anderson NG: The human plasma proteome. *Molecular & Cellular Proteomics* 2002, 1(11):845-867.

[38] Gibson DS, Finnegan S, Pennington S, Qiu J, LaBaer J, Rooney ME, Duncan MW: Validation of Protein Biomarkers to Advance the Management of Autoimmune Disorders. 2011.

[39] Atkinson A, Colburn W, DeGruttola V, DeMets D, Downing G, Hoth D, Oates J, Peck C, Schooley R, Spilker B: Biomarkers and surrogate endpoints: Preferred definitions and conceptual framework*. *Clinical Pharmacology & Therapeutics* 2001, 69(3):89-95.

[40] Saag K, Teng G, Patkar N, Anuntiyo J, Finney C, Curtis J, Paulus H, Mudano A, Pisu M, Elkins Melton M: American College of Rheumatology 2008 recommendations for the use of nonbiologic and biologic disease modifying antirheumatic drugs in rheumatoid arthritis. *Arthritis Care & Research* 2008, 59(6):762-784.

[41] Gelfand J, Gladman D, Mease P, Smith N, Margolis D, Nijsten T, Stern R, Feldman S, Rolstad T: Epidemiology of psoriatic arthritis in the population of the United States. *Journal of the American Academy of Dermatology* 2005, 53(4):573.

[42] Hueber W, Utz P, Robinson W: Autoantibodies in early arthritis: advances in diagnosis and prognostication. *Clinical and experimental rheumatology* 2003, 21(5; SUPP 31): 59-64.

[43] Aletaha D, Neogi T, Silman AJ, Funovits J, Felson DT, Bingham CO, Birnbaum NS, Burmester GR, Bykerk VP, Cohen MD: 2010 rheumatoid arthritis classification criteria: an American College of Rheumatology/European League Against Rheumatism collaborative initiative. *Arthritis & Rheumatism* 2010, 62(9):2569-2581.

[44] Ioan-Fascinay A, Willemze A, Robinson DB, Peschken CA, Markland J, Van der Woude D, Elias B, Menard HA, Newkirk M, Fritzler MJ *et al*: Marked differencesin fine specificity and isotype usage of the anti-citrullinated protein antibody in health and disease. *Arthritis & Rheumatism* 2008, 58(10):3000-3008.

[45] Sghiri R, Bouajina E, Bargaoui D, Harzallah L, Fredj H, Sammoud S, Ghedira I: Value of anti-mutated citrullinated vimentin antibodies in diagnosing rheumatoid arthritis. *Rheumatology International* 2008, 29(1):59-62.

[46] Szekanecz Z, Soós L, Szabó Z, Fekete A, Kapitány A, Végvári A, Sipka S, Szücs G, Szántó S, Lakos G: Anti-citrullinated protein antibodies in rheumatoid arthritis: as good as it gets? *Clinical Reviews in Allergy and Immunology* 2008, 34(1):26-31.

[47] Gibson DS, Finnegan S, Pennington S, Qiu J, LaBaer J, Rooney ME, Duncan MW: Validation of Protein Biomarkers to Advance the Management of Autoimmune Disorders, Autoimmune Disorders - Current Concepts and Advances from Bedside to Mechanistic Insights. *ISBN: 978-953-307-653-9, InTech* 2011.

[48] Rioja I, Hughes F, Sharp C, Warnock L, Montgomery D, Akil M, Wilson A, Binks M, Dickson M: Potential novel biomarkers of disease activity in rheumatoid arthritis patients: CXCL13, CCL23, transforming growth factor , tumor necrosis factor receptor superfamily member 9, and macrophage colony stimulating factor. *Arthritis & Rheumatism* 2008, 58(8):2257-2267.

[49] Humby F, Bombardieri M, Manzo A, Kelly S, Blades M, Kirkham B, Spencer J, Pitzalis C: Ectopic lymphoid structures support ongoing production of class-switched autoantibodies in rheumatoid synovium. *PLoS Med* 2009, 6(1):e1.

[50] Wild N, Karl J, Grunert VP, Schmitt RI, Garczarek U, Krause F, Hasler F, van Riel PL, Bayer PM, Thun M *et al*: Diagnosis of rheumatoid arthritis: multivariate analysis of biomarkers. *Biomarkers* 2008, 13(1):88-105.

[51] VanBogelen RA, Alessi D: Proteomic Methods to Develop Protein Biomarkers. *Predictive Approaches in Drug Discovery and Development: Biomarkers and In Vitro/In Vivo Correlations* 2012, 11:49.

[52] Szekely-Klepser G, Fountain S: Validation of Biochemical Biomarker Assays Used in Drug Discovery and Development: A review of challenges and solutions. *Predictive Approaches in Drug Discovery and Development: Biomarkers and In Vitro/In Vivo Correlations* 2012, 11:23.

[53] Gibson D, Blelock S, Curry J, Finnegan S, Healy A, Scaife C, McAllister C, Pennington S, Dunn M, Rooney M: Comparative ananlysisof synovial fluid and plasma proteomes in juvenile arthritis- proteomic patterns of joint inflammation in early stage disease. *Journal of Proteomics* 2009, 72:656-676.

[54] Fischer R, Trudgian DC, Wright C, Thomas G, Bradbury LA, Brown MA, Bowness P, Kessler BM: Discovery of candidate serum proteomic and metabolomic biomarkers in Ankylosing Spondylitis. *Molecular & Cellular Proteomics* 2012, 11(2).

[55] Murphy E, Roux-Lombard P, Rooney T, FitzGerald O, Dayer J, Bresnihan B: Serum levels of tissue inhibitor of metalloproteinase-1 and periarticular bone loss in early rheumatoid arthritis. *Clinical Rheumatology* 2009, 28(3):285-291.

[56] P L E M van Lent, L Grevers, A B Blom, A Sloetjes, J S Mort, T Vogl, W Nacken, W B van den Berg, Roth3 J: Myeloid related proteins S100A8/S100A9 regulate joint inflammation and cartilage destruction during antigen-induced arthritis. *Ann Rheum Dis* 2008, 67:1750-1758.

[57] de Seny D, Fillet M, Ribbens C, Maree R, Meuwis M, Lutteri L, Chapelle J, Wehenkel L, Louis E, Merville M: Monomeric calgranulins measured by SELDI-TOF mass spectrometry and calprotectin measured by ELISA as biomarkers in arthritis. *Clinical chemistry* 2008, 54(6):1066.

[58] Hammer H, Odegard S, Fagerhol M, Landewe R, Heijde D, Uhlig T, Mowinckel P, Kvien T: Extended reports-Calprotectin (a major leucocyte protein) is strongly and independently correlated with joint inflammation and damage in rheumatoid arthritis. *Annals of the Rheumatic Diseases* 2007, 66(8):1093-1097.

[59] Baillet A, Trocme C, Berthier S, Arlotto M, Grange L, Chenau J, Quetant S, Seve M, Berger F, Juvin R: Synovial fluid proteomic fingerprint: S100A8, S100A9 and S100A12 proteins discriminate rheumatoid arthritis from other inflammatory joint diseases. *Rheumatology*.

[60] Bombardieri M, McInnes I, Pitzalis C: Interleukin-18 as a potential therapeutic target in chronic autoimmune/inflammatory conditions. *Expert Opin Biol Ther* 2007, 7(1): 31-40.

[61] Raijmakers R, van Beers JJBC, El-Azzouny M, Visser NFC, Božič B, Pruijn GJM, Heck AJR: Elevated levels of fibrinogen-derived endogenous citrullinated peptides in synovial fluid of rheumatoid arthritis patients. *Arthritis Research & Therapy* 2012, 14(3):R114.

[62] Christgau S, Garnero P, Fledelius C, Moniz C, Ensig M, Gineyts E, Rosenquist C, Qvist P: Collagen type II C-telopeptide fragments as an index of cartilage degradation. *Bone* 2001, 29(3):209-215.

[63] Singer F, Eyre D: Using biochemical markers of bone turnover in clinical practice. *Cleveland Clinic Journal of Medicine* 2008, 75(10):739.

[64] van Kuijk A, Gerlag D, Vos K, Wolbink G, de Groot M, de Rie M, Zwinderman A, Dijkmans B, Tak P: A prospective, randomised, placebo-controlled study to identify biomarkers associated with active treatment in psoriatic arthritis: effects of adalimumab treatment on synovial tissue. *British Medical Journal* 2009, 68(8):1303.

[65] Gibson DS, Rooney ME: The human synovial fluid proteome: A key factor in the pathology of joint disease. *PROTEOMICSâ€"Clinical Applications* 2007, 1(8):889-899.

[66] Wilkins M, Appel R, Van Eyk J, Chung M, Görg A, Hecker M, Huber L, Langen H, Link A, Paik Y: Guidelines for the next 10 years of proteomics. *Proteomics* 2006, 6(1): 4-8.

[67] Westermeier R, Naven T, Hopker HR: Proteomics in practice: Wiley Online Library; 2002.

[68] Urbanowska T, Mangialaio S, Hartmann C, Legay F: Development of protein microarray technology to monitor biomarkers of rheumatoid arthritis disease. *Cell Biol Toxicol* 2003, 19(3):189-202.

[69] Dhamoon A, Kohn E, Azad N: The ongoing evolution of proteomics in malignancy. *Drug Discovery Today* 2007, 12(17-18):700-708.

[70] Poste G: Bring on the biomarkers. *Nature*, 469(7329):156-157.

[71] Rifai N, Gillette MA, Carr SA: Protein biomarker discovery and validation: the long and uncertain path to clinical utility. *Nature biotechnology* 2006, 24(8):971-983.

[72] Shevchenko A, Henrik Tomas JH, Olsen JV, Mann M: In-gel digestion for mass spectrometric characterization of proteins and proteomes. *Nature protocols* 2007, 1(6): 2856-2860.

[73] O'Farrell PH: High resolution two-dimensional electrophoresis of proteins. *Journal of Biological Chemistry* 1975, 250(10):4007-4021.

[74] Carrette O, Burkhard PR, Sanchez JC, Hochstrasser DF: State-of-the-art two-dimensional gel electrophoresis: a key tool of proteomics research. *Nature protocols* 2006, 1(2):812-823.

[75] Chan HL, Sinclair J, Timms JF: Proteomic Analysis of Redox-Dependent Changes Using Cysteine-Labeling 2D DIGE. *Methods in molecular biology (Clifton, NJ)* 2012, 854:113.

[76] Walther TC, Mann M: Mass spectrometry–based proteomics in cell biology. *The Journal of cell biology* 2010, 190(4):491-500.

[77] Aebersold R, Mann M: Mass spectrometry-based proteomics. *Nature* 2003, 422(6928): 198-207.

[78] Keshishian H, Addona T, Burgess M, Kuhn E, Carr SA: Quantitative, multiplexed assays for low abundance proteins in plasma by targeted mass spectrometry and stable isotope dilution. *Molecular & Cellular Proteomics* 2007, 6(12):2212-2229.

[79] Pennington S, Kitteringham N, Jenkins R, Hunt T, Webb S, Hunter C: Use of proteomics in development of biomarkers and early markers of toxicity. 2006.

[80] Hüttenhain R, Soste M, Selevsek N, RÃist H, Sethi A, Carapito C, Farrah T, Deutsch EW, Kusebauch U, Moritz RL: Reproducible Quantification of Cancer-Associated Proteins in Body Fluids Using Targeted Proteomics. *Science Translational Medicine* 2012, 4(142):142ra194-142ra194.

[81] Gibson DS, Banha J, Penque D, Costa L, Conrads TP, Cahill DJ, O'Brien JK, Rooney ME: Diagnostic and prognostic biomarker discovery strategies for autoimmune disorders. *Journal of Proteomics* 2010, 73(6):1045-1060.

[82] Low J.M. CAK, Gibson D.S., Zhu M., Chen S., Rooney, M.E., Ombrello, M.J., Moore T.L.: Proteomic analysis of circulating immune complexes in juvenile idiopathic arthritis reveals disease -associated proteins. *Proteomics Clin Appl* 2009, 3:829-840.

[83] Zhao X, Okeke NL, Sharpe O, Batliwalla FM, Lee AT, Ho PP, Tomooka BH, Gregersen PK, Robinson WH: Circulating immune complexes contain citrullinated fibrinogen in rheumatoid arthritis. *Arthritis Research and Therapy* 2010, 10(4):94.

[84] Kuhn E, Wu J, Karl J, Liao H, Zolg W, Guild B: Quantification of C-reactive protein in the serum of patients with rheumatoid arthritis using multiple reaction monitoring mass spectrometry and 13C-labeled peptide standards. *Proteomics* 2004, 4(4): 1175-1186.

[85] Baillet A, Trocmé C, Berthier S, Arlotto M, Grange L, Chenau J, Quétant S, Sève M, Berger F, Juvin R: Synovial fluid proteomic fingerprint: S100A8, S100A9 and S100A12 proteins discriminate rheumatoid arthritis from other inflammatory joint diseases. *Rheumatology* 2010, 49(4):671-682.

[86] Chang X, Cui Y, Zong M, Zhao Y, Yan X, Chen Y, Han J: Identification of proteins with increased expression in rheumatoid arthritis synovial tissues. *The Journal of Rheumatology* 2009, 36(5):872-880.

[87] Katano M, Okamoto K, Arito M, Kawakami Y, Kurokawa MS, Suematsu N, Shimada S, Nakamura H, Xiang Y, Masuko K: Implication of granulocyte-macrophage colony-stimulating factor induced neutrophil gelatinase-associated lipocalin in pathogenesis of rheumatoid arthritis revealed by proteome analysis. *Arthritis Research and Therapy* 2010, 11(1):3.

[88] Tilleman K, Van Beneden K, Dhondt A, Hoffman I, De Keyser F, Veys E, Elewaut D, Deforce D: Chronically inflamed synovium from spondyloarthropathy and rheuma-

toid arthritis investigated by protein expression profiling followed by tandem mass spectrometry. *Proteomics* 2005, 5(8):2247-2257.

[89] Giusti L, Baldini C, Ciregia F, Giannaccini G, Giacomelli C, De Feo F, Delle Sedie A, Riente L, Lucacchini A, Bazzichi L: Is GRP78/BiP a potential salivary biomarker in patients with rheumatoid arthritis? *Proteomics Clinical Applications* 2010, 4(3):315-324.

[90] Felson DT, Smolen JS, Wells G, Zhang B, van Tuyl LHD, Funovits J, Aletaha D, Allaart CF, Bathon J, Bombardieri S: American College of Rheumatology/European League Against Rheumatism provisional definition of remission in rheumatoid arthritis for clinical trials. *Arthritis & Rheumatism*, 63(3):573-586.

[91] Mullan R, Matthews C, Bresnihan B, FitzGerald O, King L, Poole A, Fearon U, Veale D: Early changes in serum type ii collagen biomarkers predict radiographic progression at one year in inflammatory arthritis patients after biologic therapy. *Arthritis and Rheumatism* 2007, 56(9):2919-2928.

[92] FitzGerald GA: Anticipating change in drug development: the emerging era of translational medicine and therapeutics. *Nature Reviews Drug Discovery* 2005, 4(10): 815-818.

[93] Fleishaker JC: The Importance of Biomarkers in Translational Medicine. *Predictive Approaches in Drug Discovery and Development: Biomarkers and In Vitro/In Vivo Correlations*, 11:1.